3|4|16
#52.95

Dance Medicine in Practice

Dance Medicine in Practice is the complete physical textbook for dance, written specifically to help dancers understand the anatomy, function and care of their bodies.

Specific chapters focus on the spine, pelvis, hips, knees, feet, shoulders and arms. Each of these covers the following key aspects:

- Anatomy: Bone structure, musculature, and function. How each part of the body moves and how it responds under pressure;
- Pitfalls: Common examples of bad practice and the effect that these can have on the body;
- Self Analysis: How to become aware of muscle groups and the capacity of each joint;
- Injury Prevention: Tips and advice on how to best avoid and prevent injury both in training and everyday life;
- Exercises: Simple and effective methods of strengthening, mobilising and relaxing joints and muscles;
- Checklists: Dos and Don'ts for the best dance technique.

The best dancers know that looking after their bodies is the key to their success, and *Dance Medicine in Practice* also covers how to ensure the best nutrition, how to plan and manage training schedules, and ensure that injuries are kept to a minimum both in frequency and impact. It is the best possible companion to a life in dance.

Liane Simmel is a medical doctor, osteopath and former professional dancer. She studied dance at the State Academy of Music and Theatre in Munich, Germany and at the Cunningham Studio in New York, USA. Today she runs her own medical practice in Munich specialising in dance medicine, osteopathy, spiral dynamics and sports medicine. As the director of the Institute for Dance Medicine "Fit for Dance" she offers dance-medical supervision for dancers and students. She is also a lecturer in Dance Medicine at the Palucca University for Dance in Dresden, the Academy of Music and Theatre in Munich and the University of Arts in Zurich.

Liane Simmel

Dance Medicine
in Practice

Anatomy,
Injury Prevention,
Training

Translated by Jane Michael and Liane Simmel

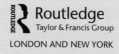

Routledge
Taylor & Francis Group

LONDON AND NEW YORK

First published 2014
by Routledge
2 Park Square, Milton Park, Abingdon, Oxon OX14 4RN

Simultaneously published in the USA and Canada
by Routledge
711 Third Avenue, New York, NY 10017

Routledge is an imprint of the Taylor & Francis Group, an informa business

Title of the original edition: Tanzmedizin in der Praxis. Anatomie, Prävention, Trainingstipps. By Liane Simmel
© 2009 by Henschel Verlag in der Seemann Henschel GmbH & Co. KG

English Language edition: © 2014 Routledge

British Library Cataloguing in Publication Data
A catalogue record for this book is available from the British Library

Library of Congress Cataloging-in-Publication Data
Simmel, Liane.
[Tanzmedizin in der Praxis. English]
Dance medicine in practice : anatomy, injury prevention, training / by Liane Simmel ; translated by Jane Michael
and Liane Simmel.
pages cm
Text in English, translated from German.
Includes index.
 1. Dancing injuries. 2. Dancers--Health and hygiene. 3. Sports medicine. I. Title.
RC1220.D35S5613 2014
617.1'0275--dc23
2013015306

ISBN: 978-0-415-80938-2 (hbk)
ISBN: 978-0-415-80939-9 (pbk)
ISBN: 978-0-203-13511-2 (ebk)

Typeset in Meta
by Saxon Graphics Ltd, Derby

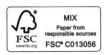

MIX
Paper from
responsible sources
FSC
www.fsc.org   FSC® C013056

Printed and bound in Great Britain by
TJ International Ltd, Padstow, Cornwall

Dance can and should be a physically and psychologically healthy practice. This perspective, the cornerstone of this publication, establishes a valuable paradigm for dance practice in all its manifestations at all levels of accomplishment.

WILLIAM FORSYTHE

Contents

Acknowledgements

Many people were involved in the production of this book, some were not even conscious of their contribution. My special thanks go to all the dancers with whom I have worked, whose questions and problems continue to prompt me to rethink, to experiment and to investigate further and further.

My grateful thanks go to:

My dear colleague D. Christian Larsen, co-founder of Spiral Dynamics, whose teaching and research have provided me with important insight into the biomechanics of movement.

My friends and colleagues Christine Baumann Leuthold, Marie-Theres Holzinger, Astrid Kiener, Bernd Klinger, Prof. Ingo Meichsner, Gerd Mittag, Dagmar Reinl, Dr Katja Schneider and Andreas Starr, who read this book during the process of writing, contributing to its present form with their comments and suggestions.

The dancers Emma Barrowman, Sophia Carolina Fernandes and Dustin Klein from the Bavarian State Ballet, Munich, Matthias Markstein from TanzTheater Munich and Caroline Geiger, who enthusiastically acted as models for the numerous photos and even willingly demonstrated mistakes as clearly as possible.

Charles Tandy, for whom no position was too tiring when it was a matter of portraying dance movements and exercises in the best possible light.

Korina Kaisershot, who produced the memorable and eye-catching drawings of anatomical details.

My editor Dr Wibke Hartewig, whose own love of dance has contributed to the success of this book.

Susanne Van Volxem, who as director of the publishing programme at Henschel Verlag made the realisation of this book possible.

The Bavarian State Ballet in Munich, for making its dance studio available for the photography.

Tanzplan Deutschland and the Schweizer Interpretenstiftung, whose support underlined the importance of this book for the international dance community.

Anna Canning, Richard Gilmore, Andrea Kozai, Jane Michael and Margot Rijven for all their effort and support in translating and proof reading the English edition of this book to make it accessible for the English-speaking dance population.

My English editor Ben Piggott, who helped through all the demanding steps to transfer the German edition into an appealing English book.

My husband Hans-Klaus, who has always supported my passion for dance. His patience, his open ear and his love gave me the necessary strength to write this book.

Dear Reader,

Here, at last, is a book aimed at the prevention and treatment of occupational injuries of dancers. You have in your hands a standard work that was long overdue, and one that, I am sure, will form an essential part of the repertoire of professional dancers as well as students and teachers of dance from now on.

In teaching, training and rehearsals, a study of and awareness for the medical basis of movement, together with an analysis of its sports-scientific background, form the basis for responsible behaviour for dancers and teachers alike, both individually and within the group. Knowledge of the physical contexts will permit broader access to the perceptual processes which are becoming increasingly important in today's dance practice. With *Dance Medicine in Practice* Dr Liane Simmel has produced a textbook that will make an important contribution to the improvement and adaptation of learning processes in a rapidly-changing dance culture, whether in the field of classical, modern or contemporary dance.

Based on her extensive experience in this field and her exchange with dancers, teachers, choreographers and doctors, the author presents with this publication the first book dedicated to applied dance medicine. It is another important contribution to the linking of practice and theory in dance training which is currently being widely discussed.

By providing support for relevant publications, Tanzplan Deutschland aims to extend knowledge in the field of dance and to make working materials available to an interested public for the encouragement of dance and especially the wide field of dance education. I am delighted that we were able to contribute to this important work. I hope you will enjoy reading it and that it will provide you with new insight and experience.

Ingo Diehl
Director of Educational Projects, Tanzplan Deutschland

Introduction

I first had the idea of writing this book many years ago, when I was a young dancer and needed help with pain I experienced while dancing. One of the doctors I consulted dismissed me with the comment: "If you carry on dancing you'll end up in a wheelchair." No further explanation, no support, and no suggestion as to how I could continue to dance with, or perhaps in spite of my physical limitations; how I should possibly change or modify my dance practice in order to avoid injury. Nor could my teachers offer me much help in my search for a better way of managing my body. Even at that time of my career I wished there had been a practical book of medicine for dancers. But I never dreamed that I would finally be the person to write it.

Some years later, when I was bold enough to attempt the balancing act of studying medicine while at the same time continuing to work in the theatre, I discovered first hand just what can happen when you understand the physiological and anatomical relationships within your own body. I spent the mornings dancing, training and rehearsing, and then went off to my anatomy lessons. The result was amazing. The pain disappeared; my extension and balance improved. I had "grasped" what was happening within my own body.

Today as a doctor and lecturer of dance medicine, I experience every day how helpful it is for a dancer to understand his or her own body. The aim of this book is to make knowledge in the fields of medicine, movement analysis and sports science, in spiral dynamics and osteopathy easily comprehensible, practical and useful for dancers.

How to Use this Book

Dancing is more than the mere learning and execution of steps and movement patterns. Dance cannot be reduced to the purely physical aspects alone. Yet: the body is the dancer's instrument. In order to be able to dance for a long time without pain, it is essential to keep your body healthy, to recognize strain at an early stage in order to avoid injury. Whatever your style of dance may be: classical, contemporary, hip hop, jazz, salsa, tap dancing (to name but a few), there is a great deal that dancers in all fields can learn from dance medicine that will provide them with essential support during their careers.

At first sight a theoretical book for dancers appears to be a problematic undertaking. Dancers are practical people who accumulate their knowledge on the dance floor; they want to transfer their knowledge directly into movement. Far be it from me to stop them! What you feel within your own body can become part of your practice during training sessions. What you have experienced yourself can be passed on to other people. With hints for self-analysis, numerous exercises and training tips, this book provides ample opportunity for the practical application of your newly-discovered theoretical knowledge.

A few words about how to work with the exercises: in most cases the exercises should be executed on both sides. It often makes sense to begin with the more "difficult" side. But there are always exceptions to this rule. If the exercise is painful when carried out on a particular side, or if the movement sequence is not clear, it can be helpful to practise it first on the "easier" side. Movement awareness and fine coordination are usually sensed more clearly, and therefore can be trained more effectively, on this side.

Try as we may, exercises are often very difficult to understand without the presence of a teacher. So be patient with yourself when trying out these exercises! Some movements may feel very unusual; time and patience are required to abandon long-established movement patterns and to train new ones to become automatic. Try imagining the movement. Forming a picture of what is happening within your body will help you in your search for the "ideal" form of movement.

In order to build up muscle, movements must be repeated several times. As a compromise between muscle strengthening and practicality in the dance studio, 25 repetitions are recommended for the majority of exercises. This number should be taken as a rough guide only since, particularly at the beginning, less is often more.

Exercises can help to prevent strain and counteract disadvantageous movement patterns in a targeted manner, but they cannot replace a medical examination. If you experience severe pain, or if pain continues over a longer period you should always consult a doctor or physiotherapist who is specialized in dance medicine.

Depending on the style of dance in question, dance steps are often called by different names. In order to avoid misunderstandings, the nomenclature and vocabulary used in this book is that of classical dance. This is not intended to exclude the other forms of dance; it was selected because many dancers are familiar with the terminology of classical dance as many of them have studied ballet, even if they perform in other dance disciplines. Furthermore, dance movements and descriptions from the field of classical dance are also often used in other dance styles.

Each reader may well use this book in a different way, depending on his or her own specific needs. If you read it from cover to cover you will get an overview of the most important aspects of dance medicine. If you need specific help for training problems, pain or injury, you will quickly find the relevant sections by referring to the chapters on the different parts of the body or dealing with specific subjects or by consulting the numerous cross-references and the index. If this book piques your curiosity and you wish to explore the various topics

in greater detail, at the end of the book you will find a list of tips for further reading that will provide a good introduction to pertinent literature in the field of dance medicine.

Despite all the knowledge presented in this book about anatomy and the science of movement, about injury prevention and training optimization, we should not lose sight of the fact that the body possesses its own specific intelligence when it comes to movement, and in dance, it is a question of using it.

Before you get started...
The medical nomenclature in this book does not follow a strict scientific system. The first time an anatomical structure is mentioned, its Latin name is added in brackets. In the text, however, Latin terms have been dispensed with as far as possible in the interest of readability. Some anatomical terms have nonetheless become part of the dancer's everyday vocabulary. The sacroiliac joint, for example, is referred to as just that.

In the description of movement, I have also followed general usage and in most cases have deliberately adopted an active form of the verb. Thus we say "the bone moves" although strictly speaking the bone is not capable of moving of its own accord. It is the muscles that move the bone. However, it is often helpful to imagine the movement originating from the relevant bones; the appropriate muscles will then expand and contract automatically.

In most cases the comments in this book apply equally to dancers of both genders. The linguistic problems arising from the need to write "he and/or she" as well as "his and/or her" cannot always be solved in an elegant manner. It seems clumsy to refer to "he and/or she" or to use the impersonal "one" each time. And so, in the interests of readability, it has been decided to use the masculine "he" and "his" for dancers of both genders when necessary. Since more than two-thirds of dancers are women, it might have made sense to adopt the feminine form throughout the book. However, this would merely have supported the widely held prejudice that dancing is primarily a female occupation. And that is not the aim of this book.

1. The Body: The Basis for Dance

Everything Needs a Name – the Anatomical Nomenclature of Movement

It is not easy to describe dance movements clearly and precisely. Different parts of the body often move completely independently of each other in different directions, and usually several joints are involved. A systematic approach is the best solution here: a clearly defined starting position and the observation of the movements in each joint separately. The anatomical nomenclature of movement, as it is used in medicine, provides exactly this. Independently of the direction in space, it permits us to precisely describe the positions and movements of the body. This is a tremendous help for the dancer. Although dance steps are laid down and are clearly named, at least within the different styles of dance, nonetheless, any attempt to describe movements in a way which is valid for all styles of dance can easily lead to discrepancies and misunderstandings. Anatomical nomenclature, with its clear system, provides a good basis for discussing and analysing dance movements across the borders of all dance genre.

The Neutral Stance – the Starting Position for Movement

The so-called *neutral* or *zero stance* serves as the starting position for movement. The movements of the individual joints are described starting from this position. This is what the neutral stance looks like: an upright standing position; the feet are parallel and pointing forward, the arms hang beside the body with the thumbs pointing outwards and the fingers extended. It is from this rather unnatural position that all movements with the same name occur in the same direction. It

makes no difference whether the movement takes place in the shoulder, elbow or hip: if we speak of bending (flexing) and straightening (extending), the joints of the body are always moved in the same plane of the body, in the case of flexion and extension in the plane which runs through the body from back to front.

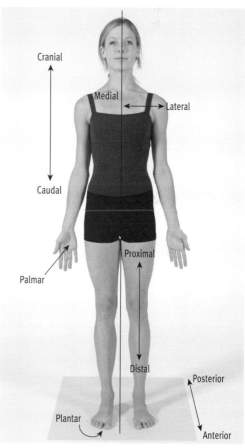

Figure 1.1 The neutral stance, with helpful terms for directions of the body.

Body Axes and Body Planes – the Geometry of the Human Body

The system of body axes and body planes is used to describe movements, from large movements within space down to small joint movements within the body. Imagine three axes running through the body. They are at right angles to each other and correspond to the three dimensions within space: the *sagittal axis* (Latin: sagittum = arrow) runs from front to back, the *horizontal axis* from one side to the other and the *vertical axis* from top to bottom.

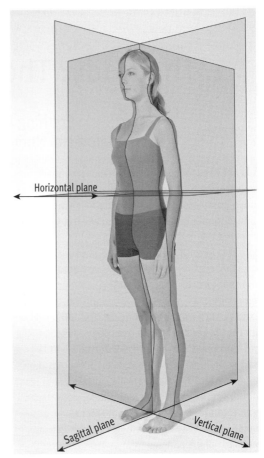

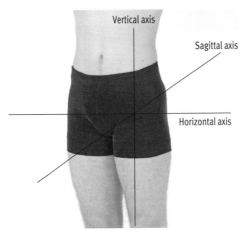

Figure 1.2 The hip joint, demonstrating the three movement axes.

Figure 1.3 The three planes of the body.

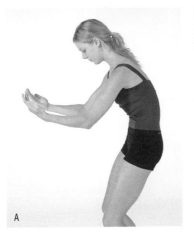

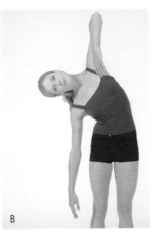

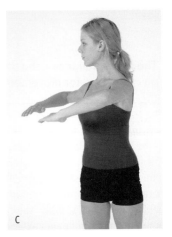

A   B   C

Figure 1.4 Dance movements of the upper body along a physical plane:
A) in the sagittal plane, B) in the frontal plane, C) in the horizontal plane.

The three planes of the body are also at right angles to each other. The *sagittal plane* runs through the body from front to back, the *frontal plane* from side to side, and the *horizontal plane* runs transversely across the body (see Figure 1.3). Movements can run exactly along these planes of the body or can consist of a combination of the different planes, for example, when the leg moves forward at an angle towards the diagonal.

The axes and planes of the body always refer to the body itself and not to its direction within the space. If the entire body or a part of the body moves within the space, then the system of axes and planes moves with it, regardless of the newly-selected direction in space. A battement devant is a movement of the leg forwards in the sagittal plane, regardless of whether the body is directed towards the front of the space or towards the diagonal.

The Nomenclature of Movement

If a part of the body moves, the movement takes place around a clearly-defined axis in the relevant plane. The axis around which the movement occurs and the plane in which the movement takes place are thus prescribed, but the direction of the movement is not. Movements around an axis can always be carried out in two opposite directions. Turning around the horizontal axis permits *flexion* and *extension*. Rotation around the sagittal axis permits *abduction* (moving away from the midline of the body) and *adduction* (moving towards the midline of the body). Movements around the

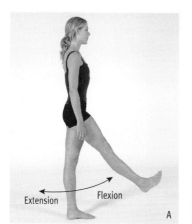
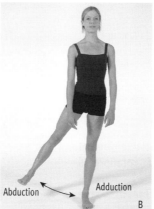
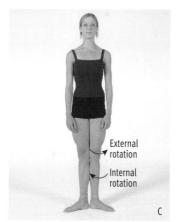

Figure 1.5 Movements in the hip joint: A) flexion and extension – around the horizontal axis, B) abduction and adduction – around the sagittal axis, C) external rotation and internal rotation – around the vertical axis.

Table 1.1 The nomenclature of movement

Axis around which the movement occurs	Name of the movement	Plane on which the movement occurs
Horizontal axis	Flexion – Extension	Sagittal plane
Sagittal axis	Abduction – Adduction	Frontal plane
Vertical axis	External rotation – Internal rotation	Horizontal plane

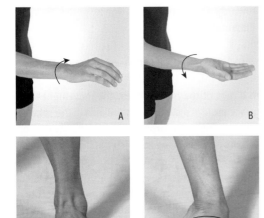

Figure 1.6 Movement of the hand:

A) pronation, B) supination.

Movement of the foot: C) pronation, D) supination.

vertical axis are described as *external* and *internal* *rotation*. Depending on its anatomical structure, each joint can carry out at least two of the six described movements.

The forearm and foot have a special movement nomenclature. Here the inward rotation is described as *pronation*, in which the back of the hand is on top (as if grasping for **b**read), or the outer edge of the foot is raised. The opposite movement is the outward rotation, known as *supination*. Here the back of the hand is underneath (like a **s**oup bowl), or the inner edge of the foot is raised.

The precise naming of the direction of movement not only helps with the description of the movement itself; it also supplies the name of the corresponding muscles and muscle groups. Thus muscles which are involved in the flexion of the hip joint are known as hip flexors; the muscles involved in the extension of the hip are known as

hip extensors. Understanding this clear system simplifies the classification and naming of the numerous muscles.

The Organization of the Body

Regardless of the position of the body within the space, and regardless of whether one is lying, standing or suspended, the anatomical nomenclature clearly defines the different areas of the body in relation to each other. This is useful because, for example, the description "this joint lies above the knee" could lead to various, possibly confusing, conclusions depending on the position of the body and its position in space. In anatomy we therefore use terms that may seem unusual at first, but their clear definition permits us to describe structures in the body and their position in relation to each other, regardless of the actual body position.

Table 1.2 Location descriptors – useful pairs of terms with opposite meanings (see Figure. 1.1)

anterior = front	posterior = rear
ventral = towards the abdomen	dorsal = towards the back
caudal = towards the coccyx	cranial = towards the head
medial = towards the midline	lateral = away from the midline
proximal = near the centre	distal = away from the centre
plantar = on the sole of the foot	palmar = on the palm of the hand

The Composition of Tissues

Training changes the body. Every dancer knows that from his personal experience. The body stature is transformed; certain areas become slimmer and others develop more strongly. The body reacts to the stress of dancing by adapting to the dance training. What can be seen externally in the body shape also takes place inside the body within its smallest building block, the cell. Its ability to divide not only serves growth but is also the basis for regeneration. Thus the body can replace used, damaged or lost cells with newly-formed ones. At the same time it adapts to take into account the current training load. By enlarging an individual cell or increasing the number of cells, the body equips itself to meet the growing demands. This adaptation is reversible. If the load is reduced, the number of corresponding cells or their size is also reduced; the body responds to the reduced workload.

Composition –
the Principle is Always the Same

One uses the term "tissue" to describe a collection of similarly formed cells with similar functional tasks. Regardless of the type of tissue, its basic structure is the same: the cells are embedded in a homogeneous amorphous mass (Greek *amorph* = formless), the intercellular substance (matrix). Depending on the tissue type, various fibres run between the cells. The tissue type is determined by the cells; its characteristics are influenced to a considerable degree by the embedded fibres.

The **intercellular substance** consists of a thick liquid in which various substances are dissolved. In quantitative terms it is composed mainly of water, protein particles, sugar, hormones and electrolytes.

In the body we distinguish between three types of **fibres**. *Collagen fibres* occur nearly everywhere within the body. It is virtually impossible to stretch them lengthways and thus they give the tissue a great deal of tensile strength. *Elastic fibres*, on the other hand, indicate a high degree of elasticity.

They can be stretched to up to 150 per cent of their original length, but immediately after completion of the traction they return to their original length. *Reticulin fibres* are the finest fibres in the human organism. They usually form microscopic nets or grids and thus provide general stability to the tissue.

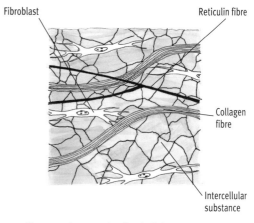

Fibroblast   Reticulin fibre

Collagen fibre

Intercellular substance

Figure 1.7 An example of typical tissue structure. In this case, connective tissue.

The Different Types of Tissue –
the Difference is in the Detail

In the human body, we distinguish between four basic types of tissue: epithelial tissue, connective and supportive tissue, muscle tissue and nerve tissue. All four differ as to the type of tissue cells, the precise structure of the intercellular substance and the number and composition of the fibres they contain.

Epithelial tissue serves to cover the inner and outer surfaces of the body. The most important example is the skin, which, depending on the size of the individual, can cover an area of up to 2m². Thus, it is considered to be the largest organ of the human body. Its job, apart from protection and temperature regulation, also includes immune defence, regulation of fluid balance through perspiration, and perception of the surrounding environment, for example, of pressure and temperature. It is also an important organ for communication. When we blush, go pale or get goose bumps we unconsciously send important messages to others.

Connective and supportive tissue is needed for the structural maintenance of the body. The **supportive tissue** includes bones, cartilage and tendons and is extremely important for the dancer as part of the movement apparatus. It is described in greater detail from page 9 on.

Connective tissue can be found everywhere throughout the body. It extends around and between the organs, vessels and nerves. Depending on the consistency, quantity and arrangement of the intercellular fibres, we distinguish between the taut *collagenous* and elastic *connective tissue*, which has a large number of fibres, determining its shape, and the looser, soft, *reticular connective tissue* which is easily movable. Connective tissue has a number of tasks to perform: these range from the protection and cushioning of the body and the storage of water and nutrients to transport and immune defence. Its metabolism is sluggish; the transport of metabolic products occurs quite slowly. Thus connective tissue is often referred to as the body's "rubbish bin". Through the increased concentration of waste products, its normally long regeneration time, is extended even further.

Fatty tissue is a special form of connective tissue. Here, fat is stored within specialized fat cells. These special storage cells have thin, elastic walls and are thus especially flexible. In this way they can adapt their storage capacity to suit requirements. It is important to distinguish between *structural* and *storage fat*. Structural fat takes on important tasks at many locations within the body: below the heel bone it serves as a "heel cushion" which pads the foot and absorbs shock. The structural fat around the kidneys secures the kidneys in place and protects them from shock and impact. Storage fat is found in particular under the skin, where it is important as an energy reserve and for temperature regulation. It is well supplied with blood vessels and is constantly

being renewed. Structural fat, on the other hand, is only made use of in times of extreme hunger. For example, in the case of eating disorders – a problem which unfortunately occurs frequently in dancers (see Chapter 9, p. 189) – the structural fat around the kidneys is partly destroyed. This has permanent consequences, as it is impossible to completely rebuild structural fat once destroyed, even with the aid of ideal nutrition.

Muscle and **nerve tissue** are essential for the performance and control of movement. They are described in more detail starting on p. 13.

Regeneration and Adaptation – Tissue is Constantly Changing

All tissues in the body are constantly changing: since all tissue is alive, old cells and fibres are destroyed and new ones are formed. The process of renewal takes place at different speeds depending on the type of tissue concerned. Muscle cells regenerate quickly in a matter of days, but ligaments, tendons and cartilage tissue need considerably longer. The regeneration process takes months or even years. The quicker a tissue can regenerate, the quicker it can adapt to external stimuli.

"Biological adaptation" is what is known in sport and dance as "trainability". The different types of tissue react very differently to the influence of training; their adaptability varies from hours to years. For instance, muscles can be trained relatively quickly; however, the growth of additional connective and supporting tissue, of bones, tendons and ligaments, takes considerably longer.

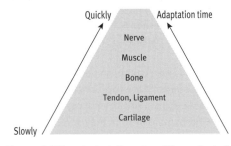

Figure 1.8 Different adaptation rates of tissues to strain.

The Skeletal System: Bones, Cartilage and Joints

The human skeleton consists of more than 200 bones. The skeleton supports the body, protects the organs and at the same time serves as attachment points for muscles, tendons and ligaments. Through its joints, it significantly influences the flexibility of the entire body. The skeleton gives the body its form and stability, although it is quite light itself: all the bones together only account for about 15 to 20 per cent of the total body weight.

Bones

Bones are characterized by their great resistance to pressure and their tensile strength as well as their breaking strength and their – often forgotten – elasticity. In addition to their obvious tasks such as support and protection, bones are also important for the production of blood cells and the storage of important mineral substances in the body. Bones owe their relatively low weight to their intelligent physical structure.

Bone tissue – bone is alive

Together, bone cells (*osteocytes*) and basic substance form the bone tissue. Ten per cent of the basic bone substance consists of water and 20 per cent of organic materials, such as protein and collagen fibres. The collagen fibres are responsible for the elasticity of the bone and for its ability to resist tension. 70 per cent of the basic substance consists of inorganic substances, minerals which are stored in the tissue – a special characteristic that occurs only in bone tissue. Calcium plays a very important role here: the calcium salts stored in the bones account for two-thirds of the bone weight; they give the bone tissue its great stability and strength.

The bone cells are supplied with nutrients and oxygen by their own system of blood vessels. A functioning metabolism is essential for the bones, as they are constantly being remodelled. Every week, 5 to 7 per cent of our bone mass is renewed;

therefore, every five months our bone tissue is completely replaced. In spite of its stability and hardness, bone is a living tissue; in a healthy person bone resorption and bone formation balance each other out. The formation is not just a matter of replacement of the bone substance; at the same time it is used for adapting bone structure to load. An increase in stress leads to an increase in the mass and density of the bone, and a decrease in stress results in loss of both strength and bone density. This shows that stress forms the bones. The function determines the form.

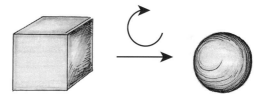

Figure 1.9 Form follows function: when a square bone rotates for a long period its corners wear out and it becomes round.

An impressive example of this is the thickening of the second metatarsal bone, which occurs frequently in dancers. On demi-pointe or pointe, the line of gravity runs between the first and second metatarsal bone. In order to adapt to this high degree of stress, the body increases the amount of bone tissue precisely where it is needed: the metatarsal bone becomes thicker (see Chapter 6, p. 123).

The "typical" bone – the structure of a long bone

The global structure of a bone will be demonstrated by the femur, a typical example of a long bone.

The long shaft, the *diaphysis*, consists of a tube-like casing (**corticalis**) of compact bone material (*compacta*). The centre of the bone is hollow. This construction provides two advantages, making the bone both more elastic and lighter in weight.

The hollow space, or *medullary cavity*, is filled with bone marrow. Both ends of the bone, the *epiphyses*, are covered with cartilage. Their interior is made up of a lattice of fine columns of bone, which, due to its sponge-like appearance, is called the **spongiosa**. This is a lightweight construction, which saves even more weight. The spongy bone tissue is very important for bone resilience. Adapting to the load, the columns of bone align themselves along the main stress lines. Thus they form a supportive structure with a high capacity for bearing loads and withstanding stress: the so-called *trabecular system* (see Chapter 4, p. 76).

The **periosteum** is a fibrous, elastic sheath surrounding the outside of the bone. It is criss-crossed by numerous blood vessels and is responsible for the nutrition and regeneration of

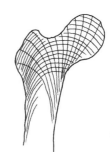

Figure 1.11 The trabecular system at the ends of the bone: the trabeculae align in order to evenly distribute the load.

the bone. If the periosteum is removed, the bone will be destroyed. Through its dense network of nerves, the periosteum has an important function in protecting the bone. If subjected to un-accustomed stress or excessive loads, the periosteum may become inflamed; the associated pain warns against further excessive stress. In some places the periosteum lies almost unprotected directly underneath the skin. These areas are especially sensitive to pain; most people are familiar with the sharp unpleasant pain caused by a blow on the shin.

Bone marrow is found in the medullary cavity and within the spongy bone tissue. In addition to filling out the cavities, its main task is the formation of red blood cells.

Cartilage

The main qualities of cartilage are high elasticity of compression, resistance to shearing forces and traction, and the ability to absorb shock.

Cartilage tissue

Cartilage tissue consists of cartilage cells and a substance in between the cells that holds water and proteins (the "intercellular substance"). It contains neither nerves nor blood vessels. Its nutrition occurs via diffusion, through the direct absorption of nutrients from surrounding tissues or from the synovial fluid. This explains the slow metabolism of cartilage and therefore its reduced ability to regenerate itself. Ideally, the alternation between weight bearing and relief on the joints

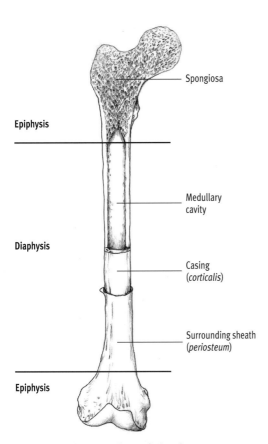

Epiphysis

Diaphysis

Epiphysis

Spongiosa

Medullary cavity

Casing (*corticalis*)

Surrounding sheath (*periosteum*)

Figure 1.10 Shape of a long bone.

results in an exchange of fluids and thus in the supplying of nutrients to the joint cartilage. If a joint is immobilized for a long time, or subjected to excessive stress, the supply of nutrients to the cartilage is interrupted; this can result in damage to the cartilage. The "critical thickness" of cartilage is considered to be 3mm; thicker layers of cartilage cannot be supplied with nutrients as effectively. Since the cartilage of the kneecap can be up to 6mm thick, this explains the frequency of cartilage irritation in this area (see Chapter 5, p. 109). During the course of life, the water content of the cartilage tissue reduces, its elasticity under compressive forces and its resistance to shearing and traction forces decreases, making it more susceptible to injury.

Cartilage types

What determines the type of cartilage is the composition of the intercellular substance and the type of fibres it contains.

In **hyaline cartilage** the intercellular substance is permeated by numerous collagen fibres. Together they form an amorphous watery mass which gives the cartilage its high elasticity under compression. Hyaline cartilage can be found everywhere where high compressive loads occur, for example, as a shiny white covering on most joint surfaces. One of its special characteristics is its high degree of adaptability. Short-term stress leads to a rapid increase in thickness of the hyaline cartilage: for a limited period, it stores additional fluid in the intercellular substance. Through this temporary swelling the cartilage is more resistant to compression and shearing forces – an ability which can be used to advantage through a targeted warm-up routine (see Chapter 12, p. 225). Long-term stress will lead to a gradual thickening of the cartilage; here the cartilage cells increase in size and number and the metabolism within the cartilage accelerates – all of which are mechanisms that increase the resistance of the hyaline cartilage. Unfortunately, the ability to regenerate after injury is very low in hyaline cartilage. Damaged cartilage cells and a damaged fibre structure cannot be reconstructed

identically. In place of the hyaline cartilage, fibrocartilage forms instead. This tissue is able to fill out the surface of the cartilage layer superficially, but its elasticity under compression is considerably less, so that the resilience of the repaired area is reduced.

Fibrocartilage is especially resistant to shearing forces. Its intercellular substance consists primarily of collagen fibres arranged in parallel rows; their number can vary depending on the stress. For example, it forms the fibrous ring of the intervertebral disc, (see Chapter 2, p. 27) and the meniscus in the knee, and serves to repair damage of the hyaline cartilage.

Elastic cartilage is particularly flexible. A network of elastic fibres runs through its intercellular substance. One familiar example of elastic cartilage is the earlobe, which can be bent in all directions without causing pain.

Joints

We use the term joint to describe the link from one bone to another. Joints have two tasks: they link together the bones of the skeleton and at the same time ensure its flexibility. The link can be immobile ("false" joints) or movable ("true" joints). Immobile joints are found, for example, in the cartilaginous zone at the front of the ribcage between the ribs and the sternum, or in the pubic symphysis between the two pubic bones. The latter permits the passive movement of the two hip bones of the pelvis towards each other, but it cannot be actively moved (see Chapter 3, p. 57). If we refer to joints, we generally mean the "true" joints, where active movement takes place.

The structure of a joint – mobility is important

Joints are basically formed from the ends of bones, the joint capsule and the joint cavity with the intra-articular space.

The **bone ends** are covered with hyaline cartilage. The smooth surface of this cartilage serves to reduce friction and absorb shocks. Each joint has at least two articular partners. If there is

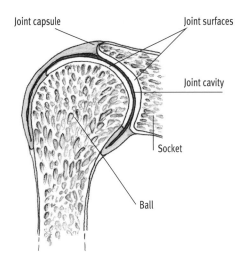

Figure 1.12 The structure of a true joint.

Table 1.3 The degree of mobility in the joint is essentially determined by three factors

Form and size of the bony joint partners	Bones
Course and strength of the joint ligaments	Ligaments
Course and number of muscles that operate the joint	Muscles

a lot of unevenness between the joint surfaces, this is balanced out by additional discs of cartilage within the joint, such as the meniscus in the knee (see Chapter 5, p. 102).

The **joint capsule** surrounds the entire joint like a casing. It consists of two layers: an inner layer with a network of numerous blood vessels and the thicker and more stable outer layer. The size and thickness of the joint capsule varies considerably from joint to joint. If stability is the most important factor, the joint capsule is fairly tight and is strengthened by numerous ligaments. If it is wide and loose the mobility of the joint is the decisive factor.

The space within the joint capsule is known as the **joint cavity**. It is filled with *synovial fluid*, a fluid with a consistency similar to that of egg white. Synovial fluid is produced by the inner layer of the joint capsule. The synovial fluid is responsible for the nutrition of the joint cartilage, for greasing the joint surfaces and for shock absorption within the joint. The consistency of the synovial fluid changes depending on its temperature and the speed of the movement. Its viscosity increases with cold and slow movements, which make the synovial fluid glutinous. Higher temperatures (e.g. after warming-up) and faster movements reduce the viscocity and with this the resistance.

Ligaments – clear instructions for the joint
Ligaments consist of taut connective tissue. The high proportion of parallel collagen fibres gives them a high degree of strength, but their elasticity is low at only 5 per cent. Most ligaments attach from bone to bone. However, there are also ligaments which increase their elasticity by penetrating the muscles with some fibres. Ligaments restrict the passive movement of joints; they give clear instructions regarding the direction of movement.

We differentiate between ligaments which lie deep inside the joint, those which run inside the capsule and thus strengthen the capsule itself, and those which cross above the outside of the joint capsule. Ligaments contain numerous receptors that provide the nervous system with information about the joint's position. Velocity, movement and joint position are registered, as well as stretching or pain. Via the ligament's receptors, there is permanent feedback on the current joint situation, which permits the body to quickly make fine adjustments and to react in a nuanced manner to each new joint position. This is essential for coordination and balance. Therefore, it is not surprising that the body's balance is greatly affected after ligament injuries.

One of the most important tasks of the ligament system is to transform compressive loads in the joint into tensile loading of the ligaments. Through optimal joint position, the compression in the joint will be transferred into a tightening of the ligaments. This relieves the joint and at the same time trains the ligaments (see e.g. Chapter 4,

p. 77). If a ligament is tightened, its inner structure is aligned according to the main direction of pull: all fibres run in the same direction. If there is no clear direction of pull, the individual fibres arrange themselves in a random pattern within the ligament; this chaotic arrangement of fibres weakens the ligament. A constant alternation of tightening and releasing encourages the metabolism within the ligament and thus increases its resilience in the long run.

Joint noises – harmless or worrying?

To this day the cause of cracking sounds in the joints, whether from a "creaking" back or pulling at the fingers, has not been fully explained. The current theory assumes that some of these cracking sounds are due to negative pressure within the joint cavity. As gases are dissolved in the synovial fluid certain movements can lead to the production of gas bubbles within this fluid. If some of these bubbles burst, we hear the typical cracking sound. The cracking sound will only be repeated when the gases have dissolved in the synovial fluid again. If a joint occasionally cracks during movement, this is not a problem. But the frequent manipulation and "setting" of joints – whether by oneself or by someone else – can lead to an over-stretching of the joint ligaments and thus to excessive local mobility, and this in turn increases the cracking. It is interesting to note that in the long term, cracking one's fingers leads to a slight swelling of the knuckles and – more notably – to a weakening of the hands. If we transfer this situation to the other joints, then the habitual cracking of joints is certainly not recommended.

The Muscles – the Motor of Movement

Whether we laugh, speak, swallow, digest, breathe or dance, the contraction of muscle cells is responsible for most movements of the body. It is the nerves which give the muscles instructions for their tasks. The nervous system is the true conductor of movement; the muscles merely execute movement. Muscle tissue is made up of millions of muscle cells. We distinguish between three different types of muscle according to their structure and their function: smooth muscles, heart muscle and skeletal muscles.

Smooth muscles are also known as involuntary muscles. Seen under the microscope they appear as a network of countless muscle cells of differing sizes and direction. Smooth muscles are found, for example, in the eyes, the blood vessels and the entire digestive system, but also as small muscles in the roots of the hair within the skin, where they contract to make the hairs stand on end and thus to give us goose bumps. As the muscles of the organs, the smooth muscles are controlled by the autonomic nervous system and by hormones. Thus they cannot be controlled by a conscious decision on our part.

As the name implies, the **heart muscle** is found only within the heart. It represents a special form, having attributes of both the skeletal muscles and the smooth muscles. On the one hand, the individual muscle cells demonstrate the typical cross-striation of the skeletal muscles, but on the other hand they are controlled, like smooth muscle, by the autonomic nervous system. The heart muscle has an unusual function with its pacemaker cells: it is able to contract independently, without receiving impulses from the nervous system.

When we refer to muscles we are usually talking about the **skeletal muscles**, the so-called striated muscles. They are attached to the bones and thus move the skeleton. As this work of the muscles can be consciously and intentionally controlled, the skeletal muscles are also known as the voluntary muscles. Looking through a microscope permits us to see the characteristic striations in the muscle fibres. The skeletal muscle system consists of about 400 individual muscles of varying size and shape, from the smallest finger muscle to the long back muscles. Together, the skeletal muscles weigh more than the entire skeleton. So, in a dancer, the skeletal muscles account for about 40 per cent of body weight, while the skeleton only accounts for 15 per cent of a person's total weight.

Because of their importance for movement and dance, the structure and function of the skeletal muscles will be described below in greater detail.

Structure

The muscle – what moves the bone

Skeletal muscles consist of long, thin muscle cells. These muscle cells can contain over a thousand cell nuclei and can be up to 40cm long; therefore, they are also described as *muscle fibres*. Several muscle fibres together form a *muscle fascicle*, and a number of muscle fascicles join together to form the *muscle belly*. Typically, the ends of the muscle belly are linked to the bone via tendons or tendon plates. The diameter of the muscle belly, the detailed architecture and composition of its muscle fibres, the relationship between muscle belly and tendon and its precise attachment point on the bone or connective tissue will largely determine the efficiency and strength of the muscle.

The muscle fibre – a closer look

The muscle fibre is the basic anatomical unit of the muscle. Within it, parallel thread-like protein structures run lengthways; these are called *myofibrils*. The smallest sub-unit of the myofibrils

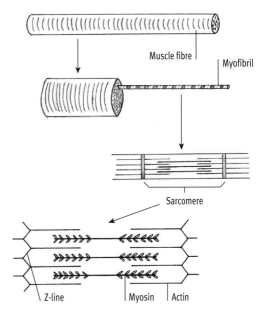

Figure 1.14 From the muscle fibre to the sarcomere, the "contractile unit" of the muscle.

is the *sarcomere*, the "contractile unit" of the muscle fibre. In a single muscle fibre several thousand sarcomeres are laid out, one after the other. Each sarcomere is framed on both sides by the so-called *Z-line*, in between which lie the chains of proteins (*myofilaments*), also known as *actin* and *myosin*. The actin is thin and attaches directly onto the Z-line, while the myosin, which is thicker, stretches between. Seen under the microscope, the alternation of these actin and myosin filaments creates the striations typical of skeletal muscles.

The muscle fibre receives the order to contract from the nervous system. Depending on the muscle, a varying number of muscle fibres are innervated by one nerve cell. The nerve cell and the muscle fibres it supplies are known as a *motor unit*. The number of muscle fibres joined together in a motor unit varies, from fewer than ten muscle fibres in the eye muscles to several thousand in the large thigh muscle (quadriceps femoris). In

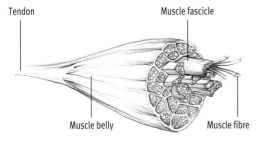

Figure 1.13 The structure of muscles.

general, the larger the motor unit, the greater the strength of the muscle. Conversely, the smaller the motor unit, the more precise the control over movement. The strength of the muscular contraction is controlled via the number of motor units which are activated. The greater the tension in the muscle, the more motor units are involved in the contraction.

The tendon – the link to the bone

Most muscles are attached to the bone via tendons. The task of the tendons is to transfer the tensile strength produced by the muscular contraction to the bone. This requires a low degree of elasticity and a large amount of longitudinal strength. The structure of the tendon allows it to fulfil both requirements optimally. It consists of collagen fibres in a parallel arrangement. When resting, they are slightly wavy. They are attached to the bone via a cartilage zone. This cartilage zone ensures a harmonious transition between the high elasticity of the muscle-tendon complex and the considerably lower degree of elasticity in the bone. With a maximum of 4 per cent stretch, the elasticity of the tendon is considerably lower than the elasticity of the muscle, which in extreme cases can stretch up to 50 per cent. With increasing age, the strength of the tendons is reduced. Fat storage and a reduction in the tendon cells reduce regenerative ability and thus lowers the resilience of the tendon tissue.

In places where tendons are subjected to high mechanical stress, special features often protect the tendon, such as sesamoid bones, synovial bursae or tendon sheaths.

Sesamoid bones are designed to strengthen the tendon and to improve the mechanics of the muscle pull. The largest sesamoid bone in humans is the kneecap.

Synovial bursae are small sacs filled with liquid which can be found wherever muscles and tendons slide across bony protuberances which make them subject to injury. Like a water cushion these bursae absorb the pressure applied to the tendon and thus prevent its being worn away. There are a large number of synovial bursae in the region of the knee. As an example, a synovial bursa directly below the kneecap cushions the patellar ligament when kneeling and thus prevents excess pressure.

Tendon sheaths are designed to ensure that tendons can glide smoothly in places where they cross over each other or run directly over bone. Forming a taut covering of tissue, they surround the tendon, permitting it to slide almost without friction within the tendon sheath. Since they are firmly anchored to the surrounding tissue they can also serve as a "deflection roller" to guide the muscle direction. For example, the tendon sheath of the long flexor muscle of the big toe passes behind and around the inner ankle, holding the muscle and tendon in their curved course (see Chapter 6, p. 129).

The fascial sheath – protection and movement

Each skeletal muscle is surrounded by a layer of connective tissue, the fascial sheath. This not only covers the entire muscle belly, but continues over the tendon tissue to the bone. It also supplies the muscle with blood vessels and nerves. The fascial sheath gives the muscle belly its characteristic form; its elasticity determines the muscle's ability to stretch. It serves as an anti-friction layer between the individual muscles, between muscle and bone or between muscle and organ. Unlimited mobility of the fascial sheaths between each other is a basic requirement for good mobility. The fascial sheaths of individual muscles are linked to each other like a chain. These fascial chains are also a metaphor for the numerous structural and functional links that run through the entire body.

Function

Contraction of the muscle – movement on the smallest level

When a muscle contracts, the sarcomeres within the muscle fibres are shortened, while the length of the individual protein chains remains the same. The shortening of the sarcomere happens as the actin and myosin slide into each other, bringing the Z-lines closer together.

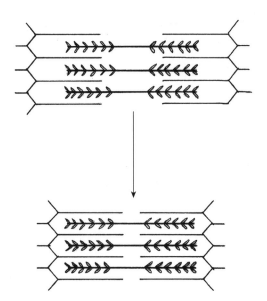

Figure 1.15 Muscle contraction – actin and myosin slide along each other shortening the sarcomere.

If a muscle fibre receives a command to contract, calcium is released within the muscle cell. The calcium precipitates a cascade of reactions, so that finally the thin actin is drawn between the thicker myosin. The Z-lines move closer together and the sarcomere becomes shorter. Although the shortening in each individual sarcomere is only a few micrometres, the contraction of several thousand sarcomeres together results in an appreciable change in the length of the muscle. The muscle contracts and becomes shorter. Calcium is an important trigger for this process.

Types of muscle work – how movement works

Through contraction, each individual sarcomere and thus the entire muscle can be shortened by about a half. The more motor units within a muscle are involved in this shortening, the easier it is to feel the tension of the muscle, even for an untrained person. It is more difficult to feel a much lower degree of tension in the muscle, a basic tension which supports posture and stability but does not limit mobility. In dance, this fine basic tension in the muscles is often required.

Contractions of the muscle can have different effects on muscle tension and muscle length:

Dynamic contraction: If the length of the muscle changes, this is referred to as dynamic contraction. A shortening of the muscle is called a concentric contraction; contraction while lengthening is described as eccentric contraction.

- In **concentric contraction** the muscle becomes shorter; both ends of the muscle come closer together and thus move the muscular anchorages on the bone towards each other. For example, the concentric contraction of the large thigh muscle (quadriceps femoris) shortens the muscle and the knee is stretched.
- In **eccentric contraction** the muscle is lengthened during the contraction; the muscular anchorages on the bone move further apart and the muscle stops the movement. For example, the eccentric contraction of the large thigh muscle (quadriceps femoris) when going downstairs. The muscle slows down the bending in the knee joint and is lengthened at the same time.

Static contraction: If the length remains the same and only the tension in the muscle changes, we refer to *static* or *isometric contraction*.

- In **static** or **isometric contraction** the muscle becomes taut without movement being visible from the outside. For example, the isometric contraction of the lower back muscles in the flat back.

The muscle in movement

The places where the muscle is attached to the bone are generally called the *origin* and *insertion*. The point of origin is usually closer to the middle of the body (proximal), and the point of insertion is further away from the middle of the body (distal). More functional are the terms *punctum fixum* (immobile end) and *punctum mobile* (mobile end). The punctum fixum is usually equated with the origin and the punctum mobile with the insertion, but allocation may be reversed depending on the movement. This can be explained using the example of the muscles in the back of the thigh. If the knee is bent in the working leg the muscles at the back of the thigh pull the lower leg back and thus bend the knee. In this movement, the origin and at the same time the punctum fixum of the musculature is the pelvis; the attachment and punctum mobile is the lower leg. In the plié it is different: here the knee is also bent, but now the thigh is brought closer towards the lower leg and the pelvis is pulled downwards. Now the punctum fixum is the insertion at the lower leg, and the punctum mobile is the pelvis.

Movement as a whole

A muscle rarely contracts in complete isolation. Mostly, several muscles work at the same time or shortly after each other, so that entire chains of muscles are involved in the movement. When muscles work together, they can fulfil different tasks depending on the movement: they can be the agonist, the antagonist, the synergist or the stabilizer.

This is explained below using the example of the raising of the parallel straight leg towards the back:

- The **agonist** – also called the prime mover – is a muscle or a muscle group which is mainly responsible for carrying out the desired movement. In our example, the muscles in the back of the thigh, the hamstrings are the agonists.
- The **antagonist** is a muscle or muscle group which counteracts the desired movement and can thus coordinate, slow down or even prevent the movement. In our example, the antagonists are the hip flexors and the rectus femoris muscle.
- The term **synergist** describes the muscles or muscle groups which support the agonist in the execution of the movement. In our example, this is the gluteus maximus in the buttocks.
- The **stabilizer** is a muscle or muscle group which contracts isometrically in order to stabilize a body part against the pull of other muscles or gravity. In our example, the stabilizer is the long muscle in the front of

the torso, the rectus abdominis muscle; it counteracts the forwards tilting of the pelvis. In this way, the pelvis is stabilized as the punctum fixum for the rear thigh muscles.

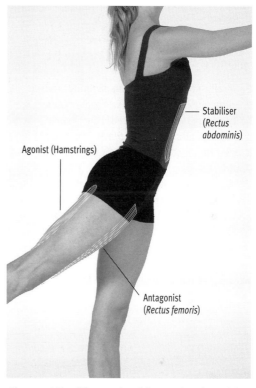

Figure 1.16 The different roles of the muscles when raising the straight leg parallel towards the back.

Certain muscles are described as **guiding muscles**. For the most part, these are muscles which do not mainly offer strength and stabilization, but rather control of movement and fine coordination. They are long and thin and mostly run across several joints, giving specific, highly-coordinated instructions for the direction of movement. They are responsible for the quality of the movement. The sartorius muscle in the upper thigh is a typical example of a guiding muscle. It is long and slender and runs across the hip and knee joints; it is not capable of very strong movements but its coordination is impressive: while it flexes at the hip joint and at the same time turns the upper thigh outwards, it ensures that the lower leg rotates inwards during bending at the knee joint. It thereby rotates the upper and lower leg in opposite directions and ensures a perfect three-dimensional spiral rotation of the leg (see Chapter 5, p. 103).

The Different Types of Muscle Fibre

Generally speaking, we can simplify matters by dividing muscle fibres into two main types:

Type 1 muscle fibres: red, thin, "slow" fibres, also known as *slow twitch fibres*. This type of fibre is used for muscle work of low intensity and long duration.

Type 2 muscle fibres: white, thick, "fast" fibres, also known as *fast twitch fibres*. They are used primarily for fast, intensive muscle tasks.

Slow, type 1 muscle fibres are organized in relatively small motor units. This allows good

Table 1.4 The different types of muscle fibre

Characteristics	Type 1 muscle fibres	Type 2 muscle fibres
Colour	red/dark	white/light
Speed	slow	fast
Strength	low	high
Fatigue resistance	high	low
Efficiency	high	low

control of the movement and improves the fine coordination. The slower the movement is carried out, the more type 1 fibres are called into action. Thus the movement can be better coordinated and more precisely trained: a good basis for technique training.

Slow, type 1 muscle fibres are about 30 per cent thinner than fast muscle fibres. This explains the usually slim appearance of endurance athletes. Dancers with type 2 muscle fibres often look quite muscular. The motor units of type 2 muscle fibres include a large number of muscles and the movements are accordingly fast and powerful, but not as easy to coordinate.

The ratio of the different fibre types within a muscle and within the body as a whole is genetically determined. Most people have a similar distribution of muscle fibre types, but there are exceptions in both directions. In a "born" sprinter, the fast type 2 fibres predominate, and in the "born" marathon runner it is the slow type 1 fibres that predominate. The unconscious choice of favourite sport and of favourite exercises by many athletes – and dancers – can probably be explained by the inborn distribution of muscle fibre types. Thus type 1 dancers find slow, restrained adagios easy while type 2 dancers are noticeable for their speed and ability to jump. Today, one thing seems certain: the genetically determined distribution of muscle fibres is virtually impossible to change, even with intensive training. Fast muscles can be changed temporarily into slow ones, but if training stops the change will rapidly be reversed. It is not possible to change slow fibres into fast ones through training. During the natural aging process the number of type 2 fibres decreases. This is one of the reasons we become slower as we get older.

The Nervous System – the Body's Conductor

Learning dance steps, understanding corrections and translating them directly into movement; remembering choreography and performing it precisely in front of an audience and with total concentration: these are all everyday demands made of a dancer, or more precisely of his nervous system. The nervous system is the body's conductor and a true miracle about which we are learning more, thanks to intensive research. It has a wide variety of tasks to perform: to absorb information, pass it on, process it, store it and repeat it. It links the different parts of the body together, communicates with the outside world and coordinates procedures within the body. The classification of the nervous system is carried out in two different ways: first, according to its position within the body and second, according to its function.

Anatomically, the nervous system is subdivided into a central and a peripheral nervous system:

The **central nervous system (CNS)** consists of the brain and the spinal cord. It is well protected against external injury by the bones of the skull and the spine. Encased in the cerebral and the spinal membranes, the CNS is surrounded by a cushion of liquid, the cerebrospinal fluid. The purpose of this fluid is to nourish the brain and the nerves and to cushion the CNS against its hard, bony casing.

The **peripheral nervous system** consists of numerous nerves which permeate the entire body. They convey impulses either from the periphery to the CNS (*sensory nerves*) or from the CNS to the periphery (*motor nerves*). The sensory pathways are also known as *afferent* (Latin: *affere* = to carry towards), and the motor pathways are called *efferent* (Latin: *effere* = to carry away).

Depending on its function, we distinguish between the somatic and the autonomic nervous system. Both systems can be further subdivided into a central and a peripheral area.

The **somatic nervous system** (Greek: *somatos* = the body) serves as a motor for the deliberate control of the skeletal muscles. It perceives stimuli and information from the periphery of the body and thus links man with his environment. It is also referred to as the voluntary nervous system.

The **autonomic nervous system** consists of two parts, the sympathetic and the parasympathetic nervous system. Together, they provide unconscious, involuntary control of the inner organs and numerous essential processes such as breathing, digestion or blood pressure regulation, for example. Therefore this system is also referred to as the involuntary nervous system.

Structure

The CNS

The central nervous system (CNS) comprises the spinal cord and the various parts of the brain (cerebrum, cerebellum and brain stem).

The **cerebrum** is the most highly-differentiated part of the CNS. It is here that our thinking, feeling and actions have their biological basis. It consists of two *hemispheres*, which are linked together via the so-called corpus callosum. The surface of the hemispheres is called the cerebral cortex; it is only a few millimetres thick. Its appearance is characterized by countless twists, crevices and furrows. These folds serve to increase the surface area of the cerebral cortex, creating the maximum surface area with a minimum space requirement, an intelligent solution.

The **cerebellum** lies below the cerebrum. It is the most important section for the learning and automatization of movements, coordination and fine control.

Within the **brain stem** lie important control centres for breathing and blood circulation; this is also the seat of the rhythm of waking and sleeping (circadian rhythm) In the medulla, one part of the brain stem, lies an important junction of nerves: this is where 90 per cent of all motor nerve fibres cross to the opposite side on their way from the brain to the spinal cord; only 10 per cent continue towards the muscles on the same side without

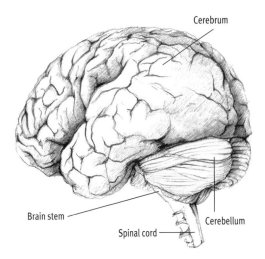

Cerebrum

Brain stem

Spinal cord

Cerebellum

Figure 1.17 The structure of the central nervous system.

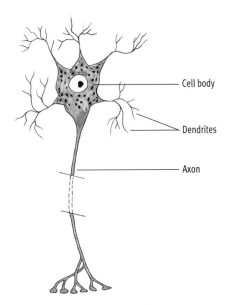

Cell body

Dendrites

Axon

Figure 1.18 The structure of a neuron.

crossing over. As a result, for example, if you learn a new movement with the right leg, the left leg learns it at the same time too. Not with the same precision, but as an appropriate copy.

The **spinal cord** is the main conduit cable for the CNS. Several million nerve fibres run through it. The extension of the nerve cells in the brain are bundled together and run through a large opening at the back of the scull along the spinal cord down to the lumbar spine. The spinal cord comes to an end roughly at the level of the second lumbar vertebra. As the spinal cord passes through the bony vertebral canal the main nerves which supply the entire torso, the arms and the legs branch off. As *spinal nerves* they emerge through little gaps between the individual vertebrae (see Chapter 2, p. 27). On their way to the periphery, they continue to divide into ever-smaller branches, thus supplying every part of the body.

The nerve cell

The basic functional unit of the nervous system is the nerve cell, or **neuron**. The entire nervous system is comprised of over 100 billion neurons. Each neuron consists of a cell body, from which a number of extensions or "processes" emerge. These little processes, or *dendrites*, serve the purpose of receiving information; they pass on impulses from the surroundings towards the cell body. A long extension, called the *axon*, transfers information from the cell body to the subsequent cells or to muscles and organs. Some of these axons are surrounded by special encasing cells; they are described as myelinated. Myelinated axons pass on nerve impulses especially quickly, and so they are often found in motor nerves. They have a conduction velocity of up to 120m/s, which works out to 432km/hr! By contrast, unmyelinated axons (which have no encasing cells) are considerably slower; they are responsible, for example, for conveying pain. Several axons together are surrounded by a casing of connective tissue. Comparable to an electrical cable, they form the nerve. Blood vessels which are responsible for supplying nutrition to the nerve run inside this casing of connective tissue.

The neurons of the nervous system are linked by more than a billion **synapses**. They are the contact points for the nerve cells. It is here that the transmission of the impulse from one neuron to the next takes place. Depending on the *neurotransmitter*, the propagation of the impulse is either encouraged or suppressed. A single nerve cell receives information from over 20,000 synapses. All this information – whether suppressive or supportive – is assessed and the perceived impulse is then finally passed on to the next nerve cell.

Function

Information processing – the nervous system remains flexible

Whether it is a corrective touch by the trainer or a hot teacup, all stimuli from the periphery are registered by the body's so-called receptors. These are nerve cells which possess specific abilities: they can change chemical or physical stimuli into electrical impulses. Temperature, pressure or pain, as well as joint position and degree of tension within the muscles are all registered by the receptors and transmitted as impulses via afferent nerves to the central nervous system. There, all impulses are switched to special centres where they are evaluated and processed. The association centres in the cerebral cortex have the task of linking the information as it arrives with corresponding memories, evaluations, emotions etc. Based on these, the brain puts together a programme of responses adapted to the situation in question. The result is then transmitted via efferent nerve fibres – once again as an impulse – to the periphery, selectively and precisely in those places where a response should take place.

By studying the distribution of the nerve pathways, we can see how important this continuous feedback is for the body. Eighty per cents of all nerves are afferent nerve fibres; they transmit information from the periphery to the central nervous system. Only 20 per cent are efferent nerves which are actually responsible for the execution of commands from the brain, transmitting impulses from the central nervous system to the periphery.

The reflex – the nervous system's automatic reactions

A reflex is an involuntary, automatic answer to a nervous stimulus. In the simplest case, the processing of the stimulus takes place in the spinal cord: afferent nerves transmit the stimulus from the periphery to the spinal cord, where the direct switching to the efferent nerve fibres takes place and transmits the response immediately to the periphery. Of special interest for the dancer is the so-called *proprioceptive reflex* (Latin: *proprius* = own; *recipere* = receive). Here the receptors in the muscles, tendons and joint capsules continuously transmit the current stance and position of the entire body to the nervous system. Hence, it is possible to act instinctively in the case of unfavourable changes in position – entirely without the involvement of the cerebrum. The *stretch reflex* is also important for the control of movement. The muscle spindles lying between the muscle fibres are the receptors which provide information at all times about the current state of muscle tension.

Plasticity – changes are desirable

The number of neurons in the body is determined before birth; it can only decrease over the course of a person's life. The exact opposite is true of the synapses. Throughout our lifetime these are constantly being renewed, each new learning process appears to be linked with the creation of new synapses. The more varied the learning content and the more varied the learning methods, the greater the stimulus for the brain. It is constantly forming new points of connection, the network of fibres becomes more dense and the area of the cerebral cortex which is involved becomes thicker and bigger.

The so-called "homunculus" (Latin: *"little man"*) provides us with insight into the distribution and representation of the individual sections of the body within the brain. Here the regions of the entire body are projected onto the area of the cerebral cortex that is responsible for them. The size of the area does not correspond precisely to the size of the area in the body. For parts of the body where fine motor coordination is particularly well trained, like the hand, relatively large areas of the cerebral cortex are available. Other parts of the body which do not execute such finely coordinated movements – such as the abdomen or back – have only relatively small areas of the

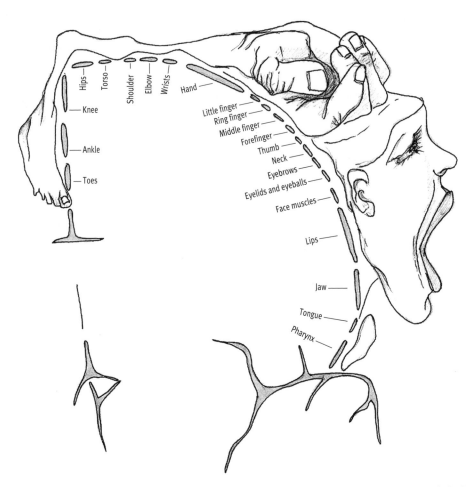

Figure 1.19 The motor "homunculus" reflects the areal distribution and representation of human body parts in the brain.

cortex. So the "homunculus" is quite distorted compared with the shape of the actual body.

It is interesting to note that musicians who play a stringed instrument have a considerably larger storage area in the brain for the fingers of the left hand than for the right hand. Whether or not this data can be transferred to the dancer and the area of the cerebral cortex relating, for example, to the dancer's feet, remains a matter for speculation.

The phenomenon of pain – the gate-control system

It's an automatic reaction; you bang your arm against the door, and experience a sharp pain. Instinctively you put your hand on the painful area and the pain subsides. This results from a sophisticated natural principle, the gate-control system for coping with pain. Painful stimuli – whether internal or external – are registered by the pain receptors and transmitted as impulses to the spinal cord. There, a large number of different neurons come together at a single neuron, a sort of control centre, a "gate" for processing pain. A large number of items of information are processed in this central neuron, items of information which may either confirm or modify each other. If the "pain" information is overshadowed in the control centre by other information such as pressure, cold

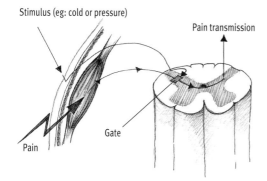

Figure 1.20 The "gate-control system" for
processing pain.

or movement, the pain stimulus is weakened. The "neutral" information blocks the "gate" and allows fewer pain impulses to pass through in the direction of the brain. The painful incident is the same, but the perception of pain is reduced.

The "channelling" – automatization of movement

If a thought process is frequently repeated in the brain, and if a movement is repeatedly carried out hundreds of times, the corresponding nerve impulses become "channelled" in their path through the nervous system. Just as a road with heavy traffic is eventually expanded to become a motorway, so the relevant nerve pathways are prepared for the increasing "through traffic". Their excitability is increased, new synapses are formed and the impulse engraves its path through the brain. The movement gets easier each time; its execution becomes more precise and more rapid, and with time, increasingly automatic. Movements that at first could only be carried out by processing at the highest level, by the cerebral cortex, become increasingly automatic over time. They are processed at a lower level, in the cerebellum, and thus take place unconsciously and without the control of the brain. Thus the cerebral cortex is relieved and can focus on other tasks and details related to movement.

We constantly make use of this automatization in our everyday lives as well as in training and dance. We can also use it as a conscious means of training our body awareness, in order to practise small corrections to the movement. By repeating them regularly, we integrate them into our subconscious. "One-second workouts" are an impressive example of this. One chooses an "anchor" that is designed to recall a special exercise repeatedly during the day. It could be the phone ringing, cleaning one's teeth, waiting at the bus stop, or an errand carried out every day. Whenever this "anchor" crops up in everyday life, the exercise is carried out immediately – the more frequently the better. Eventually, the nervous system will respond: the exercise will be channelled and the body awareness which it prompts will be engraved in the depths of the brain so that the movement becomes automatic.

In this book you will find a large number of exercises which are ideally suited for use as "one-second workouts" for the automatization of movement. One such example is the activation of the transverse arch in the forefoot (see Chapter 6, p. 149) or the awareness of the alignment of the leg (See Chapter 5, p. 118) – exercises which are important for many dancers. The steps leading to optimal body coordination are as follows: conscious integration into everyday life, a gradual automatization and finally, translation into dance.

2. The Spine: The Whole is More than the Sum of its Parts

Dancers are easy to spot not only in the dance studio but also on the street. Their erect posture radiates self-confidence. "Elongate your back", "Bring your spine in an upright position", "Centre your body above your pelvis" – these are corrections which give the spine the impulse to straighten itself. In dance, attention is paid to the correct alignment of the spine, both in lifting and in movement.

Through the integration of the two poles, head and pelvis, movements are distributed harmoniously through the entire spine; the posture is upright and nonetheless looks relaxed. The ideal image of the stable but flexible spine is equally important for dance and for everyday life. Increasing numbers of doctors and physio-therapists recommend dance as both prevention and therapy for postural defects, as good dance training improves the function of the spine by stabilizing and mobilizing it at the same time.

A high degree of flexibility and complex neuromuscular coordination throughout the entire spine are essential for dance movements. This is obvious in the cambré or arch, but even jumps, arabesques and pirouettes can only be mastered with a flexible spine. Each movement of the pelvis is continued in the lumbar spine, and each movement of the head is transmitted further via the cervical spine. In dance, sufficient flexibility throughout the entire spine and thorax, as well as the stability and dynamic strength of the trunk muscles are of decisive importance.

3D Anatomy

Consisting of 24 individual vertebral segments with more than 100 joints and a fine bracing system of over 200 small muscles, the spine is a miracle of human anatomy. Its tasks include stabilization of the torso, protection of the spinal cord and absorption of shocks as well as mobility and freedom of movement in all directions.

Structure

The chain of 33 vertebrae called the spine extends from the head to the coccyx. It is divided into five regions in each of which the individual vertebrae are counted from top to bottom: seven cervical vertebrae, 12 thoracic vertebrae and five lumbar vertebrae. Five vertebrae form the sacrum at the back of the pelvis and the four vertebrae below make up the coccyx. In adults, the vertebrae of the sacrum and of the coccyx have each grown together to form single bones, so that the spine only consists of 24 separate vertebrae (cervical, thoracic and lumbar). The vertebrae in the various regions differ from each other in size and shape, depending on their function.

If we look at the spine as a unit, it resembles a pyramid: the size and width of the vertebrae increase continuously from the top downwards, from the cervical to the lumbar vertebrae. The functional reason for this is clear: each vertebra has to bear the entire body weight above it. The last lumbar vertebra rests on the sacrum, which forms the back part of the pelvis and distributes the upper body weight across the entire pelvic

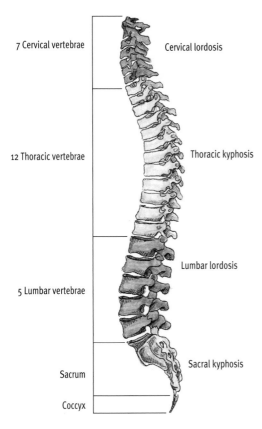

7 Cervical vertebrae

Cervical lordosis

12 Thoracic vertebrae

Thoracic kyphosis

Lumbar lordosis

5 Lumbar vertebrae

Sacrum

Sacral kyphosis

Coccyx

Figure 2.1 The structure of the spine.

Structure of a vertebra

All vertebrae are constructed the same way, but they differ in details depending on their function. The first two cervical vertebrae are the only exceptions to this general scheme (see p. 28). A typical vertebra consists of a vertebral body, the vertebral arch and seven bony processes.

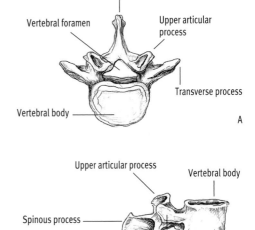

Spinous process

Vertebral foramen

Upper articular process

Transverse process

Vertebral body

A

Upper articular process

Vertebral body

Spinous process

Lower articular process

Transverse process

B

Figure 2.2 General structure of a vertebra:
A) top view, B) side view.

girdle (see Chapter 3, p. 58). The coccyx, as the bottom end of the spine, thus has no load-bearing function but it is important as the location of attachment for the pelvic floor muscles (see Chapter 3, p. 61).

The pelvis and the head form the functional poles of the spine. Their close connection is reflected in the anatomy. From the uppermost cervical joint, down to the coccyx, taut longitudinal ligaments run along the front and back of the spine. They are attached to each individual vertebra and to the intervertebral discs which lie between them. Inside the vertebral canal, the spinal cord is surrounded by the spinal membranes, which also extend from the skull down to the coccyx.

The **vertebral body** is the massive, cylindrical part of the vertebra which lies at the front. It is the load-bearing part of the spine. Its load-bearing strength is greatest when it is loaded axially. Its interior consists of a fine network of bone tissue, called the spongiosa. As the body ages, this bony lattice thins out and the compressive strength of the vertebral body declines. This is a natural aging process but it can begin in youth; given a poor diet, inappropriate stress or genetic predisposition (see Chapter 11, p. 209).

The **vertebral arch** is attached to the back of the vertebral body. Together with the vertebral body, it forms the vertebral foramen, and all the

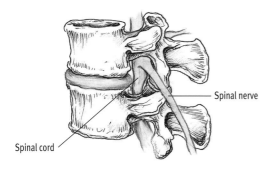

Figure 2.3 Two vertebrae together form the intervertebral foramen, through which the spinal nerves emerge.

Spinal nerve

Spinal cord

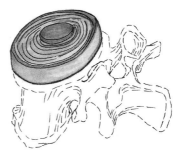

Figure 2.4 The structure of the intervertebral disc: the gelatinous core (*nucleus pulposus*) is surrounded by a strong fibrous ring (*anulus fibrosus*).

vertebral foramina together form the vertebral canal (*spinal canal*). Well protected inside the canal, runs the spinal cord with its spinal membranes, blood vessels and spinal nerves. Together, the vertebral arches of two neighbouring vertebrae form the *intervertebral foramen*, through which the *spinal nerves* emerge on the right and left.

Seven bony processes protrude from the vertebral arch: one spinous process, two transverse processes and two upper and two lower articular processes. The **spinous process** extends backwards from the middle of the vertebral arch. In many sections of the spinal column it can easily be felt through the skin. Especially prominent is the spinous process of the seventh cervical vertebra, which is therefore described as the *vertebra prominens*. The two **transverse processes** protrude from the side of the vertebral arch. This is where the ribs are attached in the region of the thoracic spine. Throughout the entire spinal column the transverse and spinous processes serve as important attachment points for muscles and ligaments. The two upper **articular processes** of one vertebra together with the two lower articular processes of the next higher vertebra form the *facet joints*. They are responsible for the flexibility of the spine.

The intervertebral disc

The intervertebral discs lie between the vertebral bodies of adjacent vertebrae. Each intervertebral disc consists of an inner gelatinous core (*nucleus pulposus*), which is surrounded by an outer ring of strong fibres (*anulus fibrosus*). The gelatinous core consists of a soft jelly-like mass, 80 per cent of which is made up of water. The cartilaginous fibre ring forms the main part of the intervertebral disc. It is made up of a large number of ring-shaped layers which together form a dense network of diagonal fibres. This intelligent construction equips the fibre ring for its important task: it counteracts the pressure of the gelatinous core and thus stabilizes the intervertebral disc during movement.

This is what it looks like in detail: in a vertically elongated spine the main load is borne by the middle of the vertebral bodies and the intervertebral discs. The gelatinous core is compressed and its height decreases while the

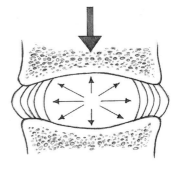

Figure 2.5 Ideal pressure distribution within the intervertebral disc under an axial load: the gelatinous core is compressed, the pressure on the fibrous ring increases and the fibres become stretched.

diameter increases. The fibre ring is tightened and thus the pressure on the gelatinous core is partly converted into traction on the fibre ring. With this mechanism the load is distributed across the entire intervertebral disc.

When bending, extending or leaning to one side, the stress on the spine is three times greater than in the axial position. Now the intervertebral disc acts like a water cushion. The gelatinous core is put under pressure on one side; it gives way and moves to the opposite direction. This locally increases the pressure on the fibre ring and the fibres become taut, thus limiting the movement.

In rotation the mechanism is different. Here the gelatinous core stays where it is and throughout the rotation, the diagonal fibres of the fibre ring tighten around the core. This increases the pressure inside the gelatinous core. The core resists the fibre ring, so to speak, and thus limits the movement.

During the course of the day the water content within the gelatinous core is reduced by the weight bearing – not a great deal, but quite noticeably. So we can lose up to 2cm in height during a single day. When we lie down and sleep at night, the reduction in pressure permits the gelatinous core to refill, so that by morning we have regained our normal height.

The Spinal Regions and their Special Characteristics

Cervical spine – the base for the head
The cervical spine carries the head, balancing it like a ball on the top vertebra and following its movements. As the seat of the sensory organs, the head was and is the centre from which the impulses for many movements originate, for the development of our evolutionary upright posture as bipeds as well as for the rapid turning of the cervical spine in the pirouette. The cervical spine acquires its remarkable flexibility through two specially shaped vertebrae: the atlas and the axis.

The first cervical vertebra, the **atlas**, possesses neither spinous process nor vertebral body. Its form resembles a ring. The skull's prominent

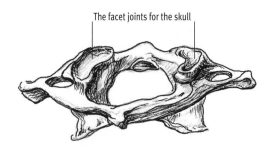

The facet joints for the skull

Figure 2.6 The atlas: the bones of the skull rest in its facet joints. The joint between the skull and the atlas is called the atlanto-occipital joint.

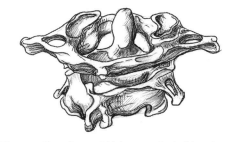

Figure 2.7 The atlantoaxial joint comprised of the atlas and the axis.

condyles sit in its two concave facet joints. This joint between the skull and the atlas, the atlanto-occipital joint, permits one direction of movement above all: the nodding of the head forwards and backwards; the "yes" movement.

The second cervical vertebra, the **axis**, also has an unusual shape. During the course of evolution it acquired the vertebral body of the atlas. This resulted in the characteristic tooth-shaped "dens" of the axis, which together with the atlas forms the atlantoaxial joint. It is to this joint that the cervical spine owes its remarkable rotational ability. It is here that most of the head-turning, the "no" movement takes place.

The transverse processes of the first to sixth cervical vertebrae demonstrate an unusual feature. Each transverse process contains an opening and all of these holes together form a channel for the **vertebral artery**, an important blood vessel supplying blood to the brain. After leaving the bony canal, the vertebral artery continues past the atlanto-occipital joint and enters the bony protection of the skull. Problems can occur at precisely this spot. Malposition of the head or tension in the muscles can constrict the blood vessel and with this reduce the blood circulation to the brain.

The thoracic spine – the ribcage

A specific feature of the thoracic spine is the set of 12 pairs of ribs which connect with the side of the vertebral bodies and the subsequent transverse processes of the vertebrae. The top ten ribs form an arch around to the front where they are attached to the breastbone (*sternum*), either directly – first to seventh rib – or indirectly – eighth to tenth rib – via a segment of cartilage. The eleventh and twelfth ribs are described as floating ribs; they are too short to be attached to the breastbone at the front. Together, all of the ribs form the ribcage, a protective case for vital structures like the heart, lungs and major blood vessels.

The ribcage reduces the flexibility of the thoracic spine, but the numerous rib joints speak for themselves. Although the movement within each individual joint is small, the ribcage as a whole is much more flexible than our everyday movements would indicate.

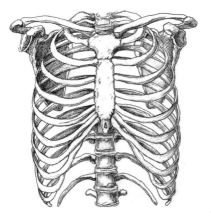

Figure 2.8 The ribcage viewed from the front.

Lumbar spine

The five lumbar vertebrae are the largest and most prominent bones in the spine. That makes sense as the entire weight of the upper body rests on

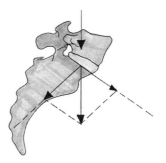

Figure 2.9 Pressure distribution in the lumbosacral joint.

them. Particular attention should be paid to the *lumbosacral joint*, the joint between the fifth lumbar vertebra and the sacrum. A complex system of ligaments stabilizes this joint, and yet the flexibility here is greater than in the rest of the lumbar spine. The reason for this is the position of the pelvis. The pelvis (and with this also the sacrum) is tilted forward at an angle of about 30° (see Chapter 3, p. 59). Unfortunately this is not a favourable position for the lower lumbar vertebra. It has the tendency to slide forward on the sacrum. This leads to unfavourable shearing forces on the intervertebral disc. So it is not surprising, that two thirds of all back problems occur in the lower section of the lumbar spine.

3D Function

The straightening of the spine, its *auto-elongation*, forms the basis for the movement of the spine and its ability to withstand stress. For this, head and pelvis have to rotate in opposite directions.

The pelvis gives the spine the movement impulse to straighten up: it curls in by turning back- and downwards on its horizontal axis (see Chapter 3, p. 58). In doing so, the sacrum, the base of the spine, straightens up and thus lengthens the lumbar spine. The stress on the small vertebral joints is reduced and the main pressure is centred on the middle of the vertebral body and the discs. The spinal canal becomes wider and the intervertebral foramina open. This creates space for the spinal nerves.

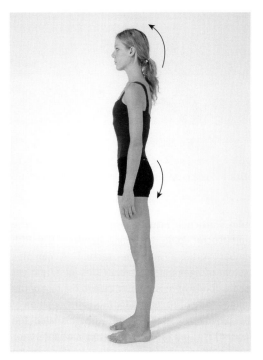

Figure 2.10 The simultaneous "rolling-in" of head and pelvis elongates the spine.

To counter the movement of the pelvis, the head rotates back- and upwards around its horizontal axis. This is a small movement with great effect. Through the almost imperceptible "yes" movement of the head, the back area of the atlanto-occipital joint is opened and vital structures like the vertebral artery and the spinal cord are given more space.

The nodding movement lengthens the nape of the neck and the movement continues down into the upper thoracic spine. The entire spine is lengthened by this minimal curling-in movement of head and pelvis; shortened structures are stretched and over-stretched ones are toned up. The straightening of the spine permits an optimal centring of the load.

Things are more complicated when we move. When walking, during the alternation between the working leg and the standing leg, the spine and the entire torso twists around an imaginary vertical line alternately to the right and to the left. On the side of the standing leg the pelvis moves back- and downwards (see Chapter 3, p. 58). The lumbar spine stretches, the intervertebral foramina are opened and give space for the nerves. The lower ribs follow the movement; with the iliac crest they are pulled backwards and downwards by the muscles. The upper part of the spine twists in the opposite direction: it rotates in the direction of the working leg and the upper ribs turn with it. The ribcage expands and so breathing automatically becomes deeper. The opposite occurs on the side of the working leg. Here the upper ribs twist backwards and the lower ones forwards. This narrows the ribcage and thus breathing out becomes easier. The alternate rotation of pelvis, spine and ribcage keeps the thoracic spine mobile and thus relieves the pressure on the cervical and lumbar spine.

Movements of the Spine

As a whole, the spine can move in three dimensions: it can bend forward, back and sideways and it can rotate. These movements are not restricted to certain sections of the spine. However, there are certain movements that, for anatomical reasons, are easier to execute in certain parts and therefore tend to be carried out in these particular sections. In general, flexibility is greatest in the cervical and lumbar spine; the thoracic spine being less mobile because of the ribcage.

Two adjacent vertebrae, the intervertebral disc between and all surrounding ligaments and muscles together form the so-called "movement segment". It is the direction of the small facet joints that defines the movement ability in each segment. This cannot be altered by training. What can be influenced, however, is the range of movement, and in the long term, this is of decisive importance for the ability of the whole spine to cope with stress.

In the **cervical spine** the joint surfaces are inclined forward at an angle of 45° from the frontal plane. This allows easy turning, flexion and extension as well as bending sideways.

Cervical spine from the side   Thoracic spine from the side   Lumbar spine from behind

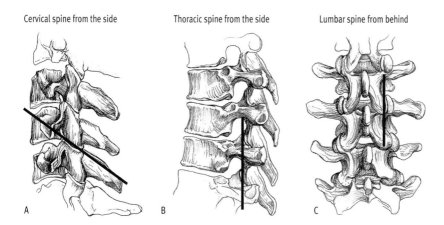

A   B   C

In the **thoracic spine**, the joint surfaces face the frontal plane. This above all enables rotation, but also allows for sidebending and flexion, albeit with restricted movement because of the ribs. Extension is limited by the spinous processes which are arranged above each other like interlocking roof tiles.

In the **lumbar spine** the joint surfaces are aligned with the sagittal plane. This restricts both rotation and sidebending. On the other hand, flexion and especially extension of the lumbar spine work very well.

Table 2.1 General mobility of the spine

Section of the spine	Flexion / Extension	Sidebending	Rotation
Cervical spine	40° / 75°	35°	50°
Thoracic spine	45° / 20°	25°	55°
Lumbar spine	60° / 35°	15°	5°

Musculature

As if by a cylindrical casing, the trunk is surrounded by the back and abdominal muscles. Referring to the direction of tension and traction, the entire trunk musculature can be subdivided into four different muscle systems: a vertical system, a horizontal system and two oblique systems running in opposite directions (see Table 2.2). Together they fill the space between the ribcage and the pelvis. They surround the trunk, provide stability for standing upright and at the same time permit a differentiated set of movements.

The muscles of the vertical and horizontal systems are responsible for the upright posture of pelvis and spine in particular, while the oblique muscles mainly work dynamically. The most important trunk muscules are described below in greater detail.

Table 2.2 The system of trunk musculature

	Vertical system	Horizontal system	Oblique systems
Abdominal Muscles	Rectus abdominis muscle	Transverse abdominis muscle	External and internal oblique abdominal muscles
Back Muscles	Vertical system of the intrinsic spinal muscles		Multifidus muscle Deep rotator muscles

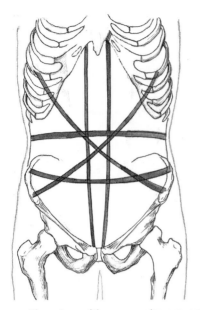

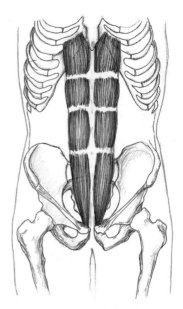

Figure 2.12 The systems of the core muscles: one vertical, one horizontal and two oblique systems.

Figure 2.13 The rectus abdominis muscle.

Abdominal muscles

The front and side walls of the abdomen are formed by large areas of muscle. The main tasks of the abdominal musculature are flexion and rotation of the spine, and straightening of the pelvis. The following muscles are distinguished from the surface inwards.

As its name suggests, the **rectus abdominis** runs vertically up and down the abdomen. It lies on both sides of the centre line extending from the lower ribs and the sternum down to the pubic bone. Along the centre line, the two muscle bellies are linked with each other through the tendinous *linea alba* (= white line). They are divided horizontally into sections by three tendinous membranes. In a highly trained muscle, each individual muscle section between the tendinous membranes shows prominently, which is why the muscle is also commonly-known as the "six-pack". The main task of the rectus abdominis is to flex the spine, for example, when the upper body is slowly rolled up from the supine position or in a contraction. If the pelvis is properly placed the rectus abdominis pulls the lower ribs down and

thus supports the position of the ribcage. Its attachment at the front of the pelvis enables it to assist in the straightening of the pelvis and thus to counteract hyperextension of the lower back.

The fibres of the **external oblique abdominal muscle** run diagonally from lateral at the top outside to medial at the bottom inside. Seen from the front it looks like a "V", with the right and left muscle each forming one side of the "V". Running at an angle of 90° from top medial to bottom lateral is the **internal oblique abdominal muscle**. In the centre, to the front, its fibres connect with the fibres of the opposite external oblique muscle. Thus the external oblique muscle on one side and the internal oblique muscle on the other side form a functional unit. Together they rotate the trunk right and left. In a rotation to the right, the left external oblique muscle and the right internal oblique muscle contract together, whereas the left internal oblique muscle and the right external oblique muscle are stretched, this being an optimal interaction for the dynamic rotation of the spine.

The **transverse abdominis muscle** forms the innermost layer of the abdominal musculature. Its

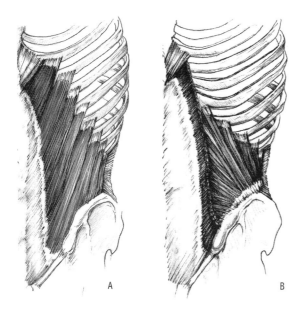

Figure 2.14 The obliques: A) the external oblique abdominal muscle,
B) the internal oblique abdominal muscle.

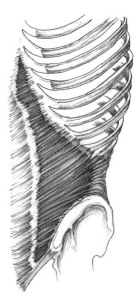

Figure 2.15 The transverse
abdominal muscle.

fibres run horizontally, thus surrounding the abdomen like a belt. In contrast to the other abdominal muscles its main task is stability. The orientation of its fibres make it into the "corset muscle". Its main task is to relieve pressure on the spine. If the transversus abdominis is active, it reduces the pressure on the intervertebral discs by up to 50 per cent. To do so, it does not even need to be pulled tight. Already about 20 per cent of muscle tension is sufficient to reduce the pressure on the spine. Unfortunately, it is not easy to become aware of such a low level of muscular activity. The details are tricky: in order to ideally stabilize spine and trunk, the transversus abdominis muscle has to be engaged just *before* the arms or legs are moved.

Spinal muscles

The spine is covered by a network of interwoven muscles. We distinguish between two sorts of back muscle: the large, superficial extrinsic muscles and the small, deep, intrinsic muscles.

During our evolution, the **extrinsic muscles** gradually moved around from our sides to take their position at the back of the spine. These include the **trapezius muscle** and the **latissimus dorsi muscle**. They are primarily responsible for the movement of the shoulder girdle and the arms. Being closest to the surface, they form the characteristic muscular relief of the back.

The **intrinsic spinal musculature, (erector spinae)**, consists of a network of numerous small muscles which are closely interwoven with each other. In their course up the spine they either run from vertebra to vertebra or skip over one or more vertebrae. Along their entire length, from pelvis to head, they link together the transverse and spinous processes of adjacent vertebrae and thus stabilize the individual segments.

The muscles which lie deepest and closest to the spine are also the shortest ones. On both sides of the spine, they mostly run obliquely from the bottom lateral to the top medial (*rotatores* and *multifidus muscles*) – from the transverse processes upwards to the spinous processes. They form the spinal musculature's important oblique system. These muscles are the deepest stabilizers of the spine and their finely coordinated adjustment is of decisive importance for the stabilization of the segments. A high density of receptors inside their muscle fibres allows this fine coordination. If the muscles on one side contract, they rotate the trunk in the opposite direction. Hence, rotation is an important movement in training for muscular stability.

Longer muscle fibres lie on top and to the side of the deep back stabilizers; they run from the iliac crest upwards to the ribs and to the transverse process of the individual vertebrae. They form the vertical system of the intrinsic spinal musculature. Their main task is the straightening of the spine.

Table 2.3 The movements of the spine and the primary muscles involved.

Back movement	Primary muscles
Flexion	Rectus abdominis muscle External and internal oblique abdominal muscles, both sides.
Extension	Erector spinae muscle, both sides.
Lateral bending	External and internal oblique abdominal muscles, one side Erector spinae muscle, one side.
Rotation	Multifidus muscle Deep rotators External and internal oblique abdominal muscle.

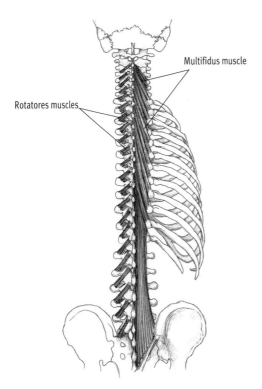

Multifidus muscle

Rotatores muscles

Figure 2.16 The deep rotators and the multifidus muscle are the deepest layer of the intrinsic spinal musculature.

The Architecture of the Spine

Man's evolution from quadruped to biped and thus adopting upright gait led to the typical double "S" form of the spine. This has produced the characteristic spinal curves in the sagittal plane (see Figure 2.1, p. 26):

- Cervical lordosis (curved forwards)
- Thoracic kyphosis (curved backwards)
- Lumbar lordosis (curved forwards)
- Sacral kyphosis (curved backwards)

The double-S shape distributes the body weight equally front and back of the point of equilibrium; the joints are centred and balanced, thus reducing the necessity of muscle work.

However, because of congenital or acquired postural faults, the spine may diverge from the ideal double-S shape. Each change has an effect on the architecture and movement ability of the entire spine. Figure 2.17 shows typical spinal

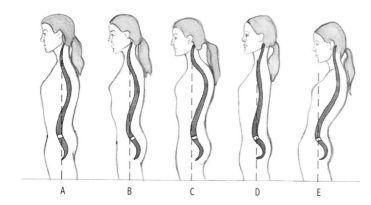

Figure 2.17 The architecture of the spine: A) balanced double-S shape, B) forward-tilted pelvis with hyperlordosis, C) increased thoracic kyphosis, D) flat back with reduction of spinal curves, E) backwards overhang of the thoracic spine, pushing the pelvis forwards.

postures which may have arisen purely functionally through postural habit or imbalance in the muscles, or which are caused by structural changes.

Breathing

The diaphragm is the most important breathing muscle. It runs diagonally through the body from the sternum across the lower ribs to the lumbar vertebrae – a large dome-shaped plate of muscle and tendon which separates the thorax from the abdomen. The diaphragm is the main motor for breathing. When it contracts, the dome shape flattens, the diaphragm sinks down enlarging the volume of the chest. Air streams into the lungs and we breathe in. The contraction of the diaphragm forces the abdominal organs downwards. The pressure in the abdomen rises and the abdominal muscles release slightly. When we breathe out, the diaphragm relaxes and returns to its dome-shaped form. The organs also slide back to their starting position. This down and up movement – diaphragmatic respiration – massages the inner organs.

The small intercostal muscles run diagonally between the ribs and support breathing. When we breathe in, they lift the ribs and expand the ribcage. The upper ribs open primarily towards the front, while the lower ones open mainly to the sides. This sideways opening of the lower ribs, is harder to see from the outside, which makes it a preferred breathing pattern in dance. In combination with diaphragmatic respiration, it is an ideal method to inhale down to the lowest part of the lungs. More air means more oxygen and thus a better oxygen supply for the entire body.

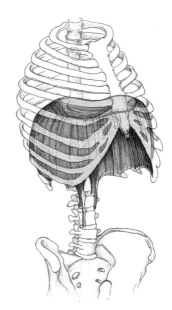

Figure 2.18 The diaphragm is the most important breathing muscle.

Dance in Focus: Load and Overload

Heavy lifting, vigorous rotations and hyper-extension of the spine are very stressful for the back, but all are regular movements in dance. Therefore, it is not surprising that many dancers complain of back pain during their dancing careers. But it is important to put this into perspective: 80 per cent of the Western population suffer from back pain during their lives, with or without physical activity.

Load

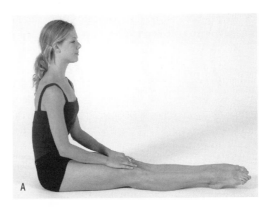

Having a mobile spine and at the same time a stable centre for arm and leg movements place high demands on the back. For a healthy back, awareness and correct performance of movements are a dancer's top priority.

The stable centre

In an optimal upright position the spine comprises an ideal and harmonious double-S shape. To achieve the stage presence desirable for a dancer, muscle tension is slightly increased and attention is focused on lengthening the spine. When dancing, the position of the spine changes constantly: it moves dynamically in three dimensions and often in complex combinations of flexion; sidebending, extension and rotation. A good dancer can find his stable centre immediately at any time from all these positions if demanded by the dance technique or choreography.

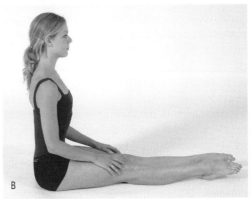

Figure 2.19 The stable centre in "long sitting": A) the risk, B) the ideal position with straight erect pelvis.

When sitting on the floor with the legs outstretched, whether in jazz or contemporary dance, attention is focused on the pelvis, which would tilt backwards if the posture were relaxed. Thus the curvature of the lumbar spine is reduced and at the same time the thoracic curve is enhanced. The pressure on the intervertebral discs increases, which can lead to overload in the long term. To avoid this, pelvis and spine should be consciously straightened. By shifting the weight directly onto the sit bones, instead of behind them, the pelvis is straightened into a neutral position. The spinal, abdominal and pelvic floor muscles all work together and thus prevent excessive flexing of the lumbar and thoracic spine.

The intrinsic spinal muscles, the deep abdominal muscles and the pelvic floor muscles play a key role in the form and function of the entire spine. Above all, it is the timing of the muscles' work that gives the spine its necessary stability and relieves stress. Even before the movement starts, the trunk muscles are switched on. The transversus abdominis, the multifidus and the deep rotator muscles contract and thus give the spine the necessary stability. This finely coordinated muscle work is difficult to perceive, often being obscured by the simultaneous contraction of larger more superficial muscle groups. But the work of these deep muscles is of decisive importance for the long-term stress resistance of the spine.

The extension of the spine

When the back is extended, either in an arch or in a cambré derrière, the coordinated use of the deep spinal and abdominal muscles reduces the strain on the intervertebral discs and the facet joints. Each time the upper body is extended, the pressure in the rear area of the intervertebral disc increases and the facet joints are compressed. If shearing forces are added, excess strain is inevitable. Coordinated muscle work can help. A harmonious arch from the head to the pelvis and the distribution of the movement over the entire spine are the best prevention for local overload. But this will not happen of its own accord. Anatomically speaking, extension is easiest in the lumbar spine; the thoracic spine being considerably less flexible in a backwards direction. Nevertheless, in order to distribute the movement harmoniously throughout the entire spine, the movement should be prepared by lengthening the entire spine and supporting the backwards movement additionally by breathing in. If the head is turned slightly to one side, the front neck muscles will prevent excessive hyperextension of the cervical spine.

Arabesque – another kind of spine extension

Beyond an angle of about 30° the backwards lifting of the leg into an arabesque leads to an extension of the spine. In this case the movement is not initiated by the head as in the arch, but by the leg moving the pelvis. The capsule and ligaments of the hip joint permit the leg only a small amount of backward movement. Therefore a characteristic evasive movement occurs in the pelvis: in order to extend the working leg up to the desired height, the pelvis tilts forward at the same time rotating towards the side of the working leg; the pelvis "opens up". But the aesthetic line of the arabesque requires a straight pelvis and a straightened spine. Thus compensation has to take place in the spine. It has to twist in the opposite direction to the pelvic rotation, towards the standing leg. The simultaneous maximal spinal extension visually reduces the tilt of the pelvis. Here care is required. As much as possible, the extension and rotation of the spine should be distributed throughout the entire lumbar and thoracic spine. In this way the movement looks harmonious and the pressure on the spine is reduced.

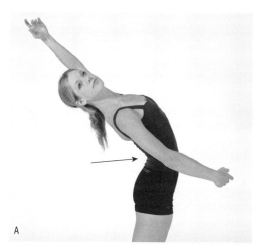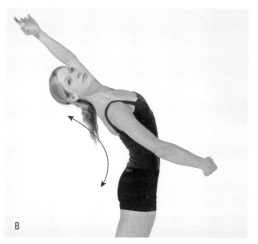

Figure 2.20 The extension of the spine: A) risk of local overload, B) harmonious motion of the entire spine.

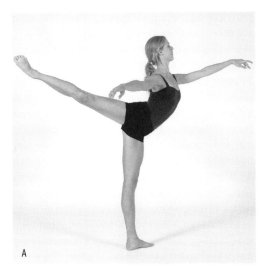

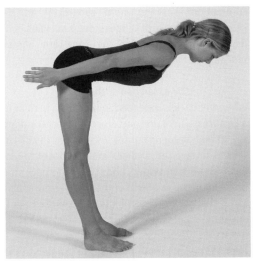

Figure 2.22 Flat back: the movement does not take place in the back, but in the hip joints.

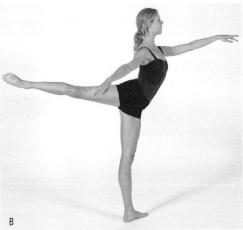

Figure 2.21 Arabesque: A) excessive lordosis of the lumbar spine with risk of local overload, B) the spine avoiding excessive tilting and rotation of the pelvis.

The flexion of the spine

Slowly rolling down the spine, vertebra by vertebra starting from the head, is part of every contemporary or jazz dance training. The flexion of the spine increases the pressure in the front part of the intervertebral discs; the back section of the fibrous ring thereby being stretched. The further the rolling down, the deeper the stretch in the deep back muscles. Ideally, the deep abdominal muscles support the movement; by contracting they reduce the pressure on the intervertebral discs. Finally, the pelvis moves too: it tilts forwards and thus visibly increases the flexion of the spine.

For flat back or in the port de bras en avant the movement is quite different. Here the forward bend is performed with a stretched thoracic and lumbar spine. The deep spinal and abdominal muscles contract and stabilize the spine; the movement takes place in the hip joints. The pelvis tilts forwards, corresponding with a bending in the hip joints. The further the upper body bends forward, the more the body's centre of gravity moves forwards. In order not to fall over, the dancer has to compensate by moving the pelvis slightly backwards. This compensation should not be too pronounced. The muscles of the buttocks and the hamstrings have to work hard to stabilize the dancer.

Pirouette

The rapid head movement during the pirouette, known as "spotting", is typical of the turning movements in dance. At the beginning of the pirouette, the dancer's eyes focus on a particular spot and the body starts to turn "below the head", with the cervical spine rotating as far as possible. Only when the spine reaches its maximum rotation

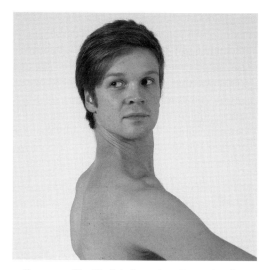

Figure 2.23 "Spotting" during a pirouette requires free movement of the cervical spine and good coordination of the muscles.

does the head begin to follow the turn. By quickly rotating the cervical spine the dancer's eyes immediately try to re-catch the spot upon which he has been focusing. The dancer is essentially trying not to let the "spot" he is focusing on out of his sight. The body follows this rapid head movement with a short delay: a feature that is necessary for balance and equilibrium occurs at the expense of the spine. In order to be able to carry out this energetic head movement without difficulty, over and over again, the head has to be perfectly positioned on the cervical spine during the entire turning process. All cervical vertebrae must be able to move freely and the thoracic spine should participate in the rotation. Furthermore, the muscles at the front and back of the cervical spine must be working in balance.

Partner work

Depending on the starting position and the lifting movement, the strain on the back can be multiplied many times: if one lifts 45kg at a distance of about 70cm from one's own centre of gravity with legs stretched, the pressure on the intervertebral discs increases to over 700kg! This is an impressive figure, which draws attention to the importance of

a good lifting and partnering technique in order to maintain a healthy back. A perfectly centred pelvis, a straight spine and optimal timing of the muscle work can considerably reduce the strain on the spine. Key to partnering that does not over-strain the back is to lift out of the bended legs and not from the back. The back should be as straight as possible; the deep abdominal and back muscles should be activated. The momentum for the lifting comes from vigorously pushing the legs against the floor. The closer the partner during the lifting movement and the straighter the pelvis and spine, the less the pressure on the intervertebral discs. Please remember: simultaneous rotation and flexion of the back during lifting are hazardous for the intervertebral discs!

Overload

Above all, it is chronic overload which leads to back problems: habitual movement patterns that lead to excessive local movement or even stress fractures of the vertebrae and unbalanced weight bearing which over-taxes the intervertebral discs. The more powerful and vigorous the movement – such movements being an integral part of today's dance styles – the greater the danger of an acute injury, ranging from a blocked joint to a pulled muscle.

Chronic overload

Chronic lumbago: Pain in the lower back region mostly occurs as a result of over-taxing the muscles or the capsular ligaments. Degeneration of the vertebrae or the facet joints may also be a factor. Shortened and hardened back muscles, weak abdominal muscles, unfavourable weight distribution on the spine or local hypermobility are frequent causes for unconscious compen-sations in posture, which in turn put an uneven strain on the spine. This is a vicious circle that requires targeted therapy to eliminate.

Chronic neck pain: Pain in the cervical spine can be caused by a number of possible factors. In dancers – especially in classical dance – the natural lordotic curve of the cervical spine is frequently completely lost, the vertebrae standing straight or even curving backwards, resulting in kyphosis. Together with the weakness of the front neck muscles and the shortening and tightening of the erector muscles of the neck, the entire cervical spine is out of balance as regards both weight distribution and movement. Sudden movements of the neck – for example, in the pirouette – can then lead to micro-injuries to the muscles, the facet joints or even to the intervertebral discs.

Spondylolysis and Spondylolisthesis: *Spondylolysis* is an interruption of the vertebral arch in the region between the articulating processes; it can either occur on one or on both sides. Most often the fifth lumbar vertebra is affected, more rarely the fourth. Although a genetic predisposition is a possible cause, spondylolysis is also regarded as a kind of stress fracture. Static factors like a prominent sway back, premature lifting before one has gained sufficient muscular stability, frequent hyperextension of the lumbar spine and also dietary shortcomings during growth will increase the risk of spondylolysis. Spondylolysis is a frequent cause of back pain in young people. The main emphasis in therapy is on local stabilization.

In case of a spondylolysis on both sides, there is a risk of the vertebra slipping towards the front. This is called *spondylolisthesis*. Here, the complete vertebra, with its transverse processes and upper articulating processes, slips forwards relative to the vertebra below. It takes with it the whole spinal column above, leaving behind only its spinous process. Gliding along the line of the spinous processes one often can feel the typical step. Most commonly, the fifth lumbar vertebra slips forward on the sacrum. The extent of the slipping determines the therapy and the ability to further stress bearing. The slipping process is usually completed by the age of 20, making further slipping in adult life unlikely. Thus it is all the more important to be careful during growth spurts and avoid movements which could exacerbate the slipping such as an excessively hyperextended posture, over-stretching of the spine without muscular support,

and partner work, at a time when the necessary stability of the upper body is still not developed.

Spondylolysis and spondylolisthesis frequently occur in dancers; fortunately, they do not necessarily force the end of a dancing career. Improvement of weight distribution and muscular support along with fine coordination permit dancers to continue to dance even after a stress fracture of the spine.

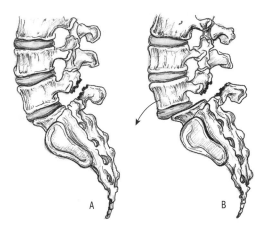

A   B

Figure 2.24 A) spondylolysis, B) spondylolisthesis of the fifth lumbar vertebra.

Scheuermann's disease: Pronounced kyphosis of the thoracic spine, referred to as "round back", is often put down to Scheuermann's disease. But Scheuermann's disease is a growth abnormality of the spine that can only be diagnosed by means of X-ray. It is important to distinguish it from a purely functional round back, the causes for which usually lie in a muscle weakness. From X-ray it is possible to recognize the specific changes to the vertebrae and intervertebral discs: the front part of the vertebral body is stunted in growth and the wedge-shaped vertebrae typical of this disorder are formed. Disc material protrudes into the still cartilaginous vertebral body, forming the typical "Schmorl's nodes", which can be seen from X-rays. The intervertebral space is reduced. In the long term, the flexibility in the affected spinal area is diminished; the other spinal regions compensating by taking over the movement. This frequently leads to over-straining in these otherwise healthy areas. Scheuermann's disease is a disease of adolescents, but the problems and pain often do not occur until adulthood.

For dancers, the location of Scheuermann's disease is of great importance. Increased thoracic kyphosis, compensated by a mobile and well-stabilized lumbar spine, can endure performance in the long term. However, if the lower thoracic spine or the lumbar spine is affected, it will be difficult to compensate sufficiently through the healthy regions of the spine. In this case dancing at a professional level is not to be recommended.

Acute injuries

Muscle injury: Pulled muscles or torn fibres occur in all sections of the spine. If the fine coordination of the supporting muscles is absent in energetic movements, rapid concentric muscle work or powerful eccentric shock absorption, the deep erector spinae muscles will be over-taxed. Muscle injuries will result.

Acute blockage: Sudden restrictions to the movement of the facet joints or rib joints occur frequently in dancers. The more flexible a joint is, the greater the range of movement to which it is used and the more energetic the movement, the greater the risk of an acute blockage. The natural play of the joint is disturbed: like a drawer that is stuck, suddenly movement is only possible in one direction. Stiffness and severe, often sharp pain during certain movements result. As a sort of protective measure, the local muscles tighten up and harden; often little muscle nodules (*myogelosis*) can be felt. The pain might even radiate into the surrounding tissues; making it difficult to differentiate between muscle pain and an irritation of the nerves. Warmth, relaxation and gentle mobilization can break the vicious cycle of a blocked joint and a compensating posture leading to even further muscle tension.

If a blockage occurs repeatedly at the same place, in addition to the statics and dynamics the organic system should also be carefully examined. Via the nervous system, each segment of the spine correlates with a specific inner organ. If there is a

restriction in organic function, even a small unspectacular movement can result in a blockage of the corresponding segment of the spine.

Slipped disc: A slipped disc usually leads to acute pain although the degeneration of the tissue happens gradually over a longer period of time. Age-related wear and tear on the intervertebral discs is a natural process. The water content of the jelly core of the disc is lessened, the fibrous ring thins out, the height of the disc is reduced and its ability to regenerate diminishes. As a result of the height reduction of the disc, the coordination within that particular segment becomes impaired. If the architecture of the spine and the muscles are not able to counteract the process, this leads to local hypermobility. The segment is too mobile and the occurring shearing forces can lead to microscopic tears in the fibrous ring. All it takes is one "wrong" movement: the fibrous ring is no longer able to withstand the pressure of the inner core, the core bulges outward (*protrusion*) or even

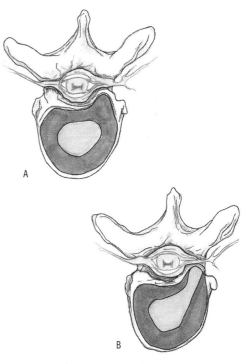

Figure 2.25 A) *protrusion* and, B) *prolapse* both differ according to the stability of the fibre ring.

breaks through the fibrous ring completely (*prolapse*). Depending on the position at which the herniated disc occurs it puts pressure on certain nerve pathways or on the spinal cord. The most typical symptom of a slipped disc is pain radiating along the entire extremity into the hand or the foot. Disturbances of sensation and weakness in the muscles point to further nerve impingement.

Slipped discs typically occur in the lumbar or the cervical spine. Here, as a result of the lordotic posture, one finds increased pressure on the back of the fibrous ring. If flexibility in the thoracic spine is lacking – a frequent problem even in dancers – movements will mainly take place in the lumbar and cervical spine, further increasing the pressure on these intervertebral discs. Ninety-five per cent of all slipped discs in the lumbar region occur between the fourth and fifth lumbar vertebrae and between the fifth lumbar vertebra and the sacrum. In the cervical spine the disc between the fifth and sixth cervical vertebrae is most frequently affected. Here, not centring the head correctly is an important contributing factor.

A slipped disc does not necessarily end a dancer's career. Almost one in four adults, even those without back pain, will show a slipped disc in examination. The size of the slipped disc, the diameter of the spinal canal, the local stability of the segment and the overall architecture of the spine are decisive factors as to whether the herniated disc will become symptomatic, and which symptoms will be present.

Pitfalls in Dance

"Stand up straight as if you have swallowed a stick." Tips like this have been heard by generations of dancers, and they are still heard in many dance studios today. Nowadays, we know that the image of the "rigid back" is of limited use when it comes to preparing the spine for dancing. But how can one avoid the typical problems in dance, such as hyperlordosis, a too-straight back or localized hypermobility? Auto-elongation and flexibility of the spine are vital for a back that is able to withstand strain.

Hyperlordosis – a Strain on the Back

When the lumbar lordosis is pronounced, this is hyperlordosis or a "sway back", irrespective of the causes for this excessive curvature. Chapter 3 (see p. 62) explains how the position of the pelvis affects the shape of the spine and consequently the lumbar lordosis. The most common reason for hyperlordosis in a dancer is forced turnout. The pelvis tilts forward, the lumbar lordosis increases, resulting in a sway back. A shortened iliopsoas muscle (see Chapter 4, p. 85) or increased tension in the lumbar erector spinae muscle can also lead to lumbar hyperlordosis. The shortening of the lumbar muscles restricts movement and is often painful; the abdominal muscles over-stretch and their strength reduce. The pelvis tilts forward and this increases the pressure on the small lumbar facet joints. With each shock-load, the articulating processes strike the vertebral arch below like a hammer. No spine can withstand this strain in the long run.

Anatomically speaking, the lumbar spine can hyperextend to a considerable degree. This explains why many dancers performing an arch or cambré derrière try to increase their range of motion by mainly extending the lumbar spine and not – as ideally is required – through using the higher sections of the spine. In the long term, this local bending is stressful to the lumbar spine and can even aggravate the lumbar hyperlordosis.

How to recognize: A sway back is most easily assessed from the side. When standing, the pelvis is tilted forward, the lumbar spine appears compressed and lumbal lordosis is prominent. The abdominal wall bulges forwards as the inner organs are falling against it.

It is important to distinguish a sway back which is musculary held from the one initiated by the

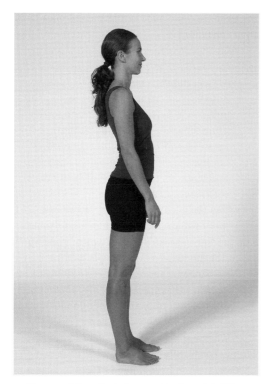

Figure 2.26 Hyperlordosis caused by the pelvis tilting forward.

tilting forward of the pelvis. To do this, ask the dancer to roll the spine down vertebra by vertebra, starting from the head. Ideally, the entire spine should form a harmonious arch: the lumbar lordosis should be completely removed and the lumbal spine rounded. If at the end of the movement a hollow-shaped indentation remains in the lumbar area, a shortening of the lumbar muscles is likely. Here, targeted stretching exercises will be necessary because, in this case, the hyperlordotic posture cannot be changed simply by correcting the position of the pelvis.

The "Overly-straightened" Back

"Extend your head towards the ceiling", "elongate your back", "keep your back straight". These are corrections which all have the same goal: to reduce the curves in the back and to actively straighten the back through muscle strength. But these corrective images run the risk of making the spine too rigid, of losing its elasticity.

The correction "Pull your chest up" is even worse. Although it is intended to help dancers to stand up straight, we often see the same mistake: they pull their shoulder blades back and push the lower ribs forward, opening the ribcage. As a result, the abdominal muscles cannot properly engage. The thoracic kyphosis is flattened, the thoracic spine is often even extended, which results in restricted movement and over-tensing of the muscles. The mobility of the thoracic spine and the ribcage is reduced.

On top of a thoracical lordosis follows a cervical kyphosis. The "kink" in the cervical spine prohibits a balanced interaction between the front and back cervical muscles. The cervical extensor muscles have to take on most of the work – with this, pain in the back of the neck is inevitable.

How to recognize: The "overly-straightened" back can best be assessed from the side. The pelvis is held in an extremely upright position and the double-S shape of the spine is almost totally diminished. The upper thoracic spine is hyperextended, the lower ribs jut out and often the shoulders are pulled backwards. The harmonious integration of the ribcage between

the pelvis and the head is lost and the back looks rigid and inflexible.

What you can do:
- Straightened spine: yes, rigid spine: no! In order to extend the spine and, at the same time, keep all segments flexible, it helps to initiate straightening through the two poles of the spine, through the simultaneous minimal rolling-in of pelvis and head.
- The distance between the lower end of the sternum and the pubic bone should be kept the same, both when standing still and when moving. While dancing it is helpful to be aware of this connecting line in order to centre the ribcage above the pelvis and to activate the abdominal muscles.
- The head should be balanced on the cervical spine like a balloon; thus being centred and requiring almost no muscle work. An imaginary line connecting the chin and the upper end of the sternum helps to experience the automatic balance of the head.

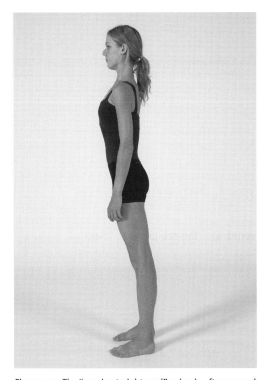

Figure 2.27 The "overly-straightened" spine is often caused by well-intentioned corrections.

The "Relaxed" Posture

Outside the dance studio, dancers, and young dancers in particular, like to adopt a posture which might be relaxing for the muscles but puts maximum strain on the joints and the capsular ligaments. The pelvis is pulled forward while the upper body protrudes backwards; thus the body's centre of gravity runs behind the pelvis. The thoracic kyphosis is increased, while the lumbar curve varies depending on the extent of the overhang. The pelvis is tilted backwards, overstretching the hip joints. The dancer hangs in his ligaments and muscle tension is almost unnecessary. In order to keep in balance, the head is pushed forward; the cervical erector muscle become firm and short. Increased pressure on the joints, increased strain on the capsule and its ligaments, strain on the spine and muscular imbalance: these are the risks of such a "relaxed" posture.

How to recognize: A "relaxed" posture can best be assessed from the side. The body's centre of gravity lies behind the midline, the pelvis is pushed forward and the thoracic spine is rounded; the upper body overhangs at the back and the arms hang unnaturally far forward.

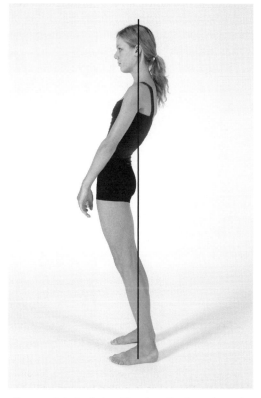

Figure 2.28 In the "relaxed" posture, the dancer hangs in his ligaments, thus increasing the pressure on the joints by relaxing the muscles.

What you can do:
- It may look relaxing on first glance, but the "relaxed" posture should be avoided by dancers if at all possible!
- Strengthening the hip flexor muscles (see Chapter 4, p. 96) and the upper erector spinae muscle, as well as raising conscious awareness of the body's own centre of gravity (see pp. 47/52), will help to break the habit of hanging in this position.

Scoliosis – Suitable for Dance?

A curvature of the spine to one side in one or more sections of the spinal column is known as scoliosis. It is usually accompanied by a rotation of the affected vertebrae. We distinguish *functional* scoliosis – which can be corrected – from *structural* or partially fixed scoliosis. The latter leads to an asymmetry of the vertebrae. Scoliosis occurs during growth and deteriorates primarily during the second growth spurt. The causes of functional scoliosis may include a difference in the leg lengths, pelvic torsion, muscle imbalance, as well as a one-sided deficiency in the stretching ability of the knee or a hyperpronated foot which is more pronounced on one side.

Depending on the location of the maximal curvature, scoliosis can be subdivided into upper thoracic (maximal curvature above the seventh thoracic vertebra), thoracic (maximal curvature between the seventh and eleventh thoracic vertebra), thoraco-lumbar (maximal curvature between the eleventh thoracic vertebra and the first lumbar vertebrae) and lumbar (maximal curvature between the second and third lumbar vertebra). The main problem with scoliosis is the increasing lack of flexibility in the affected areas of the spine. Here, the location of the main curvature plays an important role. Lumbar or thoraco-lumbar scoliosis affects the flexibility of the legs: the flexibility of the spine necessary for the arabesque or the grand battement derrière is drastically reduced. Upper thoracic scoliosis leads to a visible asymmetry of the shoulders, which can impair a dancer's aesthetic appearance. The most common form is thoracic scoliosis. Here, the thoracic spine usually curves to the right, known as right-thoracic scoliosis. Possible causes for this are "handedness" (usually right-handedness) and the position of the aorta (to the left of the centre of the body). A slightly pronounced right thoracic scoliosis is very common, much more in women than in men. It can lead to asymmetries in the ribcage, but does not usually lead to greater problems. An evenly flexible spine with moderate scoliosis is suitable for dancing. In the case of prominent scoliosis a dance-medical doctor should be consulted.

How to recognize: An experienced observer will spot signs which may indicate scoliosis even when the affected person is standing upright:

- Differences in shoulder height
- Asymmetrical position of the two shoulder blades (prominence of one shoulder blade)
- Asymmetry of the waist
- Rotation of the ribcage
- Rotation of the pelvis

If there are several indications of scoliosis when a dancer is standing upright, it is easiest to make the distinction between structural and functional scoliosis from the back. The dancer is requested to slowly roll down the spine, vertebra by vertebra, starting from the head. One looks for signs of asymmetries in the ribcage and the lumbar spine. In structural scoliosis the rotation of the spine persists even when rolling down; the typical "rib hump" can be observed.

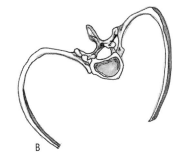

B

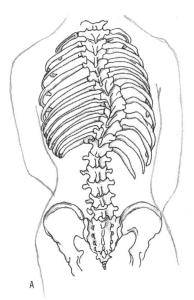

A

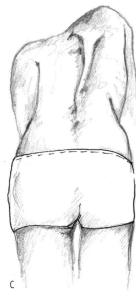

C

Figure 2.29 A right-thoracic scoliosis. A) seen from the back: lateral thoracic curve to the right, and lateral lumbar curve to the left, B) rotation of the vertebrae and their impact on the chest, C) "rib hump" on the right side while bending forward.

What you can do:

- Scoliosis does not indicate the end of a dancing career. On the contrary, no other sport trains the flexibility and fine coordination of the back in such a differentiated manner as dance. Dancing, when optimally taught and practised, is a good extension of scoliosis therapy. This may be one reason why scoliosis is so common among dancers.
- The mobility of the spine should be trained specifically where the restriction caused by the scoliotic curvature is greatest: at the point of maximal curvature. Conscious three-dimensional straightening and movement-awareness to counter the scoliotic posture will help to keep these areas mobile.

- Whether scoliosis is structural or functional, the active muscular stability of the spine and its coordinated movements are the best prerequisites for symptom-free scoliosis. Here is an example for a special dance training of a right thoracic scoliosis:
  - Active emphasis of the right standing leg (see Chapter 4, p. 71)
  - Conscious counter-rotation of the thoracic spine to the left with simultaneous extension of the left thoracic side
  - Awareness of the lengthening of the spine in the right lumbar and left thoracic sections
  - If necessary, support through arm movement (raising the left arm supports the extension of the left-hand side of the thoracic spine)

A Closer Look – Self-analysis

The optimal prerequisites for a healthy dancer's back that is able to withstand stress is an evenly curved double-S shape of the spine, good flexibility in all sections and an ideal auto-balance of pelvis, ribcage and head. Self-assessment of form, flexibility and function of the spine is best carried out with a partner.

Form and Mobility

The **form** of the spine should be assessed from the side while standing: the feet are parallel and hip-width apart, posture should be relaxed and without excessive muscle tension. The following questions will help to assess the form of the spine:

- Is the pelvis in a neutral position?
- Is the lumbar spine elongated?
- Is the head balanced easily on the cervical spine?

- Is the ribcage integrated between the two poles of the spine: the head and the pelvis?
- Both spine and abdomen should run in a harmonious line, without kinks.
- Does the body's centre line run from the middle of the ear through the middle of the shoulder joint, along the centre part of the ribcage and over the greater trochanter (see Chapter 4, p. 75), through the middle of the knee to the front of the ankle joint?

Attention should be paid to the homogeneous **flexibility** of the entire spine. Assessing from behind is one of the best ways to test this. The dancer stands with the feet parallel and hip-width apart and starting from the head, slowly rolls the spine down, vertebra by vertebra. This will allow you to check the following:

- Does the rolling down movement run straight without deviating to one side?

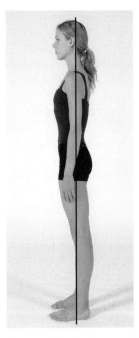

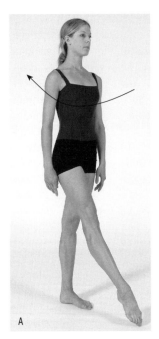

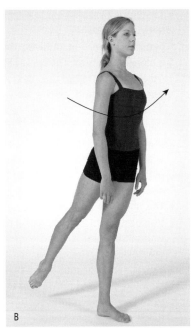

Figure 2.30 The ideal course of the body's centre of gravity.

Figure 2.31 The spiral of the spine: A) when the leg moves forwards, the spine rotates slightly towards the working leg, B) when the leg moves backwards, the spine rotates slightly towards the standing leg.

- Are the ribs on both sides of the spine at the same height?
- Is a harmonious arch formed between the head and the pelvis, without kinks? Here, special attention should be paid to the lower back: often, the lower back of a dancer will retain its lordotic curve when rolling down – a sign of excessive muscle tension.
- When extending backwards, where does most of the movement come from? Pay special attention to the lumbar spine, as typically this is where the most movement takes place – often a sign of restricted movement in the thoracic spine. Ideally, the backwards extension should be equally distributed through the thoracic and the lumbar spine.
- When bending sideways, does the entire spine, from head to pelvis, form a harmonious arch? All segments should be equally involved in the movement. NB: Watch out here for any kinks, particularly in the thoracic spine as they could indicate local hypomobility.

Function

The harmonious movement of the entire spine is of crucial importance for its functionality.

Rotation of the spine:
- The dancer sits with his back towards his partner. In response to an acoustic signal (e.g. clapping hands) he turns towards his partner without changing the position of his pelvis on the floor. Where does the main movement come from? Ideally the rotation of the cervical spine should continue harmoniously into the thoracic spine. The greater the rotational ability of the thoracic spine, the less strain is put on the cervical and lumbar spine.
- Stand upright, with the feet parallel and hip-width apart. Perform a tendu forward and backward, do this first with the right and then with the left leg. As you do this, pay attention to the upper body: does it remain

rigid or does the movement of the legs seem to continue harmoniously upwards? Can you see a small counter-rotation in the thoracic spine in relation to the movement of the working leg?

Auto-elongation of the spine: Stand upright with the feet parallel and hip-width apart or in first position. Repeat a sequence of demi-plié, stretch, relevé and lowering down several times in succession. Can the auto-elongation of the spine in the movement be perceived? Are the pelvis and the head rolled slightly inwards during the movement to extend the spine? To reinforce the auto-elongation, the dancer can put one hand on top of his head, gently pressing downwards. Thus the auto-elongation of the spine is easier to perceive.

Strength and Stability

Strength of the centre of the body: The dancer lies in a supine position with the whole spine, from head to pelvis, placed on a rolled floor mat (see Figure 2.32). The centre of the body is stabilized; the legs are bent at an angle of 90° at both the knee and the hip joint. The arms lie to the side on the floor; they are used for *gentle* support rather than stabilization. Alternately lower the right and the left leg, still bent, towards the floor. Shortly before the sole of the foot touches the floor, move the leg back towards the chest while at the same time lowering the other leg towards the floor. Dancers should be able to carry out at least 25 repetitions without losing stability in the centre of the body.

Stability of the spine: Stand upright with the feet parallel and hip-width apart or in first position. Put a (light) book on your head. Perform a tendu to the front, to the side and to the back, first with the right and then with the left leg. Notice the auto-elongation of the spine and the fine rotating movement in the thoracic spine. The stability of the spine can be assessed by the number of repetitions that a dancer can perform without the book falling to the ground.

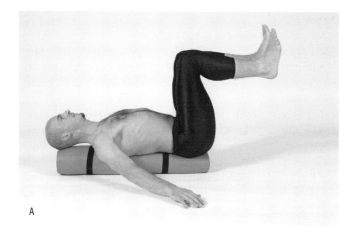

A

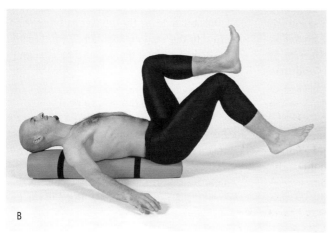

B

Figure 2.32 Test the power centre of the body: A) starting position, B) lowering the legs alternately.

Tips and Tricks for Prevention

Virtually everyone, whether a dancer or not, suffers from back pain at least once in their life. Often, poor postural habits or functional overload put stress on the back. Paying attention to one's own posture – not only in the dance studio – as well as performing specific exercises and corrections of dance technique can help to prevent back injury.

In Everyday Life

The auto-elongation of the spine through the tiny rolling-in movement of the two poles, the head and the pelvis, and the harmonious flexibility of the entire spine are the keys to a back that is optimally protected against stress. Pressure and compression – in lifting or jumping – are thus absorbed centrally in the spine and distributed equally across the vertebrae and the intervertebral discs. The flexibility of the spine can be optimally trained by walking. The alternate rotation in the thoracic spine keeps the ribcage mobile. Not only is breathing facilitated by the ribs' mobility; the cervical and lumbar spines are also subjected to less stress and the movement is harmoniously distributed across the entire back.

Tips:

- Use everyday situations to train the auto-elongation of your spine. For example, every time you pass through a door, when you are waiting at a bus stop or when you are on the phone, practise the rolling-in movement of head and pelvis at the same time and thus improve the architecture of your back. You can practice these exercises even while sitting.
- When walking, make sure that your thoracic spine remains flexible. Consciously rotate the spine to right and left. As you do so the sternum should lead the movement.
- It is especially helpful to perceive the rotation of the spine when climbing stairs. Pay attention to the extension of the lumbar spine on the side of the standing leg. Feel how the lower back muscles give way elastically.

Specific Exercises

Mobilization

 Mobilizing the thoracic spine I

Equipment: Thera-Band
Starting position: Lie on your right side. Pelvis, back and head are positioned neutrally, the right arm is stretched out upwards on the floor and your head lies on your arm. The legs are bent at a 90° angle at the hip and knee joints. Place the Thera-Band around the least moveable part of the thoracic spine; fix one end of the Thera-Band under the ribcage and grasp the free upper end with the left hand.
Action: Stabilize the left side of the pelvis at the back, down and to the outside. Turn the thoracic spine to the right towards the floor; the least moveable spinal section leads the movement. With the left hand, increase the pull on the Thera-Band; thus giving the thoracic spine the impulse for the rotational movement. Be sure to counter the movement with the left side of the pelvis! Pay attention to the opening of the left side of the ribcage – breathe in. Return to the starting position as you breathe out. Repeat several times and then change to the other side.

 Mobilizing the thoracic spine II

Starting position: Lie supine. Legs bent, feet parallel in line with the sit bones. Stretch both arms towards the ceiling with the palms of the hands touching. Shoulders and arms form a triangle that should remain throughout the entire exercise.

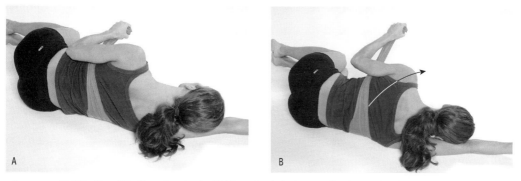

Figure 2.33 Mobilization of the thoracic spine I, with Thera-Band: the impetus for the rotational movement starts from the least moveable part of the thoracic spine. A) Starting position. B) Rotation of the thoracic spine to the right.

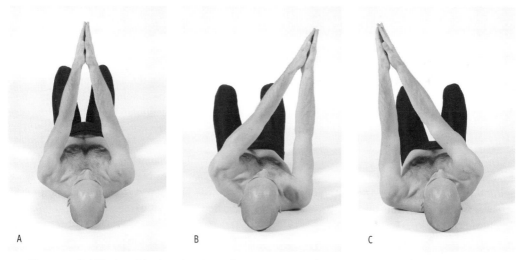

Figure 2.34 Mobilization of the thoracic spine II: A) starting position, B) rotation to the right, C) rotation to the left.

Action: Move the outstretched arms as far as possible to the right without losing the triangle shape formed by the arms and shoulders. The palms of the hands remain firmly pressed together; the movement should be taking place in the thoracic spine. Return to the starting position and repeat the movement to the other side. Carry out the rotation to right and left alternately, gradually increasing the range of motion. NB: The pelvis should be kept steady during the exercise.

E **Mobilizing the upper cervical joints – performing a "pelvic figure of eight" with the head**

Starting position: Sitting or standing. Head positioned centrally above the trunk.

Action: Make gentle nodding movements with the head, rocking it backwards and forwards on the atlas (the topmost vertebra). Now combine nodding with turning. Turn your head to the right, bending it slightly towards the left as you do so. The muscles at the back of the neck relax

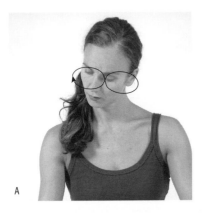

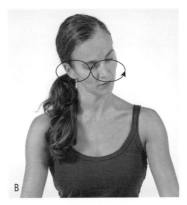

Figure 2.35 Mobilization of the upper cervical joints, performing a "figure of eight" with the head: A) right rotation, lateral bending to the left: pressure on the right atlanto-occipital joint is relieved, B) left rotation, lateral bending to the right: pressure on the left atlanto-occipital joint is relieved.

and the strain on the right upper cervical joint is reduced. Now continue the movement to the other side to perform a smooth figure of eight. Imagine you have a long nose like Pinocchio's and draw a figure of eight in the air in front of you. The chin should remain relaxed throughout the entire exercise.

Awareness

E **Auto-elongation of the spine while standing**

Starting position: Stand upright with your back towards the wall. Keep the feet parallel and hip-width apart.

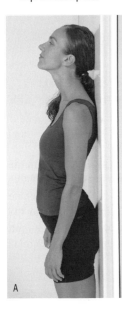

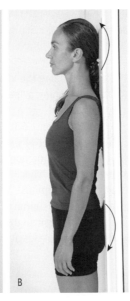

Action: The lumbar and neck muscles are tightened slightly thus increasing the curvature of the cervical and lumbar spine. When the tension is released, head and pelvis are actively rotated in opposite directions: the pelvis straightens, thereby stretching the lumbar muscles and the back area of the diaphragm. The head nods almost imperceptibly thus increasing the stretch in the cervical and thoracic spine. The spine rests against the wall, the superficial abdominal and spinal muscles remain relaxed. The exercise can also be carried out lying supine, which makes it easy to integrate it to the floor exercises of the training routine.

E **Contraction of the transversus abdominis**

Starting position: Lie supine with legs bent and feet parallel in line with the sit bones.

Action: Tighten the transversus abdominis while keeping the pelvis steady. The awareness of the fine contraction can be enhanced by various images: "stretching a silk thread between the navel and the spine", "removing the inner covering from the outer casing of the abdomen" or, "imagining the inner abdominal covering as the lining of a coat". It is best to create one's own image, which can quickly be recalled during all different sorts of movements.

Figure 2.36 Auto-elongation of the spine while standing: A) enhancement of the cervical and thoracical lordosis, B) the rolling-in of head and pelvis elongates and centres the entire spine.

Strengthening

E Strengthening the deep front neck muscles

Starting position: Lie supine with legs bent and feet parallel in line with the sit bones. Neck and chin a 90° angle.

Action: Thumb and first finger grasp the chin and pull it gently forwards. Place the other hand on the back top of your head and exert gentle pressure. Against this resistance extend the head actively away from the spine.

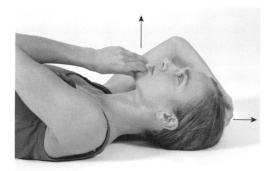

Figure 2.37 Strengthening the deep front neck muscles: active elongation of the head.

NB: The muscles at the back of the neck and the superficial front neck muscles remain relaxed; the deep front neck muscles do all the work. The contraction is supported by gently pulling the chin forward. Check the superficial front neck muscles to ensure that there is no tension.

E Strengthening the deep rotator muscles of the thoracic spine (rotatores)

Equipment: Thera-Band

Starting position: Sit upright. Place one end of the Thera-Band under the right buttock and pull taut. Pull the band diagonally forwards and hold with the right hand in front of the ribcage.

Action: Turn the upper body to the left against the resistance of the Thera-Band. The thoracic spine remains upright and the band is stretched. The deep external rotator muscles on the right side work concentrically; tightening up. When turning back, the same muscles act as a brake on the pull of the band working eccentrically. Repeat 25 times before changing sides. NB: The pelvis must remain upright and stable during the entire exercise.

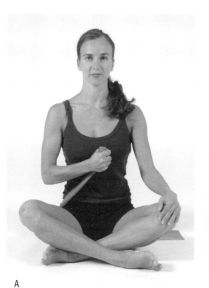

A

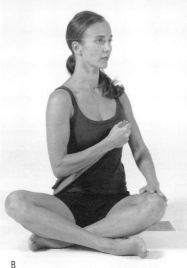

B

Figure 2.38 Strengthening the deep rotators of the thoracic spine: A) starting position, B) rotating the thoracic spine towards the left engages the deep rotators on the right side.

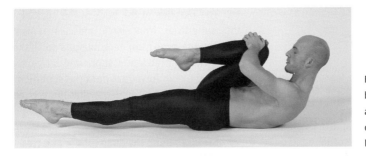

Figure 2.39 Strengthening the lower back and the abdominal muscles: alternate pulling up one leg to the chest with the other leg stretched and lifted slightly off the ground.

E   Strengthening the deep spinal and abdominal muscles (multifidus, rotatores, transversus abdominis)

Starting position: Lie supine with legs outstretched and knees pointing towards the ceiling.

Action: Simultaneously contract the transversus abdominis and the deep spinal muscles to stabilize the centre of the body. Alternately pull the bent right and left leg towards the chest, gently holding the knee with your hands without pressure. The other leg is stretched and slightly raised from the floor. Repeat 25 times. The centre of the body should remain stable throughout the entire exercise.

Action: Breathe in and tighten the lower spinal muscles until the pelvis tilts slightly forward and the lumbar spine forms a sway back. Relax as you breathe out and let the lumbar spine sink onto the floor. Simultaneously, your partner pulls the towel gently but firmly down towards the heels. This rotates the pelvis on its horizontal axis back- and downwards stretching the lumbar muscles. Each time you breathe out relax the muscles still further; the pull on the towel is made slightly stronger. NB: Do not press the lumbar spine onto the floor; the abdominal muscles should remain relaxed throughout the entire exercise.

Relaxation

E   Relaxation of the lumbar muscles I

Equipment: Towel, partner

Starting position: Lie supine with legs bent and feet parallel in line with the sit bones. The pelvis lies on a towel.

E   Relaxation of the lumbar muscles II

Equipment: Chair or edge of bed

Starting position: Lie supine with both legs bent at an angle of 90° at hip and knee joint. The lower legs are supported by a chair or the edge of the bed so that the pelvis is slightly raised from the floor.

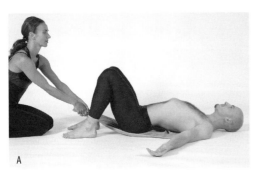

A

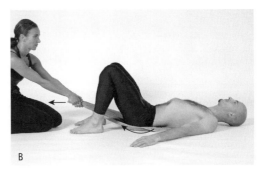

B

Figure 2.40 Relaxation of the lumbar muscles I: A) inhalation – lumbar muscles engage, tilting the pelvis forward creating lumbar hyperlordosis, B) exhalation – the towel is pulled down, helping to relax the lumbar muscles and elongate the lumbar spine.

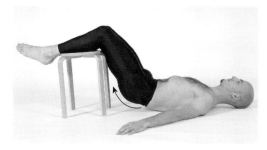

Figure 2.41 Relaxation of the lumbar muscles II: the pelvic floor leads the movement, the pelvis tilts backwards thus rounding the lumbar spine.

Action: To relax the pelvis, swing it gently to right and left. Now lengthen the back of the pelvis slowly, rolling in, starting from the bottom. The pelvic floor leads the movement. The pelvis rotates backwards around the horizontal axis; the facet joints of the lumbar spine open and the back is rounded. Slowly roll the spine back onto the floor again. Repeat the sequence several times until the relaxation can clearly be felt in your lower back.

E Relaxation through breathing

Starting position: Sit upright. Head and pelvis are slightly rolled in so that the entire spine is gently elongated.

Action: Concentrate on your breathing: as you inhale the upper ribs rise, the diaphragm contracts and sinks downwards. The thorax opens up, air streams into the farthest corners of the lungs and the "flanks" expand. When you exhale the ribcage sinks and the diaphragm relaxes. The spine gently follows the rhythm: when breathing in it lengthens and elongates, when breathing out it relaxes. The abdominal and spinal muscles remain relaxed.

In Training

- Imagining the "sit bones towards the floor" helps when positioning the pelvis. But do not forget, the opposite pole of the movement: the head and the pelvis together initiate the minimal rolling-in movement. This elongates the entire spine and the movement is harmoniously distributed, putting less pressure on each section of the spine.

- The muscular stabilization of the spine should take place via the simultaneous contraction of the small muscles of the back and the transverse abdominal muscle. Using images like "stretching a silk thread between the navel and the spine", "removing the inner covering from the outer casing" and "imagining the inner abdominal covering as a lining of a coat" can help to encourage a differentiated perception.

- The distance between the lower end of the sternum and the pubic bone should be kept the same, both when standing still and when moving. The awareness of this connecting line helps to centre the ribcage above the pelvis. The abdominal muscles seem to work by themselves.

- The head should be balanced on the cervical spine like a balloon. If it is centred, virtually no muscular effort is required. An imaginary line linking the chin and the top end of the sternum can help to enhance awareness of the auto-balance of the head.

- One of the important goals of dance training is to maintain the mobility of the entire spine. Do not fall into the temptation of carrying out movements only in those sections where you find them easiest. Do not encourage any local hypermobility! Mobilize less-flexible areas and stabilize hypermobile sections. By doing this you will be able to distribute the stress evenly across the entire spine, thereby reducing the strain on each individual section.

- Special attention should be paid to the thoracic spine. The less mobile it is, the greater the stress on the cervical and lumbar spine. A mobile thoracic spine is the best investment for a healthy back. Tiny rotations in training not only improve balance and harmonize movement but they also train the deep spinal muscles and thus stabilize the back.
- Before you begin to extend for an arch or a cambré derrière, the movement impulse should be upwards in elongation of the spine. Pay attention to forming a harmonious arch of the entire spine. The backward movement should be initiated intentionally from the thoracic spine.
- Use your breathing to stabilize your spine. When breathing in, the column of air in the lungs supports the upper body from the inside. This additional support relieves pressure on the spine.
- Stretch and relax your back after training. In order to stretch the small back muscles you need to round your back (e.g. placing your head on your knees while sitting on your heels). A flat back is not a stretch for the lumbar spine!
- Improve your lifting technique. Whenever possible, one should lift with a stable trunk which is only slightly bent forward. To improve the transfer of strength, a dancer should stand as close as possible to his partner and gather strength from his legs rather than the lower back. Breathing in before starting the lift can help stability and promotes "dynamic" lifting.

Check your dance technique:

Don't:
- Do I often stand with my pelvis tilted forward?
- Do I tend to stretch my head forward, especially when I am tired?
- Do I push the ribcage forward?
- Do my back muscles often feel hard and rigid?
- Do I usually use the regions of the spine which are already most flexible to move?
- Do I often start working from the lower back?

Do:
- Do I use the slight rolling-in movement of head and pelvis responsible for the auto-elongation of the spine when standing and moving?
- When slowly rolling down the spine, am I able to feel the flexibility between the individual vertebrae in all sections of the spine?
- Does my spine move as a harmonious whole? How flexible is it when performing an arch or a cambré derrière?
- Do I use the flexibility of my thoracic spine when dancing?
- Can I use my breathing for balance?
- Can I feel the 3D rotation of the spine in movement?

3. The Pelvis as the Centre

Stability, coupled with maximum freedom of movement for the legs, makes considerable demands on the dancer's pelvic region. It is not only in dance that the pelvis plays an important role. In the process of human evolution, the pelvis gradually straightened, permitting the body to progress from a horizontal position to a vertical one, and thus enabling mankind to evolve from a quadruped to a biped. In our time, the average human pelvis is tilted forward by about 30°.

The pelvis is regarded as the midpoint of the body and as the centre of movement. Anatomically speaking, it forms the connection between the torso and the legs. Its position and movement influences the body in both directions: upwards via the spine to the head and downwards via the hip joints and the legs to the smallest foot joint. As the central attachment point for virtually all the thigh muscles as well as the back and abdominal muscles, it is obvious that the optimal integration of the pelvis is one of the most important factors for harmonious, flowing movement. The position of the pelvis is the basis for the upright position of the entire body axis. The stability of the standing leg and the freedom of the working leg depend on the fine coordination of the pelvis.

3D Anatomy

The pelvis bears the weight of the torso and distributes it along the two hip joints. Conversely, it is through the pelvis that the repulsion force is transferred from the leg to the torso. The pelvis plays an important role in the transfer of the forces through the whole body.

The **hip bone** consists of three bones fused together: the **ilium**, the **pubic bone**, and the **ischium**. Together they form the hip socket (acetabulum), sitting diagonally tilted forwards in the pelvic girdle (see Chapter 4, p. 76).

Structure

The bony pelvic girdle consists of the two hip bones and the sacrum. Three joints provide the pelvis with elasticity: two *sacroiliac joints* at the back, between the sacrum and the ilium, and the *pubic symphysis* at the front between the two pubic bones.

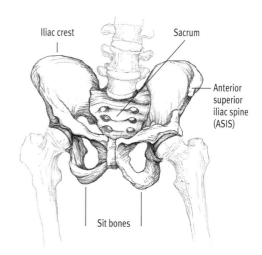

Iliac crest

Sacrum

Anterior superior iliac spine (ASIS)

Sit bones

Figure 3.1 The bony structure of the pelvis – front view.

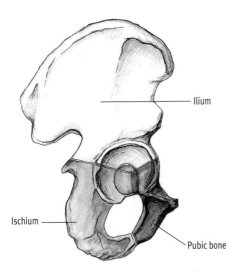

Ilium

Ischium

Pubic bone

Figure 3.2 The hip bone is composed of three bones.

The **sacroiliac joint** links the sacrum and the ilium. The two round articular surfaces on both sides of the sacrum fit perfectly together with the hollow shaped articular surfaces of the ilium. The structure of the articular surfaces, the strong ligaments and numerous muscles make the sacroiliac joint particularly stable and resilient. Its firm system of ligaments gives it a buffering/shock capacity and dynamically stabilizes the pelvic girdle.

As if it were in a basin, the lower abdominal organs rest in the bony pelvic girdle. Well-padded by connective and fatty tissue, the bladder, uterus and rectum lie in a row between the pubic bone at the front and the sacrum at the back.

The ilium offers a broad attachment site for the abdominal and back muscles. The **iliac crest** and the **anterior superior iliac spine** (ASIS) are important bony landmarks. The ischium and the pubic bone form the lower part of the hip bone. The two pubic bones are linked via the pubic symphysis; they form the front part of the pelvic girdle. The knobbly **sit bones** form the lowest part of the pelvis. As they are easy felt, for example, while sitting on a hard surface, they are also used as bony "landmarks".

The **sacrum** consists of what were originally five sacral vertebrae which have become fused to form a single bone. The sacrum has an interesting shape: it is formed like a wedge – broad at the top and narrow at the bottom. When bearing weight, it can "wedge" itself firmly in between the two hip bones, stabilizing the pelvic girdle more or less by itself. Taut ligaments link the sacrum with the tailbone, or **coccyx**. Four to five coccygal vertebrae are fused to form the coccyx. Together, sacrum and coccyx connect the spinal column with the pelvis. Forming both the end of the spine as well as the back of the pelvic girdle, the sacrum and coccyx play an important part in the transmission of force.

3D Function

The position of the pelvis is crucial for the body's balance. The straightening of the pelvis – its "rolling in" around the horizontal axis – is a continuation of the gradual movement that it underwent during mankind's evolution to an upright stance. The sit bones tilt towards the floor, the iliac crest moves backwards and the pelvis is brought upright. This straightening of the pelvis reduces the strain on the spine, centres the abdominal organs in the pelvic basin and at the same time activates the pelvic floor.

During movement, the weight of the torso has to be continuously rearranged into balancing over the standing leg. The pelvis offers an intelligent solution: on the side of the standing leg the sit bone swings forwards–upwards–inwards; it slightly moves towards the pubic bone. This moves the iliac crest backwards–downwards–outwards. The sacroiliac joint wedges itself firmly preventing undesirable shearing movements in the joint. The lumbar spine is straightened and lengthened. The pelvis "spirals" itself on top of the standing leg. Thus the load is ideally distributed across the hip joint. On the side of the working leg, the movement happens exactly the other way round: the sit bones swing backwards–

downwards–outwards, the sacroiliac joint opens up increasing the flexibility of this side of the pelvis. The continuous change between standing leg and working leg, between stress and relaxation, is an ideal training for these structures.

Movements of the Pelvis

We distinguish between two types of pelvic movement: the movement of the entire pelvis in space and the movements within the pelvic girdle.

Movement of the whole pelvis

The easiest way to understand the movement of the pelvis in space is to consider the body axes. The movement does not occur in the joints of the pelvic girdle itself, but in the two hip joints and in the lower spine. Table 3.1 shows the relationship between the axis of movement, the name of the movements and the bony landmarks which permit the pelvic movements to be assessed.

The terminology used for the tilting forward and back of the pelvis can be confusing. In medicine, the iliac crest serves as the point of

Table 3.1 The positions and movements of the pelvis

Axis	Movement	Bony landmarks
Horizontal axis	Tilting forward Tilting backward	Sit bones towards the back Sit bones towards the front
Sagittal axis	Right lateral tilt Left lateral tilt	Left iliac crest up Right iliac crest up
Vertical axis	Rotation to the right Rotation to the left	Left ASIS protrudes Right ASIS protrudes

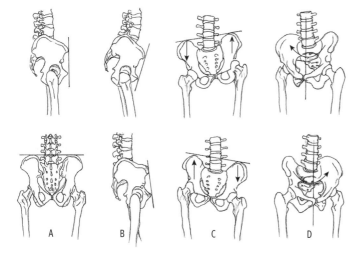

Figure 3.3 The pelvis movements around the three axes:
A) the neutral position of the pelvis,
B) tilting forward and backward,
C) tilting sideways to the right and left, D) rotation to the right and left.

reference. If the iliac crest moves forward we refer to a forward tilted pelvis: the buttocks stick out to the back, the sit bones point backwards, and the lordosis of the lumbar spine increases. However, some dancers understand a forward-tilting pelvis to mean the exact opposite: they tighten the buttocks and thereby push the pelvic floor forwards. This tilts the iliac crest backwards. In medical terms this is known as a backward-tilting pelvis.

Pelvic movements never happen in isolation; they always affect the position of the hip joints and the spine, especially the lumbar spine (see Table 3.2).

Table 3.2 Influence of pelvic movements on the hip joints and the lumbar spine

Pelvic movement	Hip Movement	Movement of lumbar spine
Tilting forward	Hip flexion	Increased extension
Tilting backward	Hip extension	Flexion
Right lateral tilt	Right hip abduction Left hip adduction	Lateral tilt to the left
Rotation to the right	Right hip Internal rotation Left hip External rotation	Rotation to the left

Movement in the sacroiliac joint

The sacroiliac joint can only be moved passively; there is no possibility to move it actively through muscle strength. If the hip joint or the lower spine moves, the movement continues through the body: every movement in the hip joint also moves the hip bone, and every movement of the lumbar spine leads to movements of the sacrum. Depending on the range of motion, the movement is transferred to the sacroiliac joint, moving it to a greater or lesser extent. Only a free and mobile sacroiliac joint will allow this movement to happen, a movement which only involves a shift of

a few millimetres, but is of crucial importance for the functioning of the pelvis.

Movement within the sacroiliac joint, at the back area of the pelvic girdle, cannot take place without mobility in the front section, in the pubic symphysis. Being built of fibrocartilage, the pubic symphysis allows the two pubic bones to passively move against each other – rather like in the spine where the vertebrae can move around the intervertebral disc. This is important for the flexibility of the pelvic girdle. This is how it works in detail: when bending your hip joint, whether slowly, as in the développé or quickly, as in the battement, the hip bone will also move sooner or later, depending on the flexibility of the hip joint. It turns backwards in relation to the sacrum. The opposite happens when the leg is moved backwards: in order to achieve the maximum range of motion, the hip bone will turn forwards.

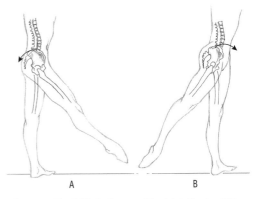

Figure 3.4 Flexibility in the sacroiliac joint: A) when lifting the leg forwards, the hip bone rotates backwards in relation to the sacrum, B) when lifting the leg to the back, the hip bone rotates forwards in relation to the sacrum.

The degree of movement within the sacroiliac joint can vary between the right and left sides and can also differ on one side between front and back. Asymmetrical flexibility like this has consequences: restricted mobility in the sacroiliac joint also restricts leg movement; achieving position involving high legs are virtually impossible without an optimally flexible sacroiliac joint.

Differences in mobility between both sides can alter the entire pelvic position. For example, if the hip bone on the right side is slightly turned forward but on the left it is turned to the back, pelvic torsion occurs. This can have far-reaching effects: if the right hip bone turns forward, the right hip socket will move downwards. The right leg, which is "suspended" from the hip joint, will be pushed downwards, as it were, and appears to be longer. In this case, the cause of a difference in leg length is not the leg itself, but the torsion of the pelvis.

Table 3.3 Possible causes of leg-length difference

Structural leg-length difference *The leg bones on one side are longer than on the other.*	Functional leg-length difference *One leg appears longer than the other, although the bones are the same length.*
Steep or flat hip on one side	Pelvic torsion
Structural discrepancy of leg axis on one side	Functional discrepancy of leg axis on one side
Growth disturbance on one side e.g. after bone fracture	Hyperpronated foot and/or flat foot on one side

Musculature

The pelvis is the central attachment point for numerous muscles. The abdominal and back muscles, coming from above, attach at the bony pelvic girdle, and almost all of the thigh muscles originate at the pelvis. The significance of the pelvic position is clear: only a stable, well-centred pelvis allows the legs to move freely. The abdominal and back muscles make an important contribution to the stability of the pelvis.

For a detailed description of the leg muscles see Chapter 4, pp. 79/104. For explanations of the abdominal and back muscles see Chapter 2, pp. 31.

The pelvic floor

Usually, in dance as elsewhere, little attention is paid to the pelvic floor, which are the muscles at the bottom of the pelvis. However, due to its central location it is ideally situated to stabilize the pelvis from below, and thus give the pelvis both stability and mobility. Like a hammock, the pelvic floor extends from the coccyx along the two sit bones to the pubic bones.

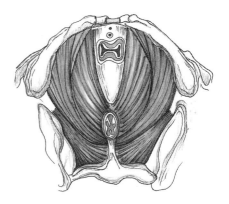

Figure 3.5 The structure of the female pelvic floor.

The pelvic floor is constructed of several layers which make it a complex and multi-functional system. The sphincter muscles of the bladder and the bowel lie in the middle of the pelvic floor and are activated automatically, while the muscle fibres at the side contract or release alternately, depending on the movement. On the side of the standing leg, when bearing weight, the pelvic floor is tightened concentrically, while it relaxes eccentrically on the side of the working leg. Prerequisite to this is a neutral pelvic position, which allows the pelvic floor to actually work as the floor of the pelvis.

Dance in Focus: Load and Overload

As the connecting point between the torso and the legs, the pelvis is equally subject to strain from both above and below.

Load

From swinging of the upper body to the isolation of the pelvis or tilting of the entire body: many dance movements cannot be performed without a stable pelvis.

The "neutral" pelvis – the pelvic position

The starting position in many dance styles is the "neutral" pelvis, the position in which the pelvis is balanced ideally on top of the hip joints like a set of scales, the muscles are almost not required to work as joints and the bones take up their positions above each other, as it were. The pelvis is upright, the sit bones are pointing downwards, the pelvic floor is actually working as the floor of the pelvis and the lower spine is optimally lengthened. The two anterior superior iliac spines are on the same plane and the iliac crests are level. The lower abdominal and spinal muscles work smoothly together and the pelvic floor is active. The economic muscle work allows for a dynamic neutral position, the ideal starting position for movements of the upper body, pelvis and legs in all directions. Even minor deviations from this ideal position can cause problems which can affect the pelvis itself, the spine, the hip joint, the knee or even the foot.

The "straight" pelvis – the pelvis in motion

The bigger the leg movement, and the more flexible the working leg, the more movement of the pelvic girdle is required. Not only is the flexibility of the hip joint utilized right up to the bony limits; the mobility of the sacroiliac joints permits the pelvic girdle to twist in itself thus providing the image of a neutral pelvic position in spite of the extreme range of motion of the legs. The pelvis functions in dance as it does in walking. As one hip bone moves in one direction, the other side counteracts the movement; the two sides of the pelvis rotate in opposite directions. Seen from outside, the pelvis hardly seems to move but a closer look is revealing: if the leg is raised to the front, the hip bone moves with it; it turns backwards in relation to the sacrum. The opposite occurs when moving the leg towards the back: then the hip bone rotates forward in the sacroiliac joint. The other side always moves the opposite way – thus creating the illusion of the "straight" pelvis. The complex mechanism shows clearly that dancers' sacroiliac joints need to be especially strong.

Stable standing leg

It is impossible to over-emphasize the importance of the standing leg in dance: only a stable standing leg ensures a stable balance and at the same time permits free use for the other leg. "Don't sit on your standing leg", "lengthen your groin": these are typical corrections which aim to help the dancer to centre the pelvis on top of the hip joint. However, the main activity of this movement does not come from the hip joint itself, but rather from the pelvic floor. As soon as weight is put on the leg, the pelvic floor starts to become active in pulling the sit bone on the side of the standing leg forwards–upwards–inwards. With this action the hip socket moves on top of the head of the femur thus centring the pelvis right on top of the standing leg. The structures on the front side of the hip joint get stretched; the "groin is lengthened". The impulse comes from the pelvic floor while the deep external rotator muscles help with the stabilization; the hip muscles are free to be used for other movements.

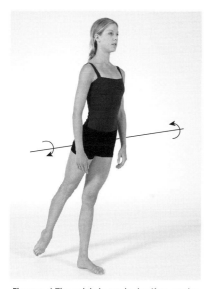

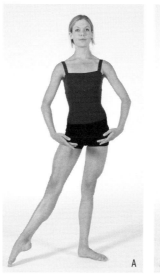

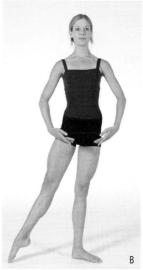

Figure 3.6 The pelvis in tendu derrière: on the working leg side, the ilium rotates forward, and on the standing leg side it rotates backwards. Viewed from the outside, the pelvis looks "straight".

Figure 3.7 A) "Sitting"on the standing leg: the pelvic floor is weak, the sit bone points backwards–downwards–outwards, B) a stable standing leg by an optimal spiral of the hip joint: the pelvic floor pulls the sit bone forwards–upwards–inwards.

Overload

The pelvic region can cause numerous, widely differing problems, from headaches to back problems to problems with the hips, knees or feet. In the pelvic region itself it is the sacroiliac joint in particular which causes problems for dancers.

Chronic overload

Irritation and instability of the sacroiliac joint: An overloading of the sacroiliac joint is common in dance. Female dancers are much more likely to suffer from inflammation and instability of this joint than their male colleagues. The reason for this is the bony structure of the joint. If the round joint surfaces of the sacrum sit deeply in the hollow articular surfaces of the ilium, as is usual in men, the joint is well stabilized and irritations seldom occur. But this stability is gained at the expense of flexibility. Because of their flatter articular surfaces, women have a much higher mobility in the sacroiliac joint. However, this

makes them more susceptible to overload and injury.

Iliopsoas Syndrome: Overloading of the iliopsoas muscle can occur simultaneously, as the cause or as the result of irritation of the sacroiliac joint. (For further information on the iliopsoas muscle, see Chapter 4, p. 81.)

Hip or knee problems: A difference in leg length, pelvic torsion or muscular imbalance can make it impossible for a dancer to neutrally position the pelvis when standing. Although this has no impact in everyday life, it can cause problems while dancing. For example, a leg which is structurally or functionally longer can prohibit optimal closing in from the tendu. When closing in the longer leg from the tendu, a dancer has two options: either bending the knee slightly or lifting the pelvis a tiny bit on the working leg side. Both compensatory actions can lead to problems if frequently repeated.

Acute injury

Blockage of the sacroiliac joint: The two parts of the joint become "locked" into each other, blocking the free movement of the joint. Movement, if at all, is only possible in one direction while movement in all other directions causes severe pain. It is essential to get out of the vicious cycle of restricted movement, pain and reflex-like muscle tension as quickly as possible by specific treatment.

Pitfalls in Dance

Whether in response to encouragement from the trainer or because of their own ambition, many dancers "cheat" in trying to achieve a greater turnout. But the exaggerated outer rotation of the legs changes the position of the pelvis and thus affects the entire posture. A forced turnout, over-straightening of the pelvis or one-sided training; some of the well-meant dance technical instructions should be questioned.

Forced Turnout – the Effect on the Pelvis

The main action in turnout takes place in the hip joints (see Chapter 4, p. 83). The hip socket is formed by the hip bone and thus is part of the pelvis. The position and flexibility of the hip joints are therefore dependent on the position of the pelvic girdle. Many dancers instinctively try to increase their turnout via the position of their pelvis. They tilt their pelvis forward around the horizontal axis. This allows the hip joint to bend slightly, releases the front joint ligaments and with this increases the passive outer rotation of the hip joint. At first sight, the turnout seems easier. But appearances are deceptive: in the long term this pelvic position makes it even harder to dance. The lumbar lordosis increases leading to a typical sway back position, which intensifies the pressure between the individual vertebrae. The balance between the abdominal and back muscles is disturbed; the back muscles become shorter and harden, while the abdominal muscles are overstretched and weaken, and so it becomes increasingly difficult to stabilize the pelvis in the neutral position.

By tilting the pelvis forward the sit bones direct towards the back and the pelvic floor ceases to function. Usually trained automatically by the constant alternation between working leg and standing leg, its dynamics are lost; it becomes weaker. Other muscles have to take over its job. This can result in muscle overload, imbalance, joint inflammation and even problems with intervertebral discs.

How to recognize: The tilting of the pelvis can most easily be seen from the side. Feet in first position, in the turnout of your choice, hands on the sit bones.

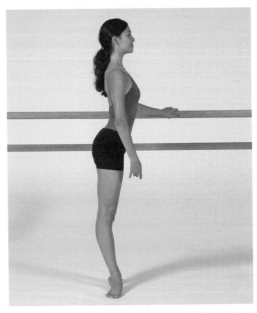

Figure 3.8 In forcing the turnout, the pelvis tilts forward and the body balance is lost.

Slow plié, the dancer should let the sit bones drop towards the floor; feeling the connection between the sit bones and the heels. The lumbar spine is elongated. Start the extension from this position. Can you keep the position of the pelvis until the knees are fully stretched? Are the sit bones still pointing downwards when the knees are fully extended? NB: If the knees are hyperextended the pelvis will automatically tilt forwards! (See Chapter 5, p. 113.)

What you can do:
- The neutral position of the pelvis is more important than the extent of the turnout. Therefore, first place the pelvis in position – sit bones towards the floor – and then turn out the legs from the hip joints.
- The legs should only be turned out to the point where the turnout can actually be held by the muscles. (see Chapter 4, p. 83).

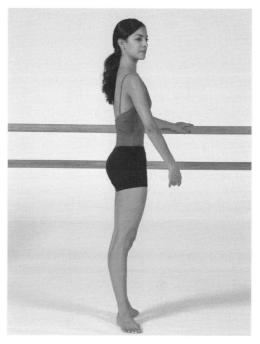

Figure 3.9 "Tucking under" is a typical overcompensation of the forward-tilted pelvis.

Tuck Under of the Pelvis

If the pelvis is rotated far backwards around the horizontal axis, this is known as "tucking under". The iliac crest tilts backwards moving the pelvis too far into an upright position. This posture can be caused by maximum tension in the gluteal muscles; by shortened abdominal muscles; or simply by over-correcting a forward-tilting pelvis. The groin is overstretched, the lumbar spine loses its elasticity and the movement looks stiff and rigid. The pelvic position and the muscle tension make efficient muscle use impossible.

"Tucking under" often occurs when in-experienced dancers perform a demi or grand plié in transferring the bending movement of the knee *en bloc* to the pelvis, losing the isolated flexion movement of the hips. The sit bones point forwards, the iliac crest tilts backwards and the lumbar spine curls.

How to recognize: The tilting backwards of the pelvis can best be seen from the side. You should put your feet in first position, in the turnout of your choice and perform a slow plié. Pay attention to the pelvic position during the movement. Can you hold the centred position of the pelvis in grand plié, or does the iliac crest tip backwards during the movement? Can you see an isolated flexion in the hip joint?

What you can do:
- The correction "tighten your buttocks" can mislead the dancer into "tucking under". This expression should not be used as training vocabulary.
- Corrective images like "create connection between sit bone and heel" or "sit bones towards the floor" help to find one's own individual neutral pelvic position.

One-sided Training – Increased Pelvic Torsion

This is familiar to many dancers: one leg can be extended almost effortlessly, while the other side is difficult and poorly coordinated. It is not surprising that a dancer will prefer to focus on the side where the movement feels better. But this increasingly one-sided effort will not only affect dance technique. After a short while the shape of the pelvis will reflect this one-sidedness and will reveal changes which can have far-reaching effects. This can be easily seen in the following example: if a dancer finds it particularly easy to raise the right leg forwards and to the side, while the left leg is easier to move backwards, this may be a sign of pelvic torsion. The right hip bone is rotated towards the back whereas the left hip bone tilts towards the front. If both hip bones are nonetheless mobile in all directions this pelvic torsion will not cause any problems. However, if the dancer subsequently prefers his "best side", the pelvic torsion may be increased. Over time, the mobility of the hip bones will be reduced: the right hip bone will be progressively more difficult to rotate forward, and the left hip bone will be more difficult to move to the back. The result is an even greater decrease in leg mobility.

If ignored, pelvic torsion will lead to increasing difficulty in performing an arabesque with the right side, and the left leg will lose height when extended to the front or side. In the long, run pelvic torsion can even lead to a change in position of the pelvic organs, which may affect the functioning of bladder, uterus and rectum.

How to recognize: It is perfectly normal for there to be differences in leg height and mobility between the two sides. What you should be wary of is if the difference between the sides continues to increase despite countermeasures in training and increased attention to the weaker side. In this case one should consult medical help for an examination of the pelvis and the hip joints.

> *What you can do:*
> - It may be tempting, but there is no point in training only the "best side". Conscious and specific training of the opposite side can reduce or even prevent pelvic torsion.
> - The sacroiliac joints should be warmed up passively (see p. 69) before putting them under stress. This can also help to prevent pelvic torsion.

A Closer Look – Self-analysis

A neutral pelvic position facilitates the body's balance and harmonizes movement, both everyday movements and when dancing.

Form and Mobility

When assessing the pelvis, its position in space is just as important as the movements within the pelvic girdle and the mobility within the sacroiliac joint.

The easiest way to assess the **pelvic position** is in front of a mirror. The feet are parallel, hip-width apart; the pelvis is relaxed. It is important that both heels stand on an imaginary line, in order not to give the wrong impression of a pelvic rotation. Now the pelvic position can be examined systematically from the front and the side by using the bony reference points, as shown in Table 3.4.

The assessment of the **mobility of the sacroiliac joints** should be carried out supine. The legs are bent with the feet parallel, and in line with the sit bones. The hands are placed on the iliac crests with the thumbs pointing backwards. Now the right hand slowly moves the right hip bone backwards–downwards–outwards. At the end of

Table 3.4 Assessment of the pelvic position

View from...	Feel	Assessment	Position	This is what it looks like
...the front	Place the hands on both sides on the iliac crests	Are the iliac crests at the same height?	lateral tilt	Picture A
...the front	Thumbs on both ASIS (anterior superior iliac spine)	Does one side protrude more than the other?	Pelvic rotation right or left	Picture B
...the side	Imagine a line through the two ASIS and the pubic symphysis	Is the line vertical to the floor?	Pelvic tilt forwards or backwards	Picture C

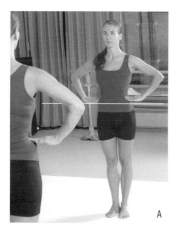
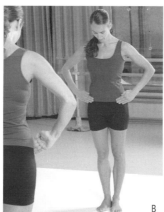
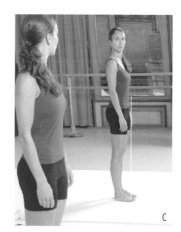

A   B   C

the movement, the left hand takes over and moves the left hip bone backwards–downwards–outwards. The movement does not need to be large but it should be smooth and harmonious on both sides. "Edges" during the course of the movement indicate that there may be a movement disorder in the sacroiliac joint (see Figure 3.13, p. 70).

Function and Stability

The three-dimensional spiralling of the pelvis helps to balance and stabilize the entire body.

The pelvic spiral in dancing: Stand straight with the feet parallel hip-width apart; hands on the iliac crests with the thumbs pointing backwards.

High passé right with the hands supporting the pelvic movement: the left hand leads the hip bone backwards–downwards–outwards and the right hand holds the right side forwards–upwards–inwards against it. The two hip bones rotate against each other. The movement is barely noticed from the outside but should be felt with the hands. Repeat the exercise on both sides alternating several times; close your eyes to increase your sense of perception. Classical dancers should also perform this movement sequence in turnout.

Stability of the pelvis: Support the body lying on the elbows with the feet on demi-pointe. Head, pelvis and legs form a diagonal which does not change during the entire test. Alternately raise the right and the left leg backwards and diagonally to

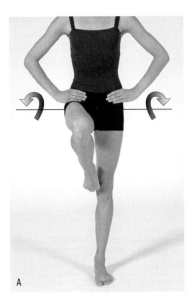
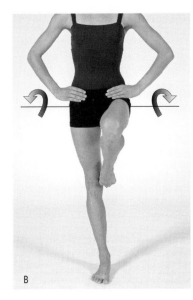

Figure 3.10 Test for the pelvic spiral: A) in the right passé the left ilium rotates backwards–downwards–outwards, whereas the right ilium holds forwards-upwards-inwards, B) in the left passé, the right ilium rotates backwards–downwards–outwards, whereas the left ilium holds forwards–upwards–inwards.

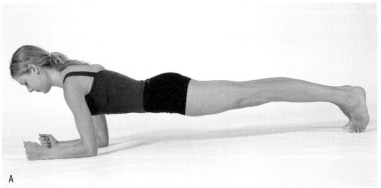

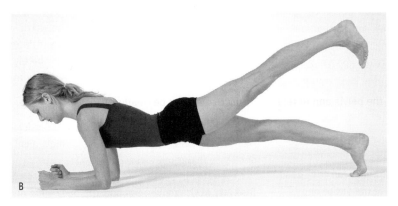

Figure 3.11 Stability test for the pelvis: A) starting position, B) the left and right legs lift alternately, and the pelvis is kept level.

the side, hold briefly and return to the starting position. You should be able to repeat the exercise 25 times without moving the pelvis from its central position. Head, pelvis and legs must always remain in a diagonal line.

Tips and Tricks for Prevention

Pain in the pelvic region is often wrongly interpreted as back pain. But a deep central pain above the sacrum or discomfort at the side in the sacroiliac joints is usually a sign of excessive stress in the pelvic girdle, a malfunction of the pelvic joints. In dance, the pelvis is subjected to considerable stress, so it is no wonder that virtually every dancer is familiar with the "deep back pain". Here even small changes can have a major effect; a pelvis which is functionally stable can take the strain in everyday life as well as in dancing.

In Everyday Life

The position and function of the pelvis can be trained in every movement: while sitting and standing, while walking, running or climbing stairs. Both the awareness of the pelvic position in standing and an optimal three-dimensional spiralling when walking are ideal everyday preparations for the increased stress in dancing.

Tips:

- Pay attention to the position of your pelvis when standing. Do the sit bones direct towards the floor? Is the pelvis upright and the lumbar spine elongated? Be aware of the work of the pelvic floor. It is only engaged when the pelvis is in an upright position.
- Never stand still. If you do have to stand for a long time, try to keep moving slightly. For example, bend your knees from time to time in order to straighten the pelvis and to relax the lower back and the sacrum. A minor adjustment of weight is scarcely noticeable but keeps your pelvis active. Your back will appreciate this.
- Especially when standing for a long time, avoid putting your weight predominantly on your favourite side. We often involuntarily sink onto the standing leg. The sacroiliac joint is then no longer firmly wedged and shearing movements occur in the joint which can lead to instability and pain in the long term.
- When walking, make a point of using your pelvic floor as the centre of the impulse. You can clearly feel the alternating activity of the pelvic floor especially when climbing stairs, thereby not only training an energetic gait but also training the muscle and thus the automatic balance of the pelvis at the same time.
- When sitting, be aware of your sit bones. Try to sit directly on your sit bones, not behind. Play with the distribution of weight. Sitting can also be dynamic!

Specific Exercises

Mobilization

E **Unilateral mobilization of the sacroiliac joint**

Starting position: Lie supine. Bend one leg at the hip and knee joint and take hold of the knee with the opposite hand. Put the other hand with the palm upwards under the side of the pelvis with the fingertips touching the sacrum, the ball of the hand lying on the hip bone and the palm of the hand just covering the sacroiliac joint.

Action: Using the opposite hand, take the bent leg and move it sideways until the back part of the iliac crests can be clearly felt on the palm of the hand lying under the pelvis. Using your hand, circle the knee for about one minute. The movement should be carried out exclusively by the hand; the leg itself remains completely passive. Important: use small, rhythmical circles; you should perceive the movement more in the sacroiliac joint than in the hip joint. Then change to the other side to repeat the action.

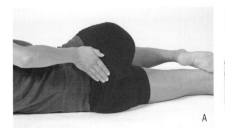
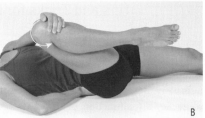

Figure 3.12
Unilateral
mobilization of the
sacroiliac joint:
A) this is how the
hand is placed on
the sacroiliac joint,
B) mobilization.

A

B

E **Bilateral mobilization of the sacroiliac joint – performing a "pelvic figure of eight"**

Starting position: Lie supine. The legs are bent and the feet parallel in line with the sit bones. The hands are placed on the iliac crests with the thumbs pointing backwards.

Action: The right sit bone moves forwards–upwards–inwards towards the left knee, with the right hand supporting the movement by guiding the right iliac crest backwards–downwards–outwards. At the end of the movement, the left side takes over. The left sit bone moves forwards–upwards–inwards towards the right knee and the left hand guides the left iliac crest backwards-downwards-outwards. The speed of the movement can be adjusted as required.

Awareness

E **Awareness of the pelvic floor**

Starting position: Lie supine. Legs bent, feet parallel in line with the sit bones; the pelvis in neutral position. If necessary, use the hands to feel the sit bones.

Action: Using only the pelvic floor muscles, slowly pull the right sit bone forwards–upwards–inwards towards the left knee, relax and return to the starting position. There should be no activity of the leg muscles; the movement is small and can hardly be seen from the outside. Repeat several times until you can clearly feel the activity of the pelvic floor. Repeat the exercise on the left side. Then alternately use the right and left sit bone: with this you imitate the pelvic movement of walking while lying on the floor.

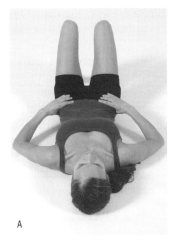
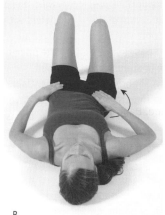
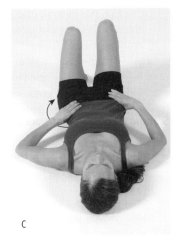

A   B   C

Figure 3.13 Bilateral mobilization of the sacroiliac joints (performing a "pelvic figure of eight"): A) starting position, B) the right ilium is turned backwards–downward–outwards, C) at the end of the movement, the left hand takes over and leads the left ilium backwards–downward–outwards.

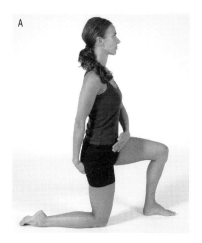

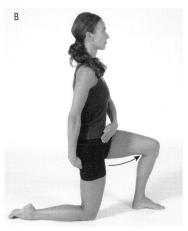

Figure 3.14 Awareness of the pelvic floor, loaded: A) starting position, B) the right sit bone moves forwards–upwards–inwards, in the direction of the left knee, the hands support the three-dimensional spiral movement of the right hip bone.

E Awareness of the pelvic floor, loaded

Starting position: Kneel on your right knee. Put the right hand on the right sit bone and the left hand on the front of the right side of the pelvis.

Action: Move the right sit bone forwards–upwards–inwards towards the left knee. The hands support the three-dimensional rotating movement of the right half of the pelvis; the sit bone initiates the movement. Notice the activity of the right half of the pelvic floor and the three-dimensional movement within the hip joint. Be aware of the lengthening in the right groin. Then change to the left leg and repeat, kneeling on the left knee.

Strengthening

E Strengthening the pelvic floor, unloaded

Equipment: Thera-Band

Starting position: Lie on your left side. Bend your legs at the hip and knee joints with the heels in line with the sit bones. One end of the Thera-Band is placed under the pelvis, running across the right sit bone diagonally forwards along the hip bone. The right hand holds taut the free end of the Thera-Band level with the navel.

Action: Against the pull of the Thera-Band the right hip bone turns backwards–downwards–outwards. The pelvic floor initiates the move-

ment: it pulls the right sit bone forwards–upwards–inwards towards the direction of the pubic bone. The spine and legs remain relaxed. The resistance can be increased or decreased by varying the amount of tension on the Thera-Band.

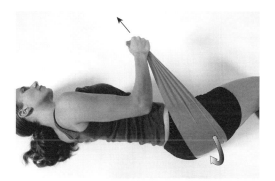

Figure 3.15 Strengthening the pelvic floor unloaded: the pelvic floor pulls the right sit bone obliquely forwards–upwards–inwards towards the pubic bone.

E Strengthening the pelvic floor, loaded – stability of the standing leg

Equipment: Barre

Starting position: Stand upright. Keep feet parallel and hip-width apart; place both hands on the barre, preferably in front of a mirror. One foot is placed on the ankle of the other foot (sur le cou-de-pied).

Action: Push the sit bone of the standing leg backwards-downwards-outwards as far as possible. Be aware of "sitting" on the standing leg. Now start the counter-movement from the pelvic floor: the sit bone swings forwards-upwards-inwards towards the direction of the pubic bone, without letting the other side of the pelvis rise high over level. Repeat the movement 25 times, change to the other leg and repeat.

Relaxation

E **Dynamics of the pelvic floor**

Starting position: Standing.

Action: Walk across the room, taking notice of the distance between the sit bone and the pubic bone: on the standing leg side, the sit bone approaches the pubic bone, whereas on the side of the working leg, the distance increases. The pelvic floor muscles alternate between concentric work on the standing leg and eccentric relaxation on the working leg.

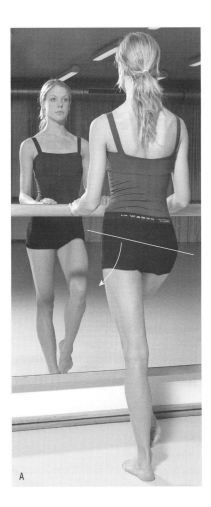

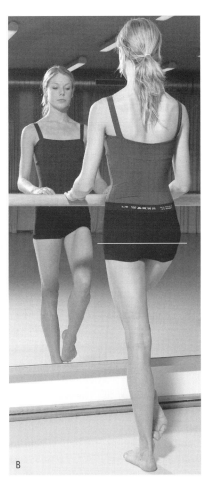

Figure 3.16 Strengthening the pelvic floor, loaded: A) the pelvic floor is inactive: "sitting" on the standing leg, B) activity of the pelvic floor on the standing leg side.

In Training

- Priority in dance is a well-centred pelvis! Images such as "feel the connection between the sit bones and the heels", "pull the sit bones towards the floor", or "imagining that the coccyx is extended down to the floor like a kangaroo's tail" can help to straighten the pelvis.
- Use your sit bones when jumping. Make sure they are always directing downwards during the takeoff, leaping and landing phases. You will notice that you can suddenly jump much higher without additional effort.
- The neutral pelvic position is more important than the degree of the turnout. Therefore position the pelvis first before turning out the legs in the hip joints.
- The correction "tighten your buttocks" might lead to an exaggerated tucking of the pelvis. It should be removed from training vocabulary.
- Warm up your sacroiliac joints specifically before you dance. By doing so you will not only protect your joints but will also increase your mobility during dancing.
- An active pelvic floor facilitates balance and reduces strain on the entire hip, back and abdominal muscles. This is the most effective muscle for pelvic stability!

- Focus your attention on the small movements within the pelvis. Awareness of the three-dimensional spiralling will help you to centre your pelvis and to keep it stable even in extreme positions.

Check your dance technique:

Don't:
- Do I tilt my pelvis forwards or backwards to force my turnout?
- Do I tilt my pelvis backwards during a demi-plié or grand plié?
- Do I "sit" on my standing leg?
- Do I raise my pelvis on the working leg side?

Do:
- Can I place my pelvis neutrally in the basic positions?
- Do I use the pelvic floor to stabilize my standing leg?
- Am I aware of the 3D spiralling of the pelvis during movement?

4. The Hip: A Joint with Consequences

"Keep your hips straight. Elongate your groin as much as you can." These are typical dance corrections which often cause confusion rather than providing help. In dance, the word "hip" is often not only used for the hip joint itself, but refers to the entire half of the pelvis, consisting of the hip bone *and* the actual hip joint. The "groin" on the other hand refers to the entire region from the iliac crest to the pubic bone.

The hip joint is a well-protected, stable joint. For dancers, its mobility is especially important. From high legs to a good turnout, above-average flexibility in all directions is required of the hip joint. In order to be able to extend the leg high into the air, however, requires more than just a flexible hip joint. Only the coordinated use of the hip muscles allows the optimum movement of the working leg and permits the dancer to hold his leg in the required position.

The turnout – the external rotation of the stretched leg in the hip joint – is part of many dance styles, albeit to a greater or lesser extent. In classical ballet a good en dehors is essential for the accurate performance of the typical dance positions and dance steps. Unfortunately, the often-attempted 180° turnout is also the cause of numerous over-stress syndromes and injuries in dance, namely when the turnout is forced beyond the limits imposed by anatomy. As a stylistic device, turnout is an essential component of dance and is also functionally useful: as a result of external rotation, the flexibility of the hip joint increases in almost all directions. But this must not be overdone.

3D Anatomy

The movement-ability of the hip joint is determined by its anatomical structure; by the form and position of the bones which form the joint.

Structure

The hip joint consists of two partners: the hip socket (*acetabulum*) and the head of the femur (*caput femoris*). The hip socket lies diagonally tilted forwards on the side of the pelvic girdle and the head of the femur forms the top end of the thigh bone (*femur*). One can feel the head of the femur: in the middle of the groin, half-way between the pubic bone and the anterior superior iliac spine (see Chapter 3, p. 57) you can feel the front part of the head of the femur through the

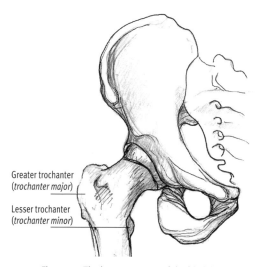

Greater trochanter
(*trochanter major*)

Lesser trochanter
(*trochanter minor*)

Figure 4.1 The bony structure of the hip joint.

layers of muscle. The hip joint is a special kind of ball-and-socket joint with the hip socket enclosing almost two-thirds of the femoral head. While this gives the hip joint its tremendous stability, it also restricts its movements.

The **hip socket** is part of the hip bone. The three bones forming the hip bone – the ilium, the ischium and the pubic bone (see Figure 3.2, p. 58) – meet precisely at the deepest point of the hip socket. The outer edge of the bony socket is enclosed by a ring of fibrous cartilage (*labrum*); it enlarges the joint surface of the socket and stabilizes the joint.

At the upper end of the thigh bone, extending from the femoral neck, is the **femoral head**. It is often confused with the **greater trochanter** (*trochanter major*) on the outer side of the femur, which can easily be felt through the skin and is often mistaken for the hip joint. The greater trochanter serves as an important attachment site for the muscles. On the inner back side of the femur lies its smaller counterpart, the **lesser trochanter** (*trochanter minor*); which also serves as an attachment point for muscles. Inside the femoral head and femoral neck can be found a system of tiny trabeculae which are arranged in spirals and with this special architecture can optimally distribute the uptaken load through the whole bone, thereby keeping the bone stable in the long term.

Position of the femoral head

Two angles serve to describe the precise position of the neck of the femur and the femoral head.

Angle of femoral inclination: The angle formed between the line drawn through the middle of the femoral neck and another one running through the shaft of the femur, is called the angle of femoral inclination. In newborn babies, this angle is about 145°; during growth it gradually decreases to around 125° to 130° in adults. In what are known as coxa valga (angle of femoral inclination more than 140°) and coxa vara (angle of femoral inclination less than 120°) there is increased stress on the hip joint, because through the resulting change in the joint anatomy, the pressure applied to the joint cannot be evenly distributed.

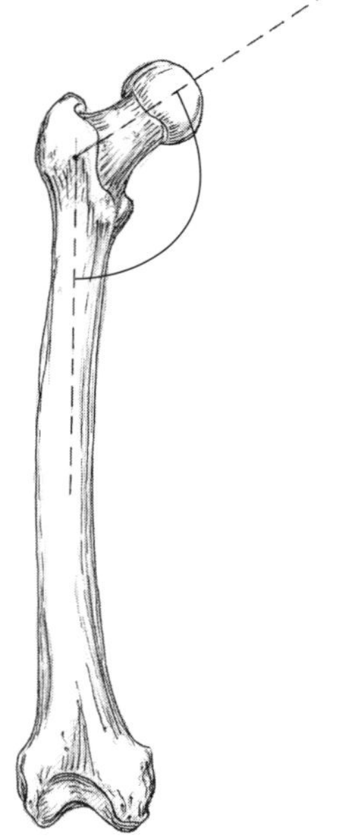

Figure 4.2 Assessing the angle of femoral inclination: draw a line through the centre of the femoral neck and another along the midline of the femoral shaft.

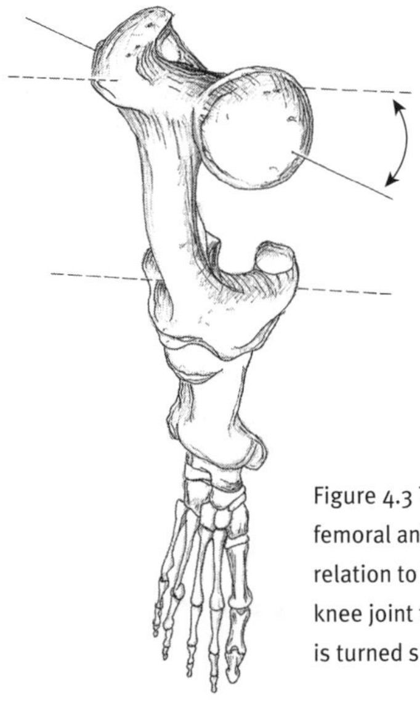

Figure 4.3 The angle of femoral anteversion: in relation to the axis of the knee joint the femoral head is turned slightly forwards.

Angle of femoral anteversion: In relation to the axis of the knee joint the femoral head is turned slightly forwards. The anteversion is the key for the rotational ability of the hip joint. It varies between 4° and 20°, with an average of about 13°. An excessive anteversion, a femoral neck which is

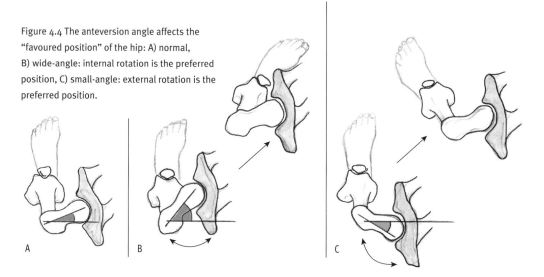

Figure 4.4 The anteversion angle affects the "favoured position" of the hip: A) normal, B) wide-angle: internal rotation is the preferred position, C) small-angle: external rotation is the preferred position.

A   B   C

rotating far forward, facilitates the internal rotation in the hip joint but restricts external rotation. A lesser anteversion leads to the opposite: the lesser the anteversion angle, the smaller the internal rotation, but the greater the natural external hip rotation.

Ligaments of the hip joint

The hip joint capsule encloses the femoral head like a cylinder and connects the hip socket with the femoral neck. Around the capsule three hip ligaments form a fan-shaped spiral: a complex ligamental system, which provides stability without too much restriction to mobility. The front pelvic ligament (*iliofemoral ligament*) is also called the "Y" ligament for the simple reason that its shape resembles an inverted "Y". It spirals across the head of the femur from the ilium to the thigh bone. Its impressive thickness of more than 1cm makes it an important stabilizer for the hip joint and the strongest ligament in the body. Whenever the hip joint rotates outwards, the Y ligament tightens; it restricts the movement and thus stabilizes both the pelvis and the hip joint.

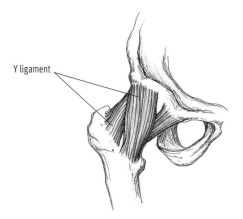

Y ligament

Figure 4.5 The Y ligament with its two components: horizontal and vertical.

3D Function

The "functional covering" is extremely important for the **standing leg**. The further the pelvis spirals itself on top of the standing leg, the more the hip socket encloses the femoral head. This increases the contact area within the joint and allows an even distribution of pressure through the whole joint. An efficient functional covering of the femoral head is therefore a top priority. In this, the ligaments of the hip joint play an important role: during weight bearing they become taut and thus redirect some of the pressure in the joint into traction on the ligaments. The prerequisite for this ideal stress distribution is optimal function: the sit bone moves forwards–upwards–inwards, spiralling the hip socket on top of the femoral head and thereby functionally enlarging the covering.

Flexibility is what counts in the **working leg**. When flexing the hip joint, the femoral head turns in the hip socket and slides slightly back- and downwards. The femur turns out and the hip joint capsule releases, thus increasing flexibility. Now the muscles are responsible for the movement. The spiralling in the hip joint, the movement between hip bone and femur, is performed in opposite directions on the working leg and the standing leg side. This alternation between load and unload is an optimal training for the hip joint.

Hip Movements

The shape of the hip socket and the femoral head determines the passive mobility of the hip joint. The deeper the femoral head is placed in the hip socket, the better the structural covering and the more stable the hip joint. But stability contradicts mobility: the better the covering of the femoral head, the less mobility there is in the joint. Basically, movements in the hip joint are possible in all directions, albeit to varying degrees (see Table 4.1).

Dancers know that when **flexing** the hip joint, external rotation increases. It is easier to position the "knee in line with the toes" in a grand plié than at the beginning of the demi-plié, when the flexion of the hips is still minimal. For turnout, however, it is precisely that which dancers require: above-average external rotation in the *stretched* hip joint. Unfortunately, we do not learn much if we measure the external rotation with a flexed hip joint.

When we look at the **extension** of the hip joint we may wonder how a dancer can extend their leg 90° in an arabesque when the extension in the hip joint itself only amounts to 30°. The answer lies in the detail: leg movements seldom occur only in the hip joint. Already before the end of the bony mobility of the hip joint is reached, the sacroiliac joint and the lower lumbar spine are brought into play.

Table 4.1 The mobility in the hip joint, measured from the neutral-zero position

Movement	Mobility
Flexion	120° active with bent knee 145° passive with bent knee
Extension	20° active 30° passive
Abduction	45°
Adduction	30°
External rotation	40 – 60°
Internal rotation	40 – 60°

The overall mobility of the hip joint in external and internal rotation amounts to approximately 90°. The greater the external rotation, the smaller the internal rotation and vice-versa.

The movement is passed on beyond the hip joint and thus the hip appears to move further. The greater the actual mobility in the hip, the later the movement is carried further into the neighbouring joints. It is therefore not surprising that dancers whose hips are less flexible will increasingly involve the sacroiliac joint and the lumbar spine in their movements and thus often encourage their own individual hypermobility in these regions.

Musculature

All muscles which move the hip joint attach at the pelvis or the lumbar spine. Thus, the position and stability of the pelvis and the lumbar spine are decisive for the mobility of the working leg and the stability of the standing leg. Numerous muscles cover the hip joint. If they are a single joint, their task lies in moving just the hip joint.

Two-joint muscles, on the other hand, which cross not only the hip joint but also the knee, serve to coordinate the entire leg. They are described in greater detail in Chapter 5.

Flexion and extension

Flexion: Many muscles are involved in the flexion of the hip joint. The main flexor muscles are the straight thigh muscle and the iliopsoas muscle (see p. 81).

The straight thigh muscle (*rectus femoris*) is the only muscle of the large thigh muscle (*quadriceps femoris*) (see Chapter 5, p. 105) that is attached to the pelvis. Passing over the front side of the femur it joins up with the three other muscles of the quadriceps femoris and runs across the kneecap to the *tibial tuberosity* on the front of the shin. It flexes the hip joint and at the same time stretches the knee. When bending the knee, the lower section of this muscle is pre-stretched, increasing its strength for hip flexion. This is one reason why it is quite easy to bring the knee up in the développé, but considerably more difficult to hold the height when it is extended.

Both actively and passively, hip flexion is considerably bigger with a bent knee than a stretched one. This is attributed to the **hamstrings** (see Chapter 5, p. 106), muscles which run all along the back of the thigh from the sit bone to the lower leg. When the hip is flexed and the knee is extended, the hamstrings are stretched along their entire length. However, if the knee is bent the hamstrings relax at the back of the knee and thus release the muscle for the hip flexion – the flexion will increase.

Extension: The amount of extension in the hip joint is considerably less than the flexion. The **gluteus maximus muscle** and the hamstrings take on most of the work during extension. The gluteus maximus muscle runs from along the entire outer surface of the ilium to the outer side of the femur, partially radiating into the iliotibial band (see Chapter 5, p. 106). As a single-joint muscle it is a particularly useful lever when extending the hip, regardless of the position of the knee joint. In addition, it can also externally rotate the femur in the hip joint.

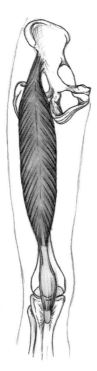

Figure 4.6 The straight thigh muscle (*rectus femoris*) runs from the pelvis to the tibial tuberosity.

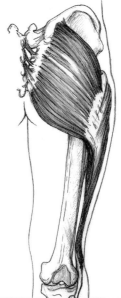

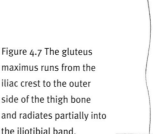

Figure 4.7 The gluteus maximus runs from the iliac crest to the outer side of the thigh bone and radiates partially into the iliotibial band.

By contrast, the **hamstrings** are two-joint muscles and therefore depend on the position of the knee: when the knee is extended they are already tensed and thus can produce higher strength for the extension in the hip joint. This is just one more reason to consciously stretch the leg in the arabesque.

Adduction and abduction

Adduction: Dancers refer to the adductor muscles as "inner thighs". The name is apt as they lie on the inner side of the thigh between the knee extensor muscles at the front and the inner knee flexor muscles at the back. Five adductor muscles of varying length pass from the lower part of the hip bone (from the pubic bone and the sit bone) to the inner back side of the thigh. The longest adductor muscle is the *gracilis muscle* which continues over the knee to the inside of the lower leg.

The main task of the adductor muscles is to pull the leg parallel towards the midline of the body (adduction). They can also serve as external or even internal rotators to the hip joint. This depends on the position of the pelvis: if the pelvis is tilted forwards, the sit bones and pubic bone move towards the back. Thus the origin of the adductor muscles lies behind their attachment point on the inner back side of the thigh. If they contract in this position they turn the legs inwards. It is important to understand that the adductor muscles can only work as external rotators when the pelvis is in a neutral and upright position. Then the sit bones direct towards the floor and the pubic bone is placed in front of the femur. Now the inner thighs can support the external rotation.

Abduction: The main abductor muscles are the **gluteus medius** and **gluteus minimus muscles**. Both pass under the gluteus maximus running from the outer surface of the ilium to the tip of the greater trochanter. In the working leg they extend the leg away from the midline of the body (abduction), in the standing leg they provide for the positioning of the pelvis: by contracting, these muscles help to prevent the pelvis from sinking

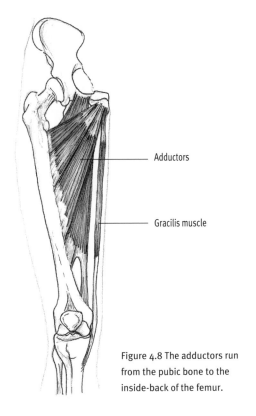

Adductors

Gracilis muscle

Figure 4.8 The adductors run from the pubic bone to the inside-back of the femur.

down on the working leg side – the undesirable "sitting" on the standing leg.

External and internal rotation

External rotation: The external rotation of the hip joint is extremely important, not only for dancers. No other movement in the hip is performed by such a high number of muscles.

The biggest and strongest external rotator is the **gluteus maximus**. It is mainly used by beginners to engage external rotation. Because of its size and exposed position its contraction is easy to feel and can even be checked visually by the teacher. In addition to its function as an external rotator, the gluteus maximus is also an important hip extensor (see p. 79).

It is much more difficult to initiate external rotation with the group of the **deep external rotator muscles**. By virtue of its close position to the joint, this sophisticated system of six small muscles is ideally suited to stabilize the turnout,

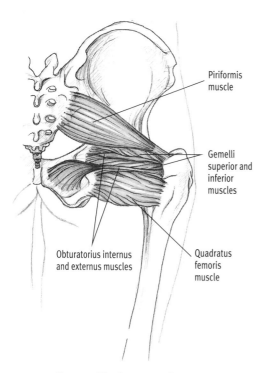

Piriformis muscle

Gemelli superior and inferior muscles

Obturatorius internus and externus muscles

Quadratus femoris muscle

Figure 4.9 The deep external rotators.

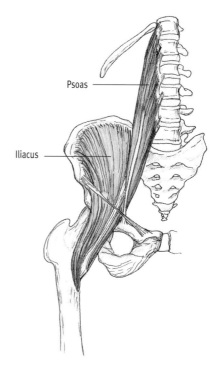

Psoas

Iliacus

Figure 4.10 The iliopsoas with its two parts.

even over a longer period. In a fan shape the muscles run across the joint capsule starting from the sacrum and the ischium, around behind the hip joint towards the greater trochanter. Their location close to the joint is the reason for their effectiveness: even a small contraction will pull the greater trochanter backwards and thus externally rotate the leg.

Internal rotation: Several muscles take part in the internal rotation of the hip joint, but for all of them the internal rotation is not their main purpose. There are no muscles whose sole function is the inner rotation of the hip joint.

The iliopsoas – The dancer's muscle

The **iliopsoas muscle** is the most important flexor in the hip joint. It is composed of two parts: the **iliacus** and the **psoas**. The iliacus muscle originates on the inside of the ilium whereas the psoas muscle starts on the front of the entire

lumbar spine up to the twelfth thoracic vertebra as well as on all the intervertebral discs which lie in between. Both muscles join into a common tendon, the **iliopsoas tendon**, which pulls across the front of the head of the femur and inserts on the lesser trochanter at the inner back side of the femur. Lying directly between the head of the femur and the tendon is a synovial bursa, which acts like a silicon cushion to protect the iliopsoas tendon from friction.

The iliopsoas muscle flexes the hip joint and at the same time turns out the leg slightly. When contracting it first, at the beginning of the flexion, pulls the femoral head slightly downwards before turning it in the hip socket and thus enlarging the flexion in the hip joint. This initial downwards pull creates space in the joint and improves mobility. Thanks to its high origin at the twelfth thoracic vertebra, the iliopsoas is the only hip flexor which enables the leg to raise higher than 90°.

The iliopsoas is one of the few muscles in the body connecting the back and the front. Running diagonally through the torso, it has close contact with important structures within the abdomen: the diaphragm, kidneys and colon all lie in the direct vicinity.

At the front of the spine, the psoas muscle is spanned by fibres of the diaphragm like an arch. The tighter and firmer the arch of the diaphragm, the less space there is for the muscle.

This can cause problems: if the diaphragm is tight – as can be the case during high concentration or superficial breathing – the psoas muscle will be trapped under the arch of the diaphragm. This restricts its function as well as its efficiency.

The kidneys lie on the muscle belly of the psoas; they use it as a surface to slide on. When inhaling, the kidneys slide downwards, when breathing out they slide upwards again. The iliacus is in close contact with the colon, which runs along the inner side of the ilium on both sides.

From this, it is easy to understand that poor functioning of the diaphragm, kidneys and colon will have a negative effect on the iliopsoas muscle in the long term because of their close anatomical location. Efficient muscle training and a good diet, sufficient fluids and awareness of breathing will contribute to the strengthening of the iliopsoas.

Table 4.2 Important movements in the hip joint and their primary muscles

Hip movement	Primary muscles
Flexion	Iliopsoas muscle Rectus femoris muscle Sartorius muscle
Extension	Gluteus maximus muscle Hamstrings (*Biceps femoris muscle, Semimembranosus muscle, Semitendinosus muscle*)
Abduction	Gluteus medius muscle Gluteus minimus muscle
Adduction	Adductors (*Pectineus muscle, Adductor minimus muscle, Adductor brevis muscle, Adductor longus muscle, Adductor magnus muscle*) Gracilis muscle
External rotation	Deep external rotator muscles (*Piriformis muscle, Gemellus inferior and superior muscles, Obturatorius internus and externus muscles, Quadratus femoris muscle*) Gluteus maximus muscle
Internal rotation	none

Dance in Focus: Load and Overload

Hip problems are common in dancing. Unfortunately, the turnout plays a somewhat ignominious role here: excessive turnout is one of the main causes of problems and pain in dancing. But there are positive aspects too: most hip pain in dancers does not originate in the hip joint itself but rather in the surrounding muscles, which means that it can be modified by adapting the dance training.

Load

Extreme mobility in the hip joint and maximal outer rotation in the turnout put great demands on the resilience of the hip joint. For the hip joint the golden rule is: one-sided overload is deadly in the long run. In effect, it is the constant alternation between load and unload, flexing and extending, outer and inner rotation that will make the hip joints resilient in dancing.

The turnout

The external rotation in the hip joint, whether it is a maximal en dehors in classical ballet or a moderate turnout in contemporary dance, is an essential position in most dance styles. This is not surprising since the general mobility of the hip is increased by the external rotation of the leg. The reason for this is the bony structure of the thigh: when extending the parallel leg to the side, the greater trochanter on the outer side of the thigh limits the mobility, jamming the muscles and soft tissues in between the greater trochanter and the pelvis. In the outer rotation it works differently: the greater trochanter rotates backwards thus permitting the turned-out leg to be extended higher to the side.

The **bony structure** of the hip joint largely determines the natural external rotation. Here, the anteversion of the femoral neck is of decisive importance. It is genetically determined and decreases during growth according to its genetic programme: from up to 40° anteversion in newborns to an average of 13° in adults.

Table 4.3 Factors which determine external rotation in the hip joint

This influences the external rotation of the hip	This increases the external rotation of the hip
Bone • Femoral head: anteversion angle (see p. 76) • Hip socket: Direction and depth	The smaller the anteversion angle, the larger the passive external rotation. The further to the side the hip socket sits in the pelvic girdle and the smaller its depth, the larger the passive external rotation.
Ligaments • Y ligament (see p. 77)	The more flexible the Y ligament, the larger the external rotation.
Muscles • Deep external rotator muscles (see p. 81) • Adductors (see p. 80)	The more differentiated the use of the deep external rotators, the larger the active external rotation. The better the use of the adductors, the larger the active external rotation.
Pelvis • Positioning	A pelvis that is neutrally placed in an upright position allows the correct use of the deep external rotator muscles and the adductors and thus enlarges active external rotation.

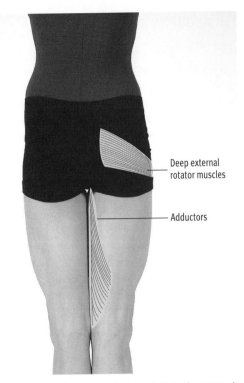

Deep external rotator muscles

Adductors

Figure 4.11 The deep external rotators initiate the turnout in the hip, the adductors supporting their work.

The external rotation of the leg occurs not only above the knee – in the hip joint – but also below the knee – in the lower leg. In order to assess the turnout ability of the entire leg, the external rotation of the hip joint *and* the bony rotation of the lower leg, the tibial torsion (see Chapter 5, p. 114), must be measured.

Anatomical turnout = external rotation in the hip joint + tibial torsion

The lesser the anteversion angle, the greater the external rotation in the hip joint. Thus the turnout is supported quite naturally by growth. Whether and to what extent the anteversion can be influenced by intensive training during the growth spurts is not fully clear even today. It is certain, however, that the anteversion of the femoral neck does not continue to change after hip growth has been completed in about the sixteenth year of life.

It may seem surprising, but contrary to expectations, professional classical dancers on average do not have a smaller anteversion angle than non-dancers. The fact that their active turnout is nonetheless so much better is primarily due to their economical **use of muscles**. The functional use of muscles helps to perform the maximum turnout prescribed by the bony limitations and to stabilize it exactly where it takes place: in the hip joint. The deep external rotators

are most suitable for doing this. They run close to the joint and exert a good lever effect in all positions of the hip joint thanks to their fan-shaped arrangement. When they contract, they pull the greater trochanter backwards and thus stabilize the hip joint in its external rotation. They are assisted by the adductor muscles, which turn the inner sides of the thigh forwards when the pelvis is in an upright position. Both muscle groups – the deep external rotators as well as the adductors – originate at the pelvis. Their function therefore depends on the position of the pelvis: only if it is in an ideal upright position does it permit the muscular stabilization of the turnout.

High extension of the legs

High legs, whether passively moved or actively extended, are a training goal for many dancers. The ideal interplay of bony structure and functional muscle work is what decides the height of the legs.

The passive mobility of the hip joint depends on its bony structure. Coxa valga, when a hip joint has a large angle of femoral inclination (see p. 76), has a strikingly high range of motion. So it is no wonder that coxa valga is found frequently among dancers.

Functional muscle work permits the optimal movement of the hip joint within its bony limits; it can be improved with specific training. Two muscles share the work involved in hip movement forwards and to the side: the rectus femoris can raise the leg to a maximum of 90°; and at this point the iliopsoas muscle has to continue the movement. Ideally, the iliopsoas takes over a large part of the lifting work already from the start of the movement. Its course makes it an optimal flexor for the hip joint: at the beginning of the movement it pulls the femoral head slightly downwards and thus creates space in the joint before introducing the hip flexion. At the same time, it rotates outwards in the hip joint, moving the greater trochanter backwards and thus permitting maximum freedom for the movement. By focusing on the work of the iliopsoas the leg is, so to speak, "lifted from below".

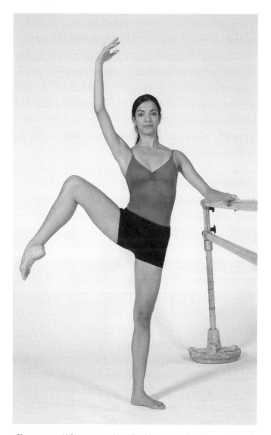

Figure 4.12 When engaging the iliopsoas the femoral head is ideally placed in the hip socket: the femoral head slides down before it turns within the hip socket.

Overload

Pain in the pelvic region has a wide variety of causes, from overworked muscles to inflammation of the tendons or irritation of the synovial bursa. Often it is the ligaments, tendons and muscles of the hip joint that cause problems for dancers.

Chronic overload

Iliopsoas syndrome: Strain on the hip flexors, especially the iliopsoas muscle, leads to a typical pain in the groin. However, it is not only increased muscle work that can lead to irritation of the muscle. With external rotation in the hip joint, the femoral head slides forward in the hip socket, pressing towards the inside of the frontal structures of the hip, including the iliopsoas. Irritation and local overstretching are the result. If the muscle lacks elasticity and length, this continuous pressure can lead to an inflammation of the muscle and its tendon. The synovial bursa directly beneath the iliopsoas tendon can also be affected.

Snapping hip: Many dancers are familiar with noises in the region of the hip. One possible cause is the gases within the synovial fluid of the joint capsule popping during large hip movements. Loud noises can be heard in the joint in particular when lowering the leg.

Noises in the groin when moving the leg to the side are often due to tension in the illiopsoas muscle. Usually there is an imbalance between the two parts of the muscle, the psoas and the iliacus. When the turned-out leg is lowered, this imbalance allows the two muscle bellies to jump over each other, producing a loud click. The iliopsoas tendon itself can produce a similar noise when it is so tightly contracted that it jumps over the femoral head during certain hip movements.

A snapping sound at the side of the hip on the outer side of the thigh indicates a shortening of the iliotibial band (see Chapter 5, p. 106). Here too, the tendon tissue is too tight and jumps over a bony protuberance, the greater trochanter, leading to a noise which is often considered unpleasant.

Tendinitis at the greater trochanter: Novice dancers in particular often complain of pain on the outer side of the thigh, in the region of the greater trochanter. This is not a pain of the hip joint! Here, the cause is the unaccustomed use of the muscles, which can lead to excessive strain and shortening of the external rotator and abductor muscles. The increased traction on the insertion at the greater trochanter leads to local inflammation.

Piriformis syndrome: The "pear-shaped" piriformis muscle of the group of the deep external rotators can be the cause of pain in the back of the thigh. Running from the lower back to the leg, the sciatic nerve, the largest nerve in the human body, runs below the piriformis muscle; in some cases it even runs directly through the muscle fibres. Tension, shortening or thickening of the muscle can thus easily lead to restriction or even compression of the sciatic nerve, resulting in pain radiating along the back side of the leg. Here the position of the pelvis plays a central role: the further forward the pelvis tilts, the higher the tension in the piriformis muscle. Add to that external rotation in the hip joint and the muscular tension is increased even further. Constriction of the sciatic nerve is inevitable.

Impingement: Depending on its cause, the impingement of the hip is subdivided into bony and soft-tissue impingement. The symptoms are similar in both cases. Maximal flexion, adduction and internal rotation of the hip joint lead to a shooting pain in the groin. We speak of a *bony impingement* when the femoral neck hits the front edge of the socket, thereby restricting the movement. The cause is usually a bony thickening of the femoral neck which can either be genetically induced or be the result of repeated microtraumas. If the muscles or the front part of the joint capsule impinge at the end of the movement, we refer to this as a *soft-tissue* impingement. A frequent cause for soft-tissue impingement is a hardening and thickening of the iliopsoas muscle.

Labral tear: The labrum is the fibrocartilage ring which surrounds the hip socket, thereby enlarging the joint surface. When maximal hip flexion is combined with adduction and internal rotation, the front area of the labrum can become trapped by the femur at the end of the movement. If this happens over and over again, it can lead to a tear in the labrum. The tissue becomes inflamed, swells and therefore becomes even more easily trapped. This is a vicious circle that must be broken as quickly as possible.

Osteoarthritis: The gradual wear and tear of the hip joint is a sign of overload. Possible causes are poor alignment of the femoral head with the hip socket (hip dysplasia, see p. 89), poor shock absorption (e.g. small plié, weak feet, frequent dancing on hard floors) or genetic predisposition. In the case of advanced osteoarthritis, it is worthwhile considering ending the professional dance career.

Acute injuries

Muscle injuries: Pulled muscles and torn muscle fibres mostly affect the inner thigh muscles directly at their attachment point on the pubic bone, as well as the hamstrings close to their attachment at the sit bone. Often the acute muscle injury is preceded by chronic muscle tension.

Pitfalls in Dance

"Tighten your buttocks", "lift your leg from below", "release the front part of your thigh". For decades these corrections have echoed through the dance studios, making dancers aware of typical mistakes in their dance technique. But not everyone knows exactly what lies behind these commands, and whether these corrections actually have the desired result, anatomically speaking. It is worth taking a closer look.

Forced Turnout – the Effect on the Hip Joint

External rotation in the hip joint can only be held and used functionally with coordinated muscle work. However, this muscle coordination is difficult to learn especially for novice dancers. Corrections such as "tighten your buttocks" are not of great help; they have exactly the opposite effect to the one intended: if the gluteus maximus contracts, it will turn the leg out, but at the same time it hinders the hip joint and prevents it moving freely. What is even worse, the tightened gluteus maximus blocks the use of the deep external rotators and thus puts out of action the very muscles which could execute the turnout properly.

If the external rotation in the hip joint is forced too far, this will also influence the joint play. During external rotation, the femoral head does not only slide forward; it is also pushed upwards. The anterior joint cavity becomes smaller and the pressure within the joint increases. This can cause problems in the long term.

When the hip joint is extended, the powerful Y ligament limits the external rotation. On the other hand, when the joint is flexed, the ligament is relaxed. Slightly flexed hip joints are therefore – consciously or unconsciously – a common trick for increasing the turnout. But there is a price to pay: the pelvis tilts forwards resulting in a sway back. In the long term this puts excessive strain on the lumbar spine, and back pain might result (see Chapter 3, p. 64). Tilting the pelvis forwards alters the interplay of the muscles: the inner thigh muscles pull the legs into an internal rotation and make it even harder for the external rotators to engage the turnout. This can lead to high muscle tension, muscle shortening and even muscle inflammation.

How to recognize: Stand in socks on a slippery floor, so that your feet do not get "stuck" to the ground. Feet parallel, with the inner sides of the

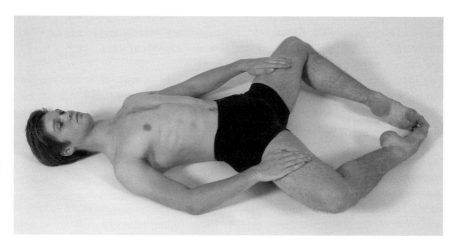

Figure 4.13
The frog position should only be performed in the supine position.

What you can do:

- The legs should only be turned out as far as the external rotation can actually be held by the muscles.
- Thinking of images like "pull the greater trochanter back" specifically engage the deep external rotator muscles. It allows one to perform the turnout more easily and efficiently.
- Avoid the "frog" position when lying prone! This position is neither suitable for testing the outer rotation in the hip joint nor for stretching or training the external rotator muscles. A flexed hip is always more mobile than an extended one. Therefore, the assessment of the outer rotation in the hip joint is only useful if the measurement is carried out with the hip extended. There is one positive effect of the "frog" position: it stretches the inner thigh muscles and can thus be used as preparation for doing the side splits. But even then the "frog" position should only be practised supine!
- Walking with legs turned out even in daily life puts unnecessary strain on the hips. A parallel gait centres the femoral head in the hip socket. The alternate load and unload of the hip joint is then an ideal training for joint and muscles.

legs touching. Turn the legs outwards from the hip with knees straight. The heels remain on the floor. Put your hand on the gluteus maximus as you do so. Can you perform the external rotation without engaging the muscle? Even from the outside, the contraction of the gluteus maximus can easily be seen. Always remember: the less tension in the gluteus maximus, the easier it is to use the deep external rotators and the more economical the muscle work will get.

High Extension of the Legs – Pain in the Groin

The biggest factor that determines the height of the legs and the strength of the movement is the optimal coordination of the muscles used to flex the hips. Often the rectus femoris muscle plays an important role in the flexing of the hips. Thanks to its size, it is easy to engage even for dancers with little training, and its contraction is easily felt. But working hard with this muscle can cause problems. Since it raises the leg from above, it presses the head of the femur firmly into the socket at the beginning of the hip flexion; the result is less mobility within the joint. Because of its origin on the anterior superior iliac spine of the pelvis it can only raise the leg up to a maximum of 90°; at that point the iliopsoas muscle has to take over. But here coordination often plays tricks: intense contraction of the rectus femoris makes it almost impossible for the iliopsoas muscle to take over its task in time. The iliopsoas is "blocked" by the strong contraction of the rectus femoris. This has an effect not only on the height of the leg but also on the dance technique. Fibres of the rectus femoris penetrate into the front part of the hip joint capsule. Thus, excessive strain on the muscle does not only lead to problems within the muscle itself, but to irritation of the joint capsule as well.

How to recognize: One can usually recognize a hard-working rectus femoris by its shape. If the belly of the muscle is prominent this usually indicates its frequent use. In this case, hip flexion is clearly initiated mainly by this muscle. A trained eye can also see this in the movement itself: if the head of the femur is pressed firmly into the socket at the beginning of the flexion, the joint loses its mobility. The increased tension in the hip joint is reflected in the movement, which appears hard and firm.

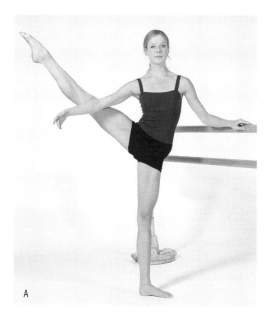
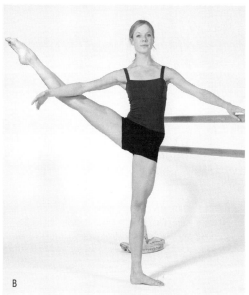

Figure 4.14 Two ways of extending the straight leg to the side: A) the straight thigh muscle does most of the work, the femoral head is pressed into the hip socket, the mobility decreases, B) the iliopsoas initiates the movement; in pulling the femoral head down first, this increases the movement ability within the hip joint; the turnout gets easier.

What you can do:
- Pay attention to the action of the iliopsoas when flexing the hip. The idea of "lifting the leg from below" can help to feel the engagement of the iliopsoas while moving and to particularly use it in dance.
- A detailed image of the course of the iliopsoas from its origins on the spine and pelvis to its connecting point on the femur can assist in awareness of the movement.
- Imagining the hip movement helps its mobility: at the beginning of the movement, the femoral head slides backwards and downwards in the hip socket, and only then should the leg start to rise.
- Due to their close contact, the kidneys and colon play an important role in the activity of the iliopsoas. Their function is largely determined by nutrition. Thus, high legs can also be a sign of good nutrition!

Hypermobility in the Hip – Hip Dysplasia

Good mobility in the hip joint is an important selection criterion in many types of dance. This means that frequently, selected dancers are those whose hip joints possess the necessary mobility, but whose bony structure might not be optimally developed to withstand the strains of dancing: dancers with hip dysplasia. This "malformation" of the hip is congenital and manifests itself in a variety of symptoms which – depending on the degree of dysplasia – vary in the severity they take. For the most part, there is a combination of a large anteversion angle, coxa valga and a steep, shallow hip socket. These are all factors which lead to a poor covering of the head of the femur, hinder an ideal distribution of pressure within the joint and thus reduce the load-bearing capacity of the joint. On the other hand it is the poor fit of the two joint partners that makes the hip joint so flexible and permits maximal mobility, especially in flexion and abduction. But there is also a price to pay for the large anteversion angle. The external

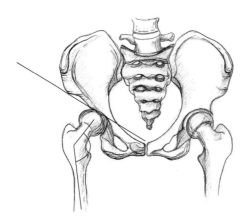

Figure 4.15 Hip dysplasia: a large anteversion angle, coxa valga and a steep, shallow hip socket lead to a poor covering of the head of the femur.

rotation is usually restricted to a considerable degree – and especially in classical dance this is a problem which should not be underestimated.

How to recognize: Whenever hip dysplasia is suspected, a precise medical diagnosis should always be carried out. The assessment of the rotation in the hip joint can provide a rough estimate in the dance studio. The dancer lies prone with the legs extended and parallel; the inner sides of the knees touching. The knee on the test side is bent at an angle of 90°; the lower leg is used as a measuring device (see Fig. 4.16). Move the lower leg passively inwards towards the floor – this corresponds with an outer rotation in the hip joint. Do not allow the pelvis to rise from the floor. For the internal rotation, move the lower leg to the outside, again making sure that the pelvis keeps stable. If the internal rotation is considerably greater than the external rotation – in other words if the lower leg can be moved considerably further outwards than inwards – this indicates a large anteversion angle. If, at the same time, hip flexion and abduction are greater than average, this might indicate a hip dysplasia.

What you can do:
- A high range of movement in the hip joint should not be the only criterion for choosing a dancer.
- The hip joint should be tested both for range of movement and for strength and stability.
- To assess the mobility of the hip joint in total, the inner rotation should also be tested. If it is noticeably bigger than the outer rotation, then further medical clarification is highly recommended.

A Closer Look – Self-analysis

A number of simple tests will help to get an impression of the shape of the hip joint even without an X-ray, to recognize one's own limits of movement and to work on them in a targeted manner.

Form and Flexibility

The **external rotation** of the hip joint is of crucial importance when working in and on the turnout. Have I already reached my anatomical limits of external hip rotation or can I improve my turnout even further with specific muscle work? Self-analysis of the external hip rotation is easiest to carry out with a partner.

The muscular external rotation of the hip: Lie prone. Both legs are extended, the inner sides of the knees touching. The knee on the test side is bent at an angle of 90°; the lower leg is used as a measuring device. The partner moves the lower leg passively inwards towards the floor – this corresponds with the outer rotation in the hip joint. Don't allow the pelvis to rise from the floor. Watch out for unwanted rotation movements in the knee. The angle between the lower leg and the vertical indicates how much external rotation the muscles of the hip will allow.

The bony external rotation of the hip: Starting position as above. Without allowing the pelvis to rise from the floor, the partner moves the dancer's lower leg passively inwards into the maximal external rotation of the hip, holding the leg in this position. Now the dancer pushes his lower leg outwards against the resistance of the partner and holds for eight seconds. With this, the hip joint rotates inwards and all internal rotator muscles are working. Release the tension and carefully further increase the external rotation ("readjust"). Repeat this sequence – tighten, release, readjust – five times. Then repeat the measurement as described above. The angle between the lower leg and the vertical line shows the bony external rotation of the hip. If the bony external rotation is

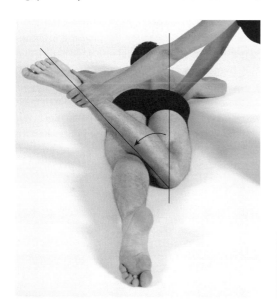

Figure 4.16 Measuring the muscular external rotation of the hip in the prone position: assessing the angle between the lower leg and the vertical line.

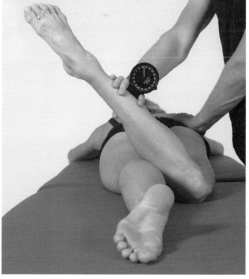

Figure 4.17 Dance-medical measurement of external rotation with a special device, the Plurimeter V.

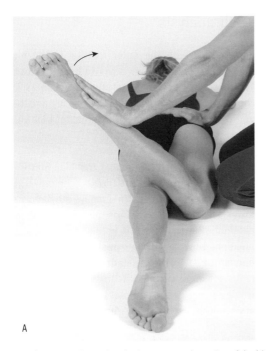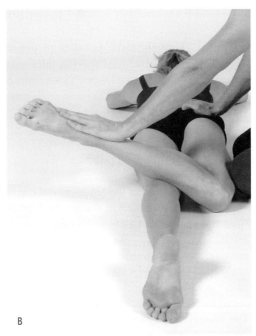

A   B

Figure 4.18 Measuring the bony external rotation of the hip in the prone position: A) the dancer pushes his lower leg outwards against the resistance of the partner, B) the dancer releases the muscle tension, the partner gently increases external rotation.

larger than the muscular one, there is a chance to improve the turnout in the hip through specific muscle training. If the bony and muscular external rotation are the same, the external rotation capacity of the hip joint is already being exploited to the full. Further improvement through training will not be possible.

Important: During hip flexion all structures at the front of the hip joint are released. Therefore, measuring the hip's external rotation when sitting or lying in the "frog" position is *not* helpful for assessing the turnout. The external rotation of the hip should always be measured in an extended hip joint.

The mobility in **flexion** can best be tested when lying supine. Bend one leg keeping the other leg stretched out on the floor. Using your hands, pull the bent knee towards the ribcage; the pelvis must remain flat on the floor. Pay close attention to the end of the movement: does the knee move outwards? Does the movement become blocked in the hip joint? Is there a pain in the groin when the leg is slightly adducted? All these are possible signs of an impingement of the hip joint (see p. 86).

Function

The working leg:
- Lie supine: legs bent, feet parallel in line with your sit bones. Put your hands on your hip joints. Raise one foot from the floor and

check the hip flexion with your hand. Do the muscles at the front of the hip joint remain relatively relaxed? Does the head of the femur sink down towards the floor during flexion? Does the leg remain parallel? Repeat the hip flexion several times.

- Stand at the barre: feet in first position, left hand on the barre, right hand on the front of the right hip joint. Slowly raise the right leg in a passé, checking the flexion in the hip with your hand: do the muscles on the front side of the hip joint remain relatively relaxed? Does the head of the femur sink downwards during the flexion? Does the external rotation increase during flexion? Repeat the passé several times.

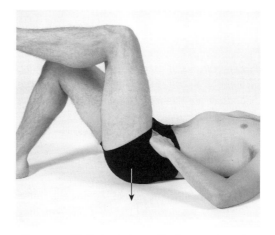

Figure 4.19 Hip flexion in the working leg, exercise in the supine position: the femoral head slides back towards the ground.

The Turnout:

- Stand in socks on a slippery floor, so that your feet do not get "stuck" to the ground. Start from a parallel position with stretched knees rotating the legs outwards from the hip joints as far as possible; the heels remain on the floor. Watch out for compensatory movements: do not tilt the pelvis forwards (sway back) or backwards ("tucking under"); do not fall on the inner side of your feet; and do not allow your knees to twist! The angle between your two feet gives the functional turnout.

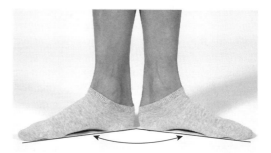

Figure 4.20 Assessment of functional turnout: with stretched knees rotating the legs outwards from the hip joints as far as possible.

Tips and Tricks for Prevention

Through specific training and a few precautions, dancers can avoid many hip problems. Ideally, such problems can be banished entirely before they affect the dancer in training or in everyday life.

In Everyday Life

Walking is an efficient way of training the three-dimensional hip movement. Conscious spiralling on the standing leg and relaxation on the working leg side, an ideal alternation between load and unload, optimally trains the hip joints. It works best with the feet parallel, when the pelvic floor and deep external rotators alternate between concentric work in the standing leg and eccentric work in the working leg; when the active shortening of the muscles is followed by their dynamic lengthening. Good timing is important here. As soon as the heel touches the ground, the deep external rotators engage to stabilize the leg in its external rotation; the pelvic floor swings the sit bone forwards–upwards–inwards and thus spirals the hip socket over the femoral head. The swinging walk, used by catwalk models, in which the pelvis is swung from one side to the other, might be visually attractive but it is not advisable for long-term load bearing and the functional muscle training of the hip joints.

Tips:

- When walking, be aware of using the deep external rotator muscles and the pelvic floor in order to optimally spiral onto the standing leg. Thus you will not only protect your hip joint, but you will also train your muscular strength. Your turnout will benefit!
- When climbing stairs, take two steps at a time. This will exercise the deep external rotator muscles in particular.

Specific Exercises

Mobilization

E **Mobilizing the hip joint**

Equipment: Chair

Starting position: Sit on the chair in second position. Put your right hand on the inner side of the right thigh; with your left hand, grasp the right iliac crest from the front.

Action: The right hand mobilizes the thigh in its external rotation, while at the same time the left hand mobilizes the right half of the pelvis forwards and thus pulls the entire pelvis into a gentle left rotation. The right hip joint is rotated three-dimensionally. Pulling with the hands intensifies the 3D movement in the hip joint.

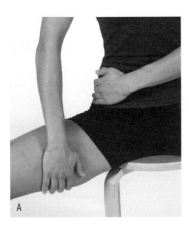 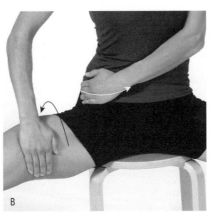

A   B

Figure 4.21 Mobilization of the hip joint: A) starting position, B) the right hand pulls the thigh in external rotation, the left hand simultaneously pulls the right half of the pelvis forward. The hip joint is spiralled three-dimensionally.

Repeat the exercise with the left hip. This exercise can also be carried out in side splits on the ground.

Awareness

E Awareness of the deep external rotator muscles in turnout

Starting position: Stand upright, feet parallel. Put the palm of your right hand on the right gluteus maximus muscle; the fingertips feel the deep external rotator muscles on the horizontal crease of the buttocks. Left hand at the front on the iliac crest.

Action: From the standing position with legs parallel and knees straight, turn out the right leg in the hip joint; the heel remains on the floor. Watch for compensatory movements: the left hand checks the neutral position of the pelvis; the right foot must not tilt inwards and the knee joint must not twist. Be aware of the movement: the greater trochanter moves backwards and closer to the sacrum. The deep external rotators initiate the movement; their tension can be felt under the fingertips. The gluteus maximus remains as relaxed as possible. Repeat on the left side.

E Awareness of the iliopsoas muscle

Starting position: Lie supine. Keep legs bent and feet parallel in line with the sit bones. The hands should be placed at the front on the groins.

Action: Lift the right leg energetically off the floor. You can easily feel the tendon of the rectus femoris muscle with your right hand; it will protrude on the front of the hip joint like a taut rope. This serves as a work indicator of the rectus femoris. Now flex the hip joint several times *without* tightening the rectus femoris muscle. Imagine you are raising the leg "from below", from the lesser trochanter, the attachment point of the iliopsoas muscle. It may help

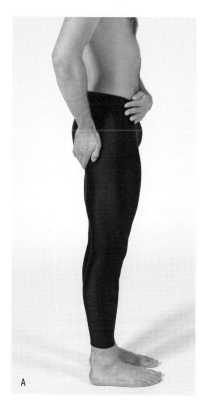

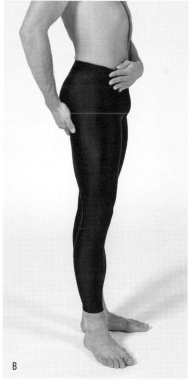

A

B

Figure 4.22 Awareness of deep external rotators in turnout: A) starting position, B) turnout the straight right leg in the hip joint.

to feel the muscle belly of the iliopsoas. This one can find in the middle between the navel and the superior anterior iliac spine. By placing your flat hand in position you can feel the muscle in the depths. This exercise requires time and patience. So persevere if it doesn't work immediately! Repeat the exercise with the other leg. Often there is one side on which it is much easier to feel the iliopsoas than on the other.

Strengthening

E Strengthening of the deep external rotator muscles

Equipment: Thera-Band
Starting position: Lie supine. Legs stretched, knees directing towards the ceiling, feet flexed. Wind the Thera-Band around the front of the right foot and hold both ends in your right hand.
Action: Push the right leg down and away from you, pushing against the resistance of the Thera-Band; the foot remains flexed; the right

side of the pelvis moves downwards. This prepares the deep external rotator for the work to come. Now change into the prone position with the inside of the knees touching. Keep the Thera-Band wound around the front of the foot with both ends in your right hand. Stretch your right arm to the side. Bend the right knee at an angle of 90°. Against the resistance of the Thera-Band pull the lower leg actively inwards towards the floor. NB: Keep the pelvis on the floor and the knee at a right angle. Repeat this part of the exercise 25 times in a row. Then repeat the entire exercise with the left leg.

E Strengthening the iliopsoas muscle

Equipment: Thera-Band
Starting position: Lie on your left side. Wind the Thera-Band in a figure of eight around both legs above the knee. Pelvis, back and head are in a neutral position, and both legs are turned out. Move the top leg into passé.

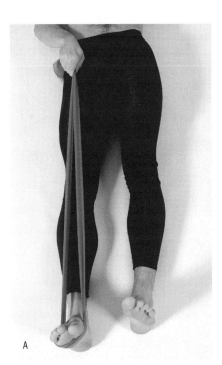

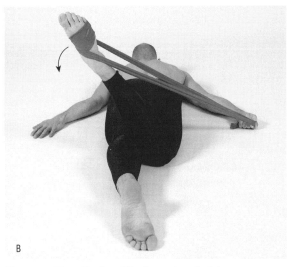

B

Figure 4.23 Strengthening of the deep external rotators:
A) preparation: push the right leg down and away against the resistance of the Thera-Band, B) action: bend the right knee at an angle of 90°. Against the resistance of the Thera-Band pull the lower leg actively inwards towards the floor.

A

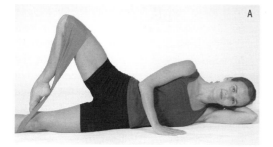

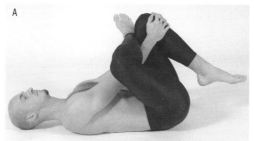

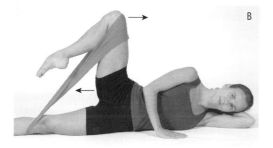

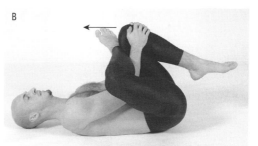

Figure 4.24 Strengthening the iliopsoas muscle: A) starting position, B) increase the passé against the resistance of the Thera-Band. Allow the femoral head to slide down in the hip socket.

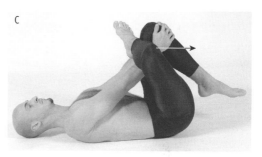

Figure 4.25 Contract-relax stretching of the deep external rotators: A) starting position, B) pull the left knee towards the chest until a stretch is felt in the right buttock, C) press the right knee down and thereby feel the muscle work in the deep external rotators.

Action: Increase the height of the passé against the resistance of the Thera-Band. Allow the hea of the femur to slide down into the hip socket; the sit bone points towards the heel. Repeat 25 times, paying attention to the position of the pelvis.

Relaxation

E **Contract-relax stretching of the deep external rotator muscles**

Starting position: Lie supine. Legs bent, feet parallel in line with the sit bones. Place the right ankle on the left knee and turn the right leg outwards. Grasp the left knee with both hands.

Action: With both hands pull the left knee towards the chest until you feel a stretch in your right buttock. Hold the stretch for eight seconds. Then actively push the right knee away from your centre, feel the deep external rotator muscles working. Hold the action for eight seconds. Release the tension and intensify the

stretch. Repeat the whole exercise five times, ending with the stretch.

E **Eccentric stretching of the iliopsoas muscle**

Equipment: Rolled towel

Starting position: Lie supine with your knees directing towards the ceiling. Place the rolled towel horizontally under your pelvis. Bend one leg, grasp the knee with both hands and gently pull it up.

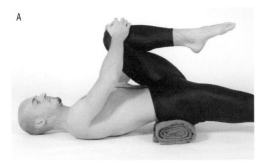

A

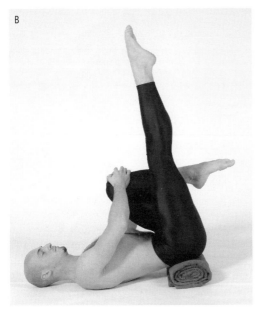

B

Action: Move the other leg through developpé 90° towards the ceiling and turn the hip joint slightly inwards; the foot remains relaxed. Now slowly lower the leg down towards the floor. NB: Keep the internal rotation; the leg remains stretched. Avoid abduction while lowering the leg. Keep the pelvis neutral; do not hyperextend the lumbar spine! The closer the leg comes to the floor, the slower the movement becomes; breathing out deeply intensifies the stretch. Relax the stretched leg on the floor. Repeat the exercise 15 times, elongating the leg further each time and feeling the stretching and relaxation of the iliopsoas. When finished, remove the towel from under your pelvis, stretch out both legs, rest on your back and be aware of any side differences. Repeat the exercise with the other leg.

In Training

* Warm up your hip joint before dancing. Lie on your back, bend one leg and pull the knee up with your hands. Now, passively mobilize your hip joint with small rhythmical circles. The hip muscles should almost completely relax.

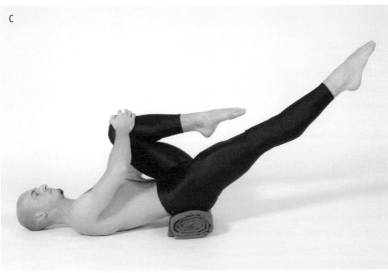

C

Figure 4.26 Eccentric stretching of the iliopsoas muscle.
A) starting position.
B) turn the straight leg slightly inwards in the hip joint. C) lower the leg slowly to the ground.

- The turnout should only be performed as much as can be actively held by the muscles.
- Use the deep external rotators for your turnout. The image of "moving the greater trochanter backwards" specifically addresses the deep external rotators and thus helps to perform the turnout more easily and efficiently.
- Try to visualize the movements within the hip joint: at the beginning of flexion, the head of the femur slides down and back in the hip socket, and only then is the leg raised.
- When flexing your hip, focus on the work of the iliopsoas. Imagine "raising the leg from below". This increases the awareness of the iliopsoas during the movement and allows dancers to use its helpful bio-mechanics in dancing.
- Imagine the exact anatomical course of the iliopsoas from its origins at the spine and the inner side of the pelvis to its insertion point on the inside of the thigh. This will help its use in the movement.
- Stretch and relax the deep external rotators while training, especially in classical dance. This is easy to do: during the demonstration of the next exercise or while your group is taking a rest, take ten seconds to stand in internal rotation.

- After training, regularly stretch your hip flexor and external rotators. Especially if your hip snaps (see p. 85), you should regularly release the muscles concerned in order to prevent irritation of the snapping tendons.

Check your dance technique:

Don't:
- Do I initiate the turnout with the gluteus maximus?
- Do I usually raise my leg engaging the rectus femoris?
- Do I tighten up my hip joint with over-strong muscle tension?

Do:
- Can I relax the gluteus maximus during turnout?
- Can I feel the deep external rotators working and the inner thigh muscles supporting when performing a turnout?
- When raising my leg, am I aware of the activity of the iliopsoas muscle?
- Am I aware of the 3D rotation of the hip joint in my working and standing leg?

5. Standing Firm: The Knee as Coordination Unit

Well-developed muscles, stability on the standing leg, and dynamism when jumping: the demands on dancers' legs are high. Hyperextended knees, also known as "sway-back knees", are particularly often found in classical dancers. Together with a high arch of the foot they result in legs following the classical aesthetics of a curved leg line. But aesthetics and function do not always match.

Being the largest joint of the body, the knee works as an important coordination centre of the leg. Located between the hip joint and the foot, it reacts to all movements and positions of its two functional partners. Rolling onto the inner side of the foot or a too small outer rotation in the hip joint puts a great deal of strain on the knee. The typical compensation strategies of a small turnout are one of the main causes of knee problems in dancing.

As more and more acrobatic movements invade the various dance styles, the strain on the knees has largely increased. Training on hard, inappropriate floors or dancing choreographies in high heels can add to the problem. Pirouettes on the knees, knee drops, and even a plié in fourth position require particular leg stability and optimal mobility in the knee. But dancers often pay little attention to their knees. They are seldom specifically warmed up, directly trained or used consciously in everyday life. Nonetheless, their functionality is a top priority if dancers' legs are to be kept fit and healthy.

3D Anatomy

The leg axis and the knee joint are directly influenced by the position of the foot and the hip. A good functional integration of the knee between foot and hip joint can have a positive influence even on structural deficits. "The function affects the form" is an important principle for healthy legs.

lower ends, both tibia and fibula together form a fork-shaped structure into which the foot is fitted. Characteristic of the tibia is its slightly spiralled

Structure

The bony leg axis is formed by the **thigh bone** (*femur*) and the lower leg. The lower leg consists of two bones: the strong **shin bone** (*tibia*) and the slender **calf bone** (*fibula*). They are linked to each other by a membrane of connective tissue. At its upper end, the head of the fibula forms an articulation with the outside of the tibia. At their

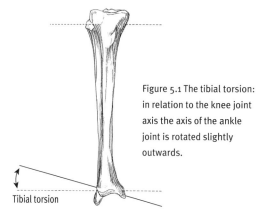

Figure 5.1 The tibial torsion: in relation to the knee joint axis the axis of the ankle joint is rotated slightly outwards.

Tibial torsion

bone structure: its lower end is slightly rotated outwards compared to the axis of the knee joint. In adults this tibial torsion averages between 10 and 15°.

Menisci

Together with the lower end of the femur, the upper end of the tibia forms the knee joint. Here, two completely different bone shapes meet: the round end of the femur from above and the flat surface of the tibia from below. Especially during movement, the two partners of the joint have only few contact points, which, in the long term, is very disadvantageous for load distribution. And yet nature has found a solution: lying between the two bones are two sickle-shaped discs of fibrocartilage called the *menisci*. The medial meniscus lies on top of the inner tibial plateau and the lateral meniscus lies on top of the outer one. It is interesting to take a closer look at the surfaces of the tibial plateaux. The inner tibial plateau forms a hollow in which the medial meniscus is embedded; the form of the outer one could best be compared with a hill on which the lateral

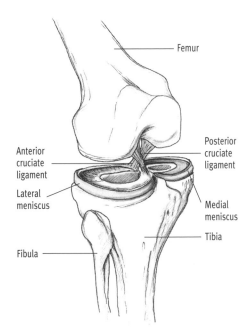

Figure 5.2 The knee bones with the two menisci and the cruciate ligaments.

Femur

Posterior cruciate ligament

Anterior cruciate ligament

Lateral meniscus

Medial meniscus

Tibia

Fibula

meniscus slides. This explains the increased mobility of the lateral meniscus compared with its medial counterpart, which is also fused with the medial collateral ligament. The task of the menisci is to increase the contact area in the knee joint and thus to evenly distribute the load throughout the entire knee, both when standing and during movement. At the same time, they help to absorb shocks and increase the mobility of the knee through their sliding mechanism.

Knee ligaments

The mechanics of the knee are supported by a complex system of ligaments. The **collateral ligaments** strengthen the joint capsule on the inside and outside. When the knee is extended, they become taut and thus give medial and lateral stability to the stretched leg. When the knee joint is flexed the collateral ligaments are also relaxed, allowing small sideways movements and the rotation of the lower leg. The **cruciate ligaments** derive their name from the fact that they cross within the knee joint. The anterior and posterior cruciate ligaments internally join the tibial plateau with the femur. The two ligaments are wrapped around each other crossing over; they are the most important ligaments in the knee. As the two collateral ligaments are relaxed in knee flexion, that is when the cruciate ligaments help to provide stability. They prevent the femur from losing contact to the joint surface of the tibia. The anterior cruciate ligament prevents the femur from sliding backwards during flexion, and the posterior cruciate ligament prevents a slide in the opposite direction.

The kneecap

The kneecap (*patella*) forms a joint with the thigh bone. Its rear side rests in a groove on the front of the femur, the femoral groove, allowing the kneecap to glide smoothly. The tendon of the quadriceps femoris muscle inserts into the upper border of the patella, and its lower pole is joined to the *tibial tuberosity* via the patellar ligament. Thus the patella is embedded in the course of the quadriceps muscle. On the one hand it serves to protect the muscle during flexion, and on the other it provides better leverage for the knee during extension movements. The movement patterns of the kneecap are dependent on the form of the femoral groove, on the shape of the patella and on the coordination of the muscles. Asymmetry in the bone structure and imbalance in the muscles can lead to disadvantageous pressure on the rear part of the patella, resulting in severe knee pain.

3D Function

Stability in the standing leg is the top priority – whether during walking, jumping or balancing. The three-dimensional spiralling is an important basic principle here. The spiral of the leg reflects in its anatomical structure in multiple ways: in the shape of the bones, the function of the knee joint, the structure of the cruciate ligaments and the

anatomy of the diagonal and spiralling muscles. The hip joint rotates outwards, the front foot rotates opposite thus turning the lower leg inwards – this is the basis for the 3D spiralling of the leg. Hip, knee and ankle are thus ideally aligned and the load is evenly distributed within the knee.

When the thigh turns outwards and the lower leg inwards, the cruciate ligaments become taut. They cross over each other thus increasing the stability of the knee. The alignment of the patella is also improved by the spiralling of the knee joint. Through the internal rotation of the lower leg, the tibial tuberosity, the attachment of the patellar ligament, is turned inwards. This allows the patellar ligament to pass almost vertically from the lower pole of the kneecap to the tibia. The patella is centred in its femoral groove, thereby optimising its direction of movement.

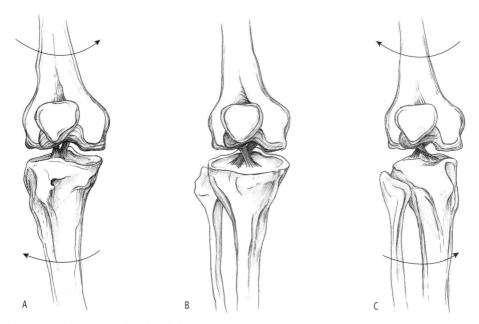

Figure 5.3 Cruciate ligaments in action: A) the femur rotates inwards, the lower leg outwards. The cruciate ligaments "un-spiral", and the stability in the knee is lost, B) neutral position, C) rotating the thigh outwards and the lower leg inwards, the cruciate ligaments become taut. The stability of the knee increases.

When the standing leg is flexed, the spiralling of the leg increases even further: the thigh rotates outwards while the ball of the big toe remains in contact with the floor and thus stabilizes the internal rotation of the lower leg. The heel is upright and the knee directly over the second toe in alignment of the axis of the foot. This is the ideal weight-bearing line for the knee during the plié.

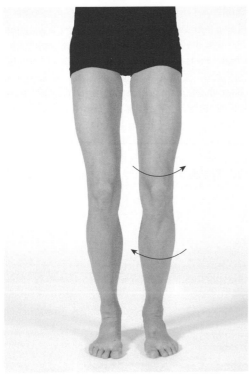

Figure 5.4 3D spiral in the bended knee: the leg spiral increases.

Movements in the Knee Joint

The knee is a modified hinge joint. It allows extension and flexion and can also rotate when flexed – but *only* when flexed. The shape of the joint surfaces provides a high degree of stability in the stretched knee; when the knee is bent mobility predominantes. The two menisci provide for an optimal load distribution.

When the knee is flexed, the menisci slide backwards, in order to compensate for the differences in the contour between the two articulating partners. When the knee is extended, they move forwards and position themselves like a placeholder between the thigh and the lower leg. During movement the alternation between load and unload kind of massages the menisci.

As in other joints, the knee joint demonstrates an obvious difference between active and passive flexibility. Actively, one can bend the knee to about 130°, whereas passively one can flex the knee up to 160°. The straight leg is described as 0° of extension; hyperextension of the knee of up to 10° is frequently seen in dancers. When the knee is flexed, the lower leg can be rotated inwards and outwards; frequently the external rotation dominates, especially in dancers. The linking of rotation with the final degrees of knee extension is termed the "locking mechanism". In relation to the lower leg, the thigh turns slightly inwards thus stabilizing the joint in the extended position.

Musculature

The guiding muscles for the 3D spiralling of the leg

The sartorius muscle and the tibialis anterior muscle are the guiding muscles for the spiralling of the leg.

The **sartorius muscle** with its long, slender muscle belly passes across two joints, the hip joint and the knee joint. It runs from the front of the pelvis – from the anterior superior iliac spine – to the inner side of the tibia. Thanks to its diagonal course, it rotates the thigh outwards and at the same time holds the inner rotation of the tibia to counter the movement.

The **tibialis anterior muscle** follows the same diagonal course, originating from the lower leg and inserting on the foot. It runs from the lateral front part of the tibia to the inner side of the hind- and midfoot and thus stabilizes the lower leg in its inner rotation when the foot is optimally positioned.

muscle bellies (*vastus medialis, vastus inter-medius* and *vastus lateralis*) origin on the front side of the thigh bone; the fourth, the *rectus femoris*, has its origin on the pelvis, on the anterior superior iliac spine. All four sections of the muscle join together above the kneecap to form a tendon which inserts into the superior border of the patella. As an extension of this tendon the patellar ligament runs from the lower pole of the kneecap to the tibial tuberosity. Well-coordinated muscle work in the quadriceps femoris is essential in order to achieve optimal alignment of the patella. Here the balance between the inner and outer muscle belly is of particular importance. If the outer muscle dominates during the movement, the patella will be pulled to the outside, resulting in unequal load on the kneecap or even dislocation of the patella.

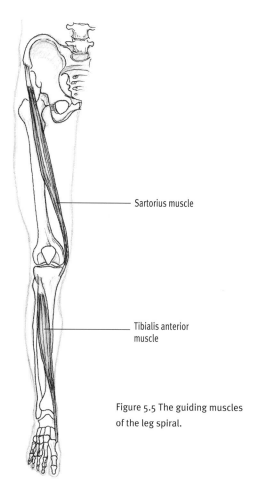

Sartorius muscle

Tibialis anterior muscle

Figure 5.5 The guiding muscles of the leg spiral.

Flexion and extension

Flexing and extending are the main movements in the knee joint. It is interesting to compare the differing structure of both, the knee flexor and extensor muscles. Most of the knee flexor muscles are two-joint muscles: not only do they flex the knee, but at the same time they also move the hip or the ankle joint. Fine coordination is required here. Most knee extensor muscles, on the other hand, are single-joint muscles and thus only move the knee. Here strength is the main requirement.

Extension: The main extensor in the knee joint is the **quadriceps femoris muscle**. Three of its

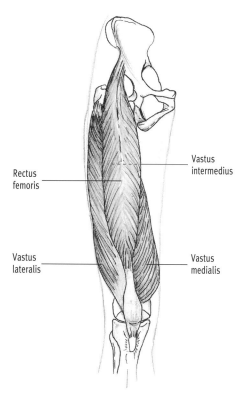

Rectus femoris

Vastus intermedius

Vastus lateralis

Vastus medialis

Figure 5.6 The quadriceps femoris.

Flexion: The **hamstrings** on the rear of the thigh are responsible for bending the knee. Because of their position they are also termed as the *ischiocrural musculature*: they run from the sit bone (*ischium*) to the lower leg (*crus*). The hamstrings consist of three muscles; all of them originate on the sit bones and run either to the inside of the lower leg (*semitendinosus*, *semimembranosus*) or to the outside (*biceps femoris*). Together they bend the knee. The muscles on the inner side of the knee also function as internal rotators, whereas the outer muscle operates as an external rotator. In the plié the coordinated use of the hamstrings helps to achieve the optimal alignment of the knee. As two-joint muscles, the hamstrings extend the hip joint while simultaneously flexing the knee joint. When the hip is flexed, e.g. during the battement devant, the hamstrings are stretched at their upper portion. This increases their traction on the knee. The knee will automatically bend slightly if no other muscles actively work against it.

Some of the **calf muscles** also work as knee flexors. Their course and function are described in more detail in Chapter 6, p. 128.

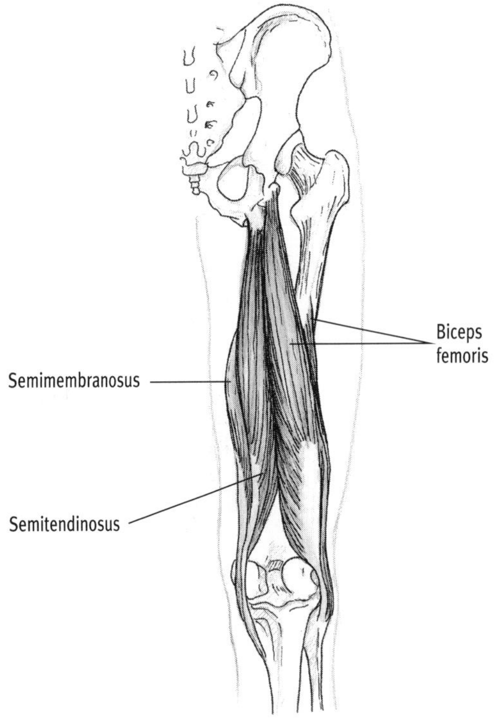

The **iliotibial band** is a strong, tendon-like fascia that runs along the outer side of the thigh. It is tensed from above by fibres of the gluteus maximus and the tensor fasciae latae muscle; at its lower end it is anchored on the outer side of the tibia and the fibula. When standing on one leg it tenses the outer side of the thigh. With this, it counters the "sitting on the standing leg" – the dropping of the pelvis towards the working leg side – as well as preventing a one-sided overload of the knee joint.

Figure 5.7 The hamstrings are comprised of three muscles, running from the sit bone to the inside and outside of the lower leg.

Table 5.1 Important movements in the knee and the muscles involved

Knee movement	Primary muscles
Flexion	Hamstrings (*biceps femoris muscle*, *semimembranosus muscle*, *semitendinosus muscle*) Gastrocnemicus muscle Sartorius muscle
Extension	Quadriceps femoris
External rotation with knee bent	Lateral hamstring (*biceps femoris muscle*)
Internal rotation with knee bent	Medial hamstrings (*semimembranosus muscle*, *semitendinosus muscle*) Sartorius muscle Gracilis muscle

Leg Shapes

When assessing leg shapes we distinguish between malalignment, which is determined by the bony anatomy, and functional malalignment. The shape of the bones of the upper and lower leg influences form and axis of the whole leg. A bony malalignment cannot be corrected by dance training alone. But good muscle coordination and a conscious spiral of the leg can have a positive effect on the malalignment.

The best-known malalignments of the leg, **bowed legs** and **knock knees**, are also common in dancers. The characteristic deviance of the knee can be seen when examined from the front: a deviance in the frontal plane, outwards in bowed legs and inwards in knock knees. These malalignments of the leg are often the result of an "un-spiralling" of the leg, in which the thigh turns inwards and the lower leg outwards – exactly the opposite direction to the functionally stable 3D leg spiral. In consequence the kneecaps point inwards. Depending on the position of the lower leg and feet, this results in functional bowed legs or "knock knees".

Hyperextension of the knee, also known as **sway-back knees**, is frequently found in dancers. This can most easily be seen from the side. It is important to pay attention to the maximal hyperextension in the knee joint. In classical dance a hyperextension of the knee of about 10° is what dancers are aiming for.

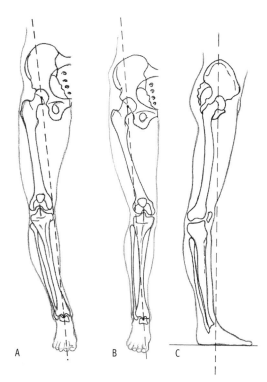

Figure 5.8 Typical deviations of the leg axis, even in dancers: A) bowed legs, B) knock knees, C) sway-back knees.

Dance in Focus: Load and Overload

The optimal alignment of the legs is the key to healthy knees. The correction "knee in line with the toes" contains everything needed for the stabilization and alignment of the leg axis. It is one of the most effective preventions of knee problems, and not only in dance.

Load

Regardless of which type of dancing we refer to, the strain on the knee is considerable. A great deal of this strain can be avoided through precise dance technique that takes one's own physical make-up into account.

The turnout

The main movement of turnout takes place in the hip joint. It can, and should, only be trained at this point (see Chapter 4, p. 83). Nonetheless, the turnout as a whole is assessed not only by the rotational ability of the hip joint but also by the bony alignment of the leg. The torsion of the tibia is particularly important. With a range of between 0° and 40° in adults, this can vary considerably. Dancers with a large tibial torsion can stand fairly relaxed with their feet in fifth position, and even a pretty small external rotation in the hip joint can be partly compensated for by a large tibial torsion. But there are disadvantages: dancers with a large tibial torsion have difficulty positioning their knees above the toes at the beginning of the demi- plié, when the hip is only barely flexed.

   Working in turnout changes the alignment of the entire leg musculature. By the external rotation in the hip joint, the muscles on the inside of the thigh (adductors) are turned forwards; the iliotibial band on the outside turns backwards and the lateral hamstring also turns towards the back. This can lead to muscle imbalance: the inner thigh muscles lose their tension and get weaker; the lateral hamstring and the iliotibial band get tense and shorten. If, instead of the deep external

rotator muscles, the gluteus maximus is used to produce external rotation in the hip joint – something that is frequently seen in beginners – the traction of the gluteus maximus muscle will tighten the iliotibial band even more. The economic equilibrium of the muscles is disturbed.

The plié

Plié is one of the most frequent movements in dance. Every jump, every landing begins or ends in plié. Here the knee flexor muscles initiate the flexion concentrically and the quadriceps femoris resists eccentrically, contracting against the flexion. Both muscle groups originate on the pelvis, whose centred position is a prerequisite for a well-coordinated plié. Ideally, the three-

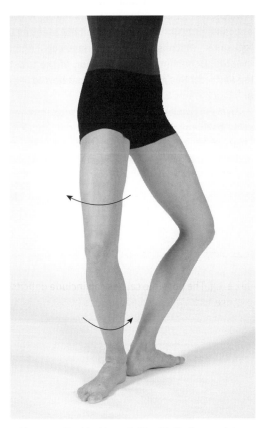

Figure 5.9 The ideal leg spiral in plié: the femur rotates outwards, the lower leg remains in internal rotation.

dimensional spiral of the leg is retained in the flexion and even increased: external rotation in the hip, internal rotation in the lower leg – in this way the load is evenly distributed between the medial and lateral meniscus, the cruciate ligaments are wound around each other optimally stabilizing the knee, and the kneecap is centred in its femoral groove. The spiralling of the knee joint is independent on the posture of the leg, whether it is in first, fifth or parallel position. Ideally, the knee bends along the axis of the foot directly over the second toe.

Stretched knees

Many dance styles call for legs to be stretched to the maximum extension. The greater the passive hyperextensibility of the knee, the easier it is for the dancer to stretch the knee actively. Hyperextended knees are therefore considered to be the ideal leg form, especially in classical dance. But they also harbour a danger: in hyperextension, the three-dimensional spiralling of the leg can become lost; the thigh turns slightly inwards, the cruciate ligaments relax and the kneecap is subject to one-sided pressure; the stability of the knee is reduced. In the standing leg a knee hyperextension of about 10° seems to be a good compromise between a stable leg axis and an aesthetic line. In the working leg, full hyper-extension can be used.

Overload

Knee pain in dancing is usually a sign of incorrect loading, often as a result of poor statics in the entire leg. The possible causes can include deficits in dance technique, compensations resulting from hip or foot problems as well as dancing on hard floors or in unfamiliar shoes. The knee often suffers the consequences.

Chronic overloading

Patellofemoral pain syndrome: Patellar chondropathy is a general term for pain on the rear of the kneecap. The cause is an overloading of the cartilage at the back of the patella. This results in irritation, cartilage swelling and even destruction of the cartilage. The problem arises when the patella does not move in the ideal alignment within its femoral groove; then the pressure in the joint is unevenly distributed. Usually, the outer area of the kneecap is subjected to the most pressure. In the long term, high pressure on a relatively small area leads to an overloading of the cartilage. If the shape of the patella and the femoral groove do not optimally fit together, this might lead to additional stress. Functional malalignments can also give rise to problems. If the thigh turns inwards when the knee is flexed, the femoral groove of the patella will be rotated inwards underneath the kneecap. During flexion, the kneecap follows the traction of the patellar ligament pulling the patella to the outside. The pressure in the outer area of the kneecap increases considerably. Pain after sitting for a long period, at the beginning of the movement or after long training sessions may result. High tension in the thigh muscles can worsen the pain through constantly pressing the kneecap against the femoral groove.

Outside   Inside

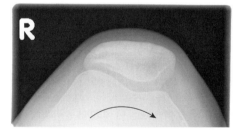

Figure 5.10 X-ray of a flexed knee (view from below): the patella is tilted; the main pressure is on the outer side of the kneecap. If the thigh rotates further inward, the imbalance in the joint increases even more.

Meniscus degeneration: Meniscal wear usually affects the medial meniscus, especially the back area known as the posterior horn. Compared with the lateral meniscus, the medial meniscus is less mobile and thus more susceptible to shearing forces. Maximal knee flexion compresses the posterior horn of the medial meniscus and can lead to slow degeneration of the cartilage; the vulnerability of the meniscus increases.

Patellar Tendonitis (jumper's knee): An inflammation of the patellar ligament directly at the lower pole of the kneecap is known as jumper's knee. The possible causes for this range from extremely hyperextended knees, to forced rotation in the knee joint caused by insufficient turnout of the hips, jumping on a hard floor, sudden increase of training intensity or inadequate warm-up. As part of the therapy, a temporary load reduction is necessary.

Osgood Schlatter disease: Tension on the patellar ligament at its insertion on the tibial tuberosity can lead to inflammation in this area, especially in young male dancers. During growth, the patellar ligament is linked to the tibia by an area of cartilage. This area is sensitive to excessive traction: the cartilage gets irritated and the tibial tuberosity becomes swollen. Physical stress on this area must be reduced. Even years later, a prominent tibial tuberosity may be a sign of the early stages of Osgood Schlatter disease.

Bursitis: There are numerous bursae in the knee region. Their task is to protect the muscles, tendons or ligaments from pressure or friction. Direct mechanical pressure, for example, through tightly fitting leggings or during dynamic floor work, can lead to inflammation, especially of the bursae lying on or below the kneecap. Swelling, redness and pain are typical signs of a bursitis. It calls for reduced load and avoidance of further pressure.

Acute injuries

Tear of the anterior cruciate ligament: When the knee is flexed, the cruciate ligaments take over the stabilization of the knee. If during knee flexion there is a sudden forceful rotation on the lower leg, the anterior cruciate ligament is put under a maximum strain. Given insufficient muscular stabilization, the ligament will not be able to withstand the tension: a partial or complete tear will result. The posterior cruciate ligament is much less frequently torn. There are numerous causes for a rupture of the cruciate ligament: acute trauma during landing or in dynamic floor work, as well as collisions with others.

Acute meniscal tear: A complete tear of the anterior cruciate ligament is often accompanied by other injuries. Typical for a major knee trauma is an injury combination of a torn anterior cruciate ligament, a torn medial collateral ligament and a tear in the medial meniscus. However, injuries to the meniscus can also occur in isolation. Often it is the back area of the medial meniscus which is affected, as it is there that the greatest shearing forces occur.

Patellar dislocation: A dislocation of the kneecap from its femoral groove usually happens while landing or turning on an unstable leg axis. The forced external rotation of the lower leg pulls the kneecap sideways. If the muscles fail to counteract the movement, the patella may glide out of its groove. If the kneecap dislocates repeatedly even under minor strain, we speak of a *recurrent patellar dislocation*. In this case a professional career in dance is not recommended.

Pitfalls in Dance

The three-dimensional spiral of the legs is essential in dance, but it is difficult to apply consistently. If the turnout is forced from the knees, if the plié is not stabilized by the muscles, or if the dancer is in the habit of hyperextending the knees, an optimal coordination of the knee is impossible. Then, far from relieving the pressure on the knee, the exact opposite will take place: the thigh turns in, the lower leg turns out and the knee will become "un-spiralled". That is not a good starting point for healthy dancers' knees!

The Forced Turnout –
the Effect on the Knee Joint

The maximal turnout from the feet upwards and not from the hips downwards is responsible for many knee problems in dance. Biomechanically speaking, a rotation in the extended knee joint is not possible. On the other hand, in the hyper-extended knee, mobility is increased through the instability of the ligaments and the lack of muscular stabilization: to a minor degree the knee joint can be passively rotated.

This is a dangerous mechanism, because through the forced rotation in the extended knee excess pressure will be put on the medial collateral ligament, and the muscles and tendons attached on the inner side of the knee will get over-stretched. The medial meniscus will be subjected to dangerous shearing forces. The external rotation in the lower leg pulls the kneecap to the outer side of its femoral grove: one-sided strain on the patellar cartilage or even dislocation of the patella (see p. 110) may occur. The lateral hamstring and the iliotibial band shorten and hold the lower leg in a slight external rotation – even outside the dance studio. Thus the knee continues to "un-spiral" even when walking. The pull of the lateral muscles blocks the head of the fibula, which passes on its lack of mobility further down the leg: even the ankle joint loses some of its mobility.

How to recognize: The spiral of the extended leg can be assessed from the position of the kneecap and the location of the tibial tuberosity. Ideally the midline of the patella and the midpoint of the tibial tuberosity should lie more or less directly in a vertical line. A minor deviation of the

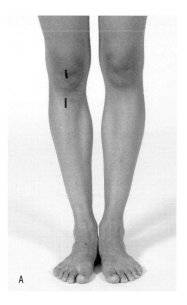
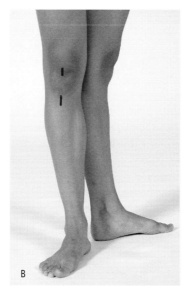

Figure 5.11 Assessing the rotations in the extended knee: A) parallel: The midline of the patella and the centre of the tibial tuberosity should be almost perpendicular to each other, B) turnout: the distance of the lines should remain unchanged from the parallel state.

tibial tuberosity to the outside is normal, especially in women. The knee position is examined in standing with the legs first in a parallel position, then with the legs turned out. The distance between the midline of the kneecap and the midpoint of the tibial tuberosity should stay the same regardless of the position. If the distance gets bigger in the turnout position, this indicates the turnout being forced from the knees.

What you can do:
- The legs should only be turned out as far as the external rotation can actually be held by the muscles of the joint (see Chapter 4, p. 83).
- The first position should always be performed with stretched knees turning out from the hip joint. Taking the first position with flexed knees will start the turnout from the feet upwards and is risky for the knees.
- Walking with feet turned out outside the dance studio places unnecessary strain on the knees. The leg spiral can best be trained when walking with feet parallel and this also strengthens the knee for dancing.

The Uncontrolled Plié

One of the most common mistakes in dance is when the knees fall inwards during the demi-plié, whether with feet parallel or in turnout. There are many causes for this, from the bony restriction of hip mobility, to weakness or imbalance of the muscles or a lack of fine coordination. This has serious consequences for the knee: with every knee movement, the menisci passively move along, in flexion they slide backwards together with the femur. If the knee falls to the inner side

during the plié, the menisci will also be carried along by the movement. While the lower leg bends, the femur rotates inwards, or – looked at it the other way round – the lower leg turns outwards in relation to the femur. Now the menisci follow the backwards sliding of the thigh on one side and the external rotation of the tibia on the other. This is especially hazardous for the medial meniscus, which for anatomical reasons has only a limited mobility. Its lower part glides forwards with the plateau of the tibia whereas its upper part is pulled backwards with the thigh. This leads to shearing forces that no meniscus will be able to withstand for long.

With every plié, the quadriceps femoris muscle works eccentrically. The deeper the plié, the more forcefully the kneecap, which is embedded in the course of the thigh muscle, will be pressed into the femoral groove. One can imagine how high the pressure will rise at the rear of the patella when performing a grand plié. An optimally aligned knee axis is crucial here.

How to recognize: "Keep the knee in line with the toes". The implementation of this correction can be easily recognized: is the kneecap aligned with the second toe? When the knee is bent, is it possible to draw a vertical line down to the gap between the first and second toes?

What you can do:
- "Knee in line with the toes" applies to every position, whether standing with feet parallel or in turnout, whether in demi or grand plié.
- Fourth position grand plié should only be performed – if at all – if your dance technique is good and when you are sufficiently warmed up. Only if the leg axis is optimally positioned, is it possible to evenly distribute the high pressure on the entire rear side of the kneecap.

Hyperextended Knees

Hyperextended knees are an inevitable part particularly of classical dance; functionally, however, they are anything but ideal. Hyperextended knees hinder the stable leg spiral: the thigh turns inwards, the cruciate ligaments "untwist" and the knee becomes unstable. Damage to the meniscus can be caused by rotation in the knees, the muscle and tendons lying at the back of the knee joint are subject to excessive stress. Hyperextended knees increase the hyperextension of the lumbar spine, the pelvis tilts forwards and balance becomes more difficult. The classical foot positions can no longer be executed accurately. First and fifth position are only possible with knees bent. Hyperextended knees often lead to the weight being transferred backwards, so that the heel takes the main weight. This can cause excess stress in the entire leg, leading to painful overload.

A hyperextension of the knee of up to 10° is tolerated in dancing. This is a compromise that is not easy to achieve. Many dancers find it difficult to *never* fully straighten the standing leg or to never use the feeling of the full extension as a signal for the optimal leg axis. It gets even more complicated when full use is made of the maximal knee hyperextension in the working leg. Here, the brain has to learn to clearly distinguish between the working and the standing leg.

How to recognize: Typical hyperextended legs are best assessed from the side, with feet parallel and legs extended. Draw an imaginary line from the hip joint to the middle of the ankle joint. If the knee is positioned behind this line, we speak of hyperextended legs.

In dance medicine, to assess the amount of hyperextension of the leg, the hyperextension angle of the knee itself is measured. This should be carried out both passively, when lying down, and actively, when standing.

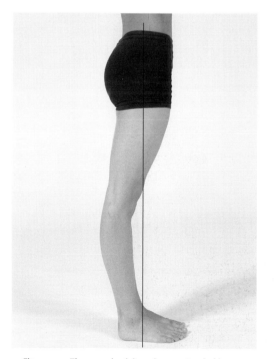

Figure 5.12 The sway-back leg – hyperextended knees.

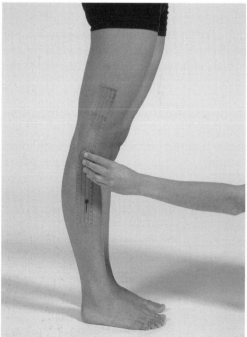

Figure 5.13 Dance-medical measuring of hyperextended knees with the help of a goniometer.

What you can do:
- Do not passively sink into the hyperextension. A hyperextension of over 10° in the standing leg must be counteracted in training.
- Think of the straight leg axis in the standing leg. The entire muscles surrounding the knee should be used to stabilize the knee. Do not pull the kneecap upwards when straightening the leg! This is the only way to allow the front and back thigh muscles to work together evenly.
- Imagining the three-dimensional spiral of the leg might help a dancer to achieve the optimal leg extension. When the femur starts to turn inwards, the knee hyperextends. Even when standing with feet parallel, only extend the knee to the point where a slight external rotation in the hip joint can still be felt.

A Closer Look – Self-analysis

A well-coordinated leg axis is the basis for a long period of injury-free dancing. Shape, flexibility, function and strength of the entire leg can be most easily assessed with a partner.

Form and Flexibility

The leg axis is determined by the bony structure of the thigh and lower leg on the one hand and by the mobility of the hip, knee and ankle joints on the other.

The **bony torsion of the tibia** is an important factor in determining turnout. Assessment of the tibial torsion is carried out with the dancer lying prone. Both knees are kept straight with the inner sides of the knees touching. Bend the knees at an angle of 90°; the feet should remain relaxed. By exerting light pressure on the soles of the feet a partner gently pushes the feet into a flexed position (dorsiflexion of the feet). Be careful not to force the movement in any direction, the feet are moved gently in the ankle joint only. Imagine a line from the middle of the heel to the second toe, each of these lines forms an angle with the centre line, which permits an estimate of the tibial torsion to be made. The greater the angle, the greater the tibial torsion. It is not uncommon for there to be a difference between the two sides.

In dance medicine the tibial torsion is measured when a dancer is kneeling. He should kneel on the examination table, with the knees bent at a right

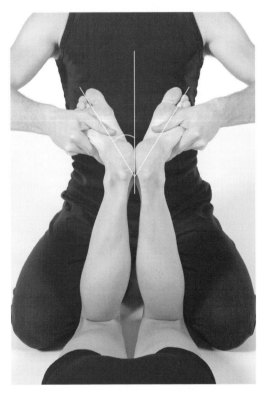

Figure 5.14 Assessment of bony tibial torsion: the angle indicates the tibial torsion.

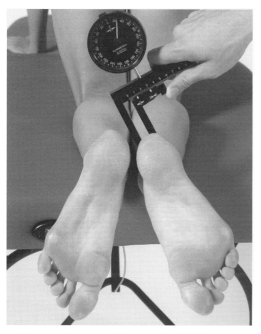

Figure 5.15 Dance-medical measuring of tibial torsion with a Pluritor T.

Maximal flexion: Lie supine. One after the other, flex your knees as far as possible. At the end of the movement does the bending feel soft and flexible? Is it the same feeling in both knees?

Passive hyperextension: Lie supine with both legs softly stretched and the knees pointing towards the ceiling. A partner raises one foot off the floor until the back of the knee starts to lift from the ground. The distance between the heel and the floor serves to estimate the passive hyperextension of the knee.

Rotation: Sit with one knee bent at an angle of 90°, the foot slightly flexed with the weight on the heel. Both hands take hold of the lower leg directly below the knee joint. They actively support to turn the lower leg outwards and inwards. The foot shows the degree of movement. Ideally the amount of internal and external rotation should be the same (see Figure 5.16).

Function and Strength

A precise **analysis of the knee position** provides information about the three-dimensional spiralling of the leg:

1. When sitting with your knee relaxed, take a pen and mark the midline of the kneecap and the midline of the tibial tuberosity. The two lines serve as guidelines for the assessment of the functional axis of the leg (see Figure 5.11, p. 111).
2. Stand upright with relaxed muscles in front of a mirror, with your feet parallel and hip-width apart. How big is the gap between the two guidelines?
3. Keep your feet parallel pointing straight in front of you. Now actively turn the femur outwards in the hip joint; make sure that your big toe joint keeps contact on the floor. Does the gap between the two lines get smaller?
4. Demi-plié in parallel position. Can you bring the two lines directly into a vertical line with each other while performing the demi-plié?
5. Repeat steps three and four in turnout.

angle and the feet hanging relaxed over the edge of the table. A special angle-measuring device (Pluritor T) is positioned at the back of the medial and lateral malleolus, used to take a direct reading of the tibial torsion.

To assess the **axis of the legs** you should stand in front of a mirror with the feet parallel, hip width apart. The leg muscles should be as relaxed as possible. Check for the following:

- Do the kneecaps point inwards?
- Do the inner sides of the knees touch each other?
- Do you show bowed legs or "knock knees"?

Turn sideways to the mirror, with feet parallel, hip-width apart, the knees extending as far as possible. Now imagine a line running from the hip joint to the middle of the ankle joint. You will identify hyperextended legs if the knee joint is placed behind this line (see p. 113).

The **mobility of the knee** should be tested when the knee is not weight bearing:

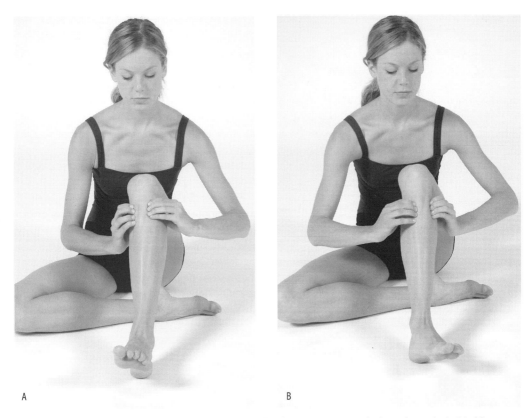

A   B

Figure 5.16 Assessment of rotation of the knee: both hands support to rotate the lower leg to the inside (A)
and the outside (B). The foot indicates the range of rotation.

The **strength of the functional leg axis** is tested while standing. The feet are parallel, hip-width apart; both hands on the barre, preferably in front of a mirror. Put the weight on one leg with the other foot touching the ankle of the standing leg (sur le cou-de-pied). Repeatedly perform a demi-plié on one leg with the leg axis optimally aligned.

It should be possible to repeat this 25 times without the guidelines for knee positioning – midline of the kneecap and midline of the tibial tuberosity – deviating markedly from each other in plié or extension. Classical dancers should also repeat this test in turnout.

Tips and Tricks for Prevention

Knee pain is common in dance. Overload and incorrect dance technique are the most common causes for problems of the knee. Special awareness during and outside training sessions can help to cope with knee problems or – ideally – to prevent them in the first place.

In Everyday Life

In everyday life, as in dance, the knee should always be positioned in line with the toes, whether you are standing, walking or running. The spiral-ling of the leg can best be trained when climbing stairs. When flexing the knee the femur turns slightly outwards in the hip joint; the foot is positioned parallel, as is the lower leg and the knee is aligned with the second toe. Thus the knee is optimally stabilized, the load evenly distributed, and the structures are released. When the knee extends, the spiral reduces, keeping the directions of the rotation – the thigh outwards and the lower leg inwards – until the end of the extension. NB: If the knee is hyperextended, the directions of the rotation are reversed: the patella, the cruciate ligaments and the menisci are put under one-sided strain and will suffer from overload in the long term, thereby losing the stability of the knee.

Tips:

- When walking, make sure that your knee is always in line with your toes. You can practise this particularly well when climbing stairs. Choose some stairs that you pass every day and make this your daily routine for practising the "three-dimensional stair climbing".

- Even when standing, pay attention to the direction of your knees. If the thighs are slightly turned inwards in your hip joints with the kneecaps pointing to the inner side, you will tend to passively hang in your knees. Imaging the active leg spiral can help to consciously align your leg axis in everyday situations; this will help to functionally improve bowed legs or "knock knees".

- Hyperextended knees are problematic even in everyday life. Pay attention to the functional spiralling: the kneecaps should always be aligned with the toes.

- When sitting, do not cross your legs on a regular basis; in crossing the legs the lower part of the leg which lies on top hangs in a slight external rotation thus "un-spiralling" the knee. In the long term that is not an ideal position for relaxing the knee joint.

- Avoid wearing high heels in everyday life. High heels are a strain on the knee and can lead to pain and overload, especially in the front part of the knee.

Specific Exercises

Mobilization

E **Mobilizing the menisci – relaxation of the biceps femoris muscle – "windscreen wiper"**

Starting position: Sit with one knee bent at an angle of 90°. The opposite hand should touch the inner side of the lower leg. The foot is slightly flexed or relaxed on the floor.

Action: Rotate the lower leg inwards with the hands supporting the movement: the outer hand smoothes along the outside of the thigh and extends the biceps femoris muscle, while the inner hand supports the internal rotation. Repeat the exercise each time slightly increasing the range of motion. Focus on the relaxation and extension of the biceps femoris while performing the internal rotation.

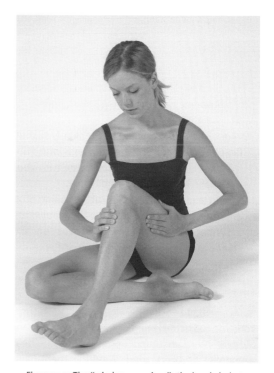

Figure 5.17 The "windscreen wiper": the hands help to rotate the lower leg inwards.

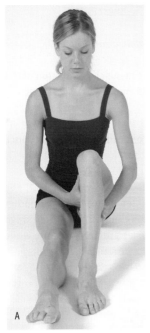
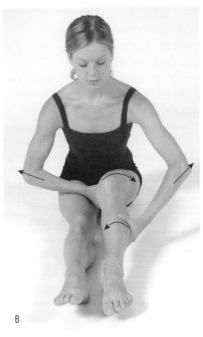
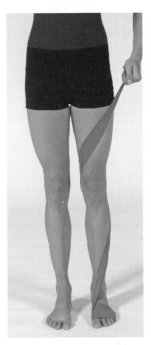

A   B

Figure 5.18 Awareness of the 3D leg spiral, non weight bearing: A) starting position, B) pull both arms outwards while extending the knee, so that the upper leg rotates outwards and the lower leg inwards.

Figure 5.19 Awareness of the 3D leg spiral, weight bearing.

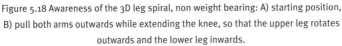

Awareness

E **Awareness of the 3D leg spiral, non weight bearing**

Starting position: Sit with the right leg slightly flexed. Take hold of the right thigh with your left hand and of the right lower leg with your right hand both holding from below.

Action: Extend your right knee while pulling both arms outwards thus turning the thigh outwards and the lower leg inwards. Focus on the spiralling action. Repeat the exercise with the left leg.

E **Awareness of the 3D leg spiral, weight bearing**

Equipment: Thera-Band

Starting position: Stand upright with your feet parallel hip-width apart. Wind the Thera-Band around one leg as shown in Figure 5.19.

Action: Perceive the spiral of your leg: press the ball of the big toe into the floor and increase the outer rotation in your hip joint by pulling on the Thera-Band. Test the leg with the Thera-Band in various positions as working leg and standing leg. Be aware of the spiral: the thigh turns outwards and the lower leg counters the movement with an internal rotation. The spiral increases in the plié and decreases when the leg is extended.

Strengthening

E **Strengthening the knee muscles**

Starting position: Stand upright with the feet parallel, hip-width apart; both hands on the barre, preferably in front of a mirror. Stand on one leg with the Thera-Band wound around it (see Figure 5.19), the foot of the working leg should touch the ankle of the standing leg (sur le cou-de-pied).

Action: Perform 25 demi-pliés on the standing leg keeping the optimal leg axis. Be aware of the spiral of the leg: the thigh turns outwards and the lower leg counters with an internal rotation. Actively increase the spiral in the plié and slightly relax it when extending the leg, but never giving up completely. Repeat the exercise on the other leg.

Relaxation

E **Contract-relax stretching of the quadriceps femoris muscle**

Starting position: Lie prone with both legs extended and the inner sides of the knees touching.

Action: Bend one knee and grasp your foot with your hand; pull the leg to a maximum knee flexion; press the pelvis towards the

floor to increase the stretch. NB: Do not hyperextend the lumbar spine! Hold the stretch for eight seconds. Then actively press your foot against your hand being aware of the muscle activity in the thigh; hold the muscle contraction for eight seconds, release afterwards. Repeat the exercise five times, ending with the stretching. Then repeat the exercise with the other leg.

E **Contract-relax stretching of the hamstrings**

Starting position: Lie supine, legs extended and your knees directing towards the ceiling. Raise the straight right leg, keeping the pelvis level. Depending on your mobility, hold the leg around the thigh or the lower leg with both hands. The left leg remains extended on the floor.

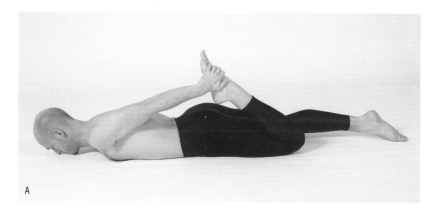

A

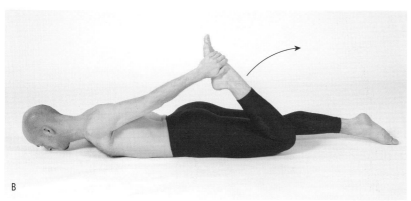

B

Figure 5.20
Contract-relax
stretching of the
quadriceps femoris:
A) pull the leg to the
maximum knee
flexion, B) actively
push the foot against
the hand.

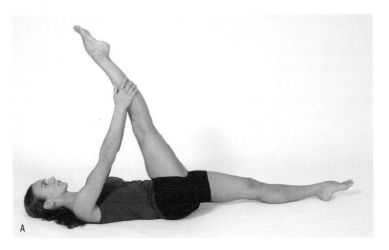

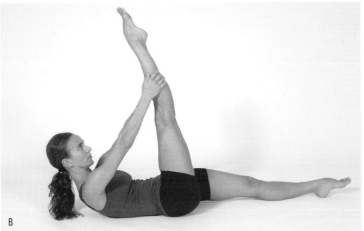

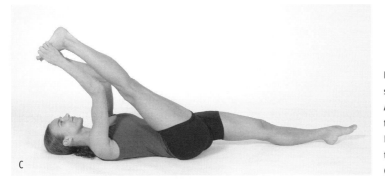

Figure 5.21 Contract-relax stretching of the hamstrings:
A) the hands lead the right leg in the stretch position,
B) press the straight leg against the resistance of your hands,
C) deepen the stretch.

Action: Use your hands to stretch the leg and hold the position for eight seconds. Then press the stretched leg against the resistance of your own hands; be aware of the muscle activity on the back of the thigh. Hold the stretch for eight seconds. Release the tension, then extend the stretch position further. Repeat the exercise five times, ending with the stretch. Change to the other leg.

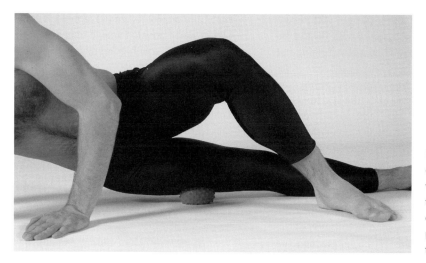

Figure 5.22 Relaxation of the iliotibial band, with massage ball: roll the outer side of the extended leg from the pelvis to the knee over the massage ball.

A tip for dancers who mainly work in turnout is that through the external rotation the biceps femoris muscle is subject to increased strain. In order to relax this muscle specifically, perform this exercise with the leg turned in. You might notice the stretch on the outer back side of the thigh.

E Relaxation of the iliotibial band I

Equipment: Massage ball

Starting position: Lie on your side with both legs extended. Bend the top leg and place the foot in front of the other leg. Position the massage ball under the outer side of the thigh of the extended leg. Support yourself with your hands distributing the weight between the arms and the bend leg.

Action: Along the outer side of the thigh roll the straight leg over the massage ball covering the whole distance from the pelvis (origin of the iliotibial band) to the knee joint (insertion of the iliotibial band). Vary the pressure as required. Repeat the exercise on the other side.

E Relaxation of the iliotibial band II

Starting position: Sit with your right leg slightly bent and the lower leg slightly turned inwards.

Action: Using your right hand, massage the lateral side of the thigh muscles backwards and outwards, as if you could wind the loose muscles around the femur. At the same time the left hand supports the lower leg in its internal rotation. Increase the intensity of the massage. Then change to the other side.

In Training

- Warm up your knees before the training session. It is best to work the knee with no weight on. Cycling (e.g. cycling on the way to the training session) or lying on your back and cycling on the floor are ideal warming-up methods. Pay attention to the leg axes as you do so: knees and toes should be held in parallel alignment and this optimal axis should be kept when flexing.
- Do not initiate your turnout from the knees! In order to avoid twisting in the knee joints, the external rotation must always be held by the external rotator muscles of the hip. Do

not position yourself in turnout with flexed knees. The first position should always be performed with stretched knees turning out from the hip joint.

- Pay attention to your leg axes! Always be aware of the 3D spiral of the leg: external rotation in the hip joint countered by anchoring the ball of the big toe on the floor. Thus you can improve your leg axis functionally and avoid excessive hyper-extension in your knee joints.

- Do not pull up your kneecap. This considerably increases the pressure on the patella and may lead to irritation of the cartilage. Be aware of the length and the spiral of your leg rather than the maximal extension in your knee.

- Do not place your feet too wide apart when standing with feet parallel, as an unfavourable muscle imbalance can result: the lateral thigh muscles will become hard and shortened and the inner muscles get overstretched and weak. Position your feet under your hip joints, not under the outer sides of the pelvis.

- Actively hold the leg spiral in plié: the thigh turns outwards and the lower leg counters the rotation. The knees align with the second toe. Watch out for tension in the biceps femoris muscle. For an ideal spiral of the leg, the muscle has to give way eccentrically. This is only possible if it is not abused to force the turnout.

- Perform the grand plié only after warming up fully! Avoid grand pliés at the beginning of training before you have warmed up properly. When the muscles are still cold and lacking flexibility, the kneecap will be pressed forcefully against its femoral groove. A grand plié in fourth position should only be carried out – if at all – with good muscular control and healthy knees!

- "Rolling in" increases the strain on the inner side of the knee. Pay attention to the 3D spiralling of the foot (see Chapter 6, p. 125). The more stable the foot, the less stress on the knee.

- Stretch and relax your thigh muscles after training. If you feel any pain around the patella relax the quadriceps femoris muscle in particular, in order to reduce the pressure on the kneecap.

- Wear knee protectors during training and rehearsals where you have frequent floor contact with your knees.

Check your dance technique:

Don't:
- Am I forcing the turnout from my knees?
- Do my knees fall inwards during demi-plié?
- Am I hyperextending my standing leg?
- When I stretch my legs do I pull up my kneecaps?

Do:
- In the plié do I always position my knee directly in line with the toes?
- Can I stretch my leg and still feel the "width" in my knee joint?
- Am I aware of, and capable of, holding the 3D spiral of the leg in all positions?

6. The Foot as a Base

By and large, our society pays little attention to feet. From an early age we squeeze them into shoes which are often not particularly supportive, and restrict mobility. Hard asphalt adds to the problem, so that healthy, mobile and strong feet are unfortunately the exception in our civilization.

But healthy feet are the basis for a dancer's body. Whether in jumps, pirouette or while dancing on pointe: only a healthy foot can absorb shock, can elastically react to any unevenness of the floor and provide dynamic support for the dancer's movements. Therefore dancers have to pay special attention to their feet, not only in the dance studio. More than any other form of "sport", dance makes demands on the feet. Where else do we put such strain on the transverse arch of the foot by training for hours

on demi-pointe, not to mention forcing the feet into hard pointe shoes?

Dance is often held accountable for a number of foot injuries and deformities. There is no doubt about it: dance puts strain on the foot, but it also strengthens it. Good training supports dancers to stand on stable feet.

High priority for dancers' feet is flexibility: whether standing on demi-pointe or pointe, or in demi-plié, a mobile foot improves the flow of the movement. A dancing shoe seldom provides protection and support. High heels, pointe shoes, slippers or barefoot dance generally demand that the foot has sufficient stability of its own. A combination of stable statics, great flexibility and dynamic muscular strength is therefore essential for healthy feet.

3D Anatomy

The foot is an anatomical masterpiece when it comes to flexibility, strength and stability.

Structure

The foot consists of 26 separate bones. It is subdivided into three sections: the hindfoot, the midfoot and the forefoot.

The hindfoot – also known as tarsus – consists of the **talus**, the **calcaneus** (heel bone), the **navicular,** the **cuboid** and the three **cuneiforms**. The midfoot is composed of the five tube-shaped **metatarsals**. Here we always count from the inside outwards, from the medial to the lateral: the metatarsal of the big toe counting as "no. 1", and the metatarsal of the little toe as "no. 5". The second metatarsal has a special status. It is firmly

anchored deep in the tarsus and thus is the most inflexible of all metatarsals. When dancing, especially on pointe or demi-pointe, it is placed under considerable strain and reacts by a typical thickening of the cortical bone which can be clearly seen on X-ray (Figure 6.2., p. 124).

The toes form the forefoot. All to**es** consist of three phalanges. Only the **big toe** (*hallux*) has a special status – like the thumb: in spite of its dominant shape it is formed out of only two phalanges. The flexibility of the foot is a result of its numerous joints. The large number of ligaments gives it its elastic strength.

The **talus** is a very special bone. It is covered with numerous articular surfaces and is stabilized by a complex system of ligaments, but it has no muscle attachments of its own. It transfers the body's weight to the foot, and conversely

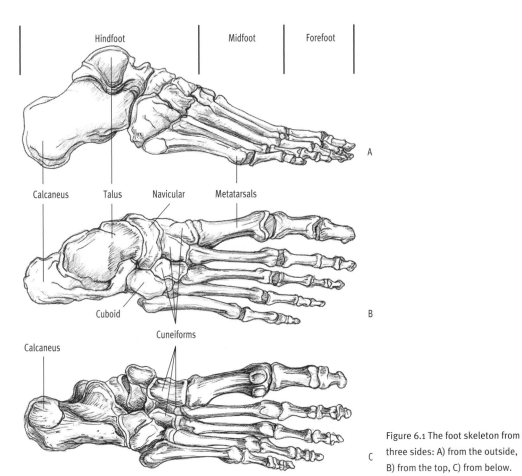

Figure 6.1 The foot skeleton from three sides: A) from the outside, B) from the top, C) from below.

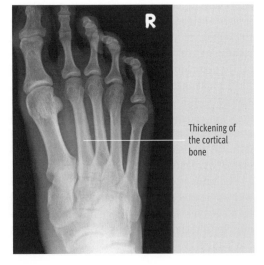

Thickening of the cortical bone

transmits impact from the foot upwards. Thanks to its trapezoidal form, it fits well into the ankle "mortise" formed by the tibia and the fibula. The muscles running past it and the large number of adjoining joints influence the flexibility of the talus.

Figure 6.2 Thickening of the corticalis of the second metatarsal in a dancer: a typical reaction of bone to the increased load.

3D Function

Feet have to be stable, but at the same time flexible and elastic. The foot meets these high requirements through its optimal construction principle. Its general design can be compared to a spiral. The two ends of the spiral – forefoot and heel – rotate in opposite directions: the forefoot turns inwards (pronation) and the heel counteracts the movement by rotating outwards (supination). The calcaneus is positioned vertically and the forefoot lies horizontally on the ground. The ball of the big toe has firm contact with the ground and the toes relax on the floor. This is how the dynamic, three-dimensional structure of the healthy foot results. The cuneiforms live up to their name. Their triangular form – broad on top and narrow underneath – recalls the keystone of a Roman arch. When bearing weight, they act as wedges thus forming the stable foot arches.

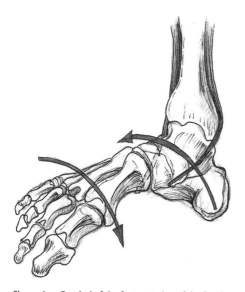

Figure 6.3 3D spiral of the foot: rotation of the forefoot inward (pronation), rotation of the hindfoot outward (supination). The forefoot and the hindfoot are rotated towards each other at an angle of 90°.

The Arches of the Foot

The 3D spiral of the foot leads to the well-known transverse and longitudinal arch. The longitudinal arch runs from the calcaneus to the ball of the big toe, while the transverse arch extends between the metatarsal no.s 1 to 5. Bearing the spiral in mind, the two arches can also be combined to a three-dimensional arch structure. This extends from the outside of the heel to the ball of the big toe. The transverse arch can mainly be found in the non weight-bearing foot. When bearing weight it yields, cushioning the movement. When putting weight on it while walking it is flatly pressed onto the ground, permitting an even distribution of the pressure. Each time it contacts the floor the foot is pre-stretched like a spring, in order to push away from the ground dynamically.

This alternation between holding and giving way, between stretching and contracting, is a prerequisite for a healthy foot. It becomes progressively stronger through the strain: the weight bearing improves both the circulation and the flow of nutrients to the tissue; the pressure builds up the bones; the tension strengthens the ligaments; and regular exercise trains the muscles.

Terminology of Foot Movement

While dancers widely agree as to what is named "flexing" and "pointing" the foot, medical terminology often leads to misunderstandings. To describe the movements of the ankle joint in

Point or stretch in dance = lowering down the top of the foot; in medical terms = plantar flexion.
Flex in dance = bringing the top of the foot up; in medical terms = dorsiflexion.

medical terminology the terms "plantar flexion" and "dorsiflexion" are used. Plantar flexion refers to the motion of bringing the sole of the foot, the plantar surface, further away from the shin, such as in "pointing the foot". All muscles engaged in moving the foot into the plantar flexion are termed as *flexor muscles*. So, for example, the long muscle which points the big toe is called the flexor hallucis longus muscle. Conversely, dorsiflexion refers to bringing the top of the foot, the dorsum, and the shin closer together such as in "flexing the foot". This is where confusion easily starts: as all muscles which initiate the dorsiflexion are called *extensor muscles*, e.g. the long muscle which pulls the big toe up in a flexed position in dance is named the extensor hallucis longus muscle. One has to be careful to avoid confusing the terminology of the motion with the naming of the muscles engaging the movement.

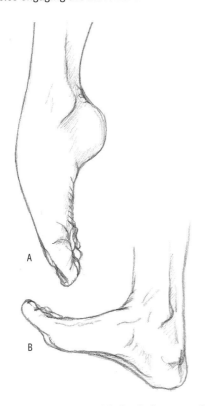

Figure 6.4 The movement of the foot in the upper ankle joint: A) plantar flexion, in dance: Point, B) dorsiflexion, in dance: Flex.

The Joints of the Foot

The joints between the midfoot and the hindfoot as well as within the hindfoot itself cannot be actively moved. Their main tasks are shock absorption, dynamization and balance of the whole foot.

Metatarsophalangeal joints

The front end of the metatarsals, the so-called *metatarsal heads*, together with the proximal phalanx of the toes form the *metatarsophalangeal joints*. These are known as **MTP** for short, and are numbered from inside to outside in the same way as the metatarsals. Accordingly, the metatarsophalangeal joint of the big toe is known as MTP 1. Beneath it, lie two small flat bones, each about the size of a lentil, known as the sesamoid bones.

The ankle joint

The joint between the foot and the lower leg, the ankle joint, is of particular interest because of its large mobility. Anatomically speaking, the ankle joint is divided into two sections: the lower and the upper ankle joint. The **lower ankle joint** lies between the talus, calcaneus, navicular and cuboid bones. Its intricate shape makes it a very complex joint. This is where the rotation of the foot around the sagittal axis takes place: *supination*, the raising of the inner side of the foot, and *pronation*, the raising of the outer side of the foot (see Chapter 1, p. 6).

The **upper ankle joint** is the joint between the talus and the lower leg and is located between the two bony prominences (*malleoli*) on either side of the ankle joint. The outer malleolus is formed by the end of the fibula, the inner malleolus by the end of the tibia. Together, the two bones form the ankle "mortise", into which the talus fits. With each plantar flexion the talus turns in the mortise thereby slightly gliding forward. In dorsiflexion the opposite occurs: the talus turns while sliding backwards. The sliding movement increases the range of movement and is thus of particular interest for dancers.

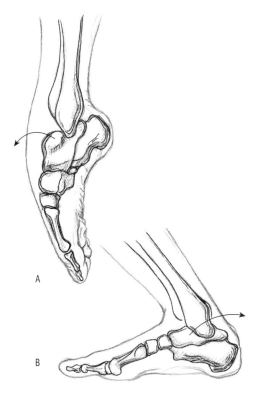

A

B

Figure 6.5 The motion of the upper ankle joint:
A) in plantar flexion the talus slides forwards,
B) in dorsiflexion the talus slides backwards.

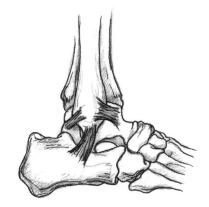

Figure 6.6 The lateral ligaments of the foot: three lateral
ligaments stabilize the ankle joint.

The form of the talus is also interesting. Its articular surface is broader at the front than at the back. This explains the increased joint mobility on demi-pointe compared to when standing with one's foot flat on the ground. When the talus turns and slides forward, the narrower back part of the articular surface contacts with the ankle mortise and the joint has more play; bony stability in the upper ankle joint is thus lower in plantar flexion. In a deep plié or when the foot is maximally flexed it is exactly the opposite. Then the ankle mortise is slightly expanded by the broader articular surface of the frontal part of the talus. Part of the pressure within the joint is transformed into traction on the ligaments thus elastically stopping the movement. This intelligent construction relieves pressure on the joint.

An ingenious **system of ligaments** protects and stabilizes the upper ankle joint. On the outside, three external lateral ligaments run radially forwards and backwards from the outer malleolus to the talus as well as directly downwards to the calcaneus. These ligaments contain a large number of receptors which are responsible for the balance and stability of the ankle joint. On the medial side of the ankle joint lies the broad deltoid ligament, which extends fan-like from the inner malleolus to the bones of the hindfoot. Because of the fan-shaped arrangement of the lateral and medial ligaments the movement in the ankle joint is optimally guided in every position, regardless of whether it is a high demi-pointe or a deep plié.

The hinge movement, the raising and lowering of the foot, takes place in the upper ankle joint, while the sideways movements happen in the lower ankle joint. Together, both joints permit full mobility to the foot in all directions; this is why they are regarded as a functional unit. The axis of the upper ankle joint – between the medial and lateral malleolus – is slightly turned outwards relative to the axis of the knee joint (see Chapter 5, p. 101). It runs diagonally from back–top–outside to front–bottom–inside. This oblique position explains the tendency of the foot to sickle in the pointed position, while by contrast, in the plié, the tibia turns inwards on the talus thus intensifying the typical "rolling in" of the foot. In dance it is essential to actively counteract these biomechanics.

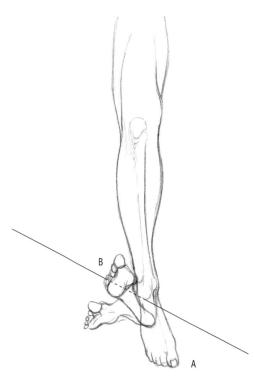

Figure 6.7 Preferred direction of foot movement as a result of the oblique axis of the ankle joint: A) on pointe: caution! "sickling", B) in flex: caution! "rolling in".

Musculature

The muscles permit the active, powerful and dynamic movement of the foot. Basically, they are divided into two groups: the intrinsic muscles, which are located within the foot, and the extrinsic muscles, which extend from the lower leg across the ankle joint into the foot.

Intrinsic muscles – short foot muscles
The intrinsic muscles are the local muscles of the foot itself. They have both their origin and insertion on the foot and thus have no influence on movements within the ankle joint. It is their task to stabilize the foot and to support the three-dimensional arch structure. They play a major role in the formation and dynamics of the transverse arch. Of particular importance for the dancer are the **short flexor** and **extensor muscles of the toes**. They run from the hindfoot to the proximal phalanges and flex or extend the toes. Together with the long flexor and extensor muscles they are responsible for the movement and strength of the toes.

Extrinsic muscles – long foot muscles
The extrinsic foot muscles originate at the lower leg and cross as tendons over the ankle joint to their insertions on the bones of the foot. Some of these long muscles are attached to the hindfoot or midfoot; they move the foot at the ankle joint and affect the position of hind- and midfoot. Other muscles, like the long flexor and extensor muscles of the toes, continue past the hind- and midfoot to the distal phalanges of the toes. Their main task is to move the toes.

The calf muscle: The most impressive extrinsic muscle of the foot is the calf muscle. Its job is to lower the front of the foot which makes it responsible for concentrically extending the foot in the ankle joint and eccentrically gently yielding the movement in the plié. It not only acts as a plantar flexor, but at the same time lifts the inner side of the foot upwards, thus causing the foot to sickle, which is not desirable in dance. The calf muscle consists of two muscles which meet at their insertion on the calcaneus: the **gastrocnemius muscle** attaches on the back of the femur just above the knee, while the **soleus muscle** starts on the back of the lower leg.

The gastrocnemius muscle is a two-joint muscle. It passes over the knee and ankle joint. In addition to moving the foot within the ankle joint it also bends the knee. The soleus muscle, in contrast, is a single-joint muscle. It moves the foot within the ankle joint, but has no effect on the knee. Both muscles join together at the Achilles tendon, which is the strongest tendon in the body with a diameter of 1cm. It is remarkably resistant to tearing – it can withstand 12 to 15

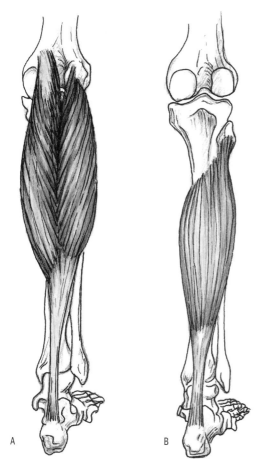

Figure 6.8 The calf muscle consists of two muscles:
A) gastrocnemius, B) soleus.

is to stabilize the ankle joint and prevent it from twisting outwards. This is especially important on demi-pointe or on pointe, since in these positions the bony architecture does not provide adequate stability.

The inside of the sling is formed by the **anterior** and **posterior tibial muscles**. The anterior tibial muscle runs from the outer front side of the tibia diagonally down and inwards to the inner side of the midfoot. It flexes the foot or pulls the lower leg forwards into a plié, when the foot is firmly resting on the floor. The posterior tibial muscle also runs diagonally from the entire back of the lower leg to the inner side of the sole of the foot, inserting at the navicular and the cuneiforms. It is an important initiator for pointing the foot.

The muscular sling supports the 3D spiral of the foot. The long peroneal muscle rotates the forefoot inwards – it pronates – thereby ensuring the firm contact of the ball of the big toe with the floor. This is functionally important. By rotating outwards – or supinating – the calcaneus, the anterior and posterior tibial muscles you can ensure that the hindfoot remains in an upright position.

The long flexor muscle of the big toe: The *flexor hallucis longus* muscle is regarded as one of the most important muscles of the dancer's foot; in literature it is often referred to as **FHL**. Its fame in the dance world is due not only to its function, but also to the problems which it can typically cause in dancers. Its muscle belly originates at the outer rear side of the lower leg running down towards the inner malleolus. There it turns into a strong tendon which, encased in a fibrous sheath, runs around the back of the medial malleolus. It continues along the inner side of the sole of the foot, passes between the two sesamoid bones beneath the ball of the big toe attaching at the end phalanx of the big toe. The main job of the FHL is the plantar flexion of the big toe and the ankle joint. Working concentrically it is important for the powerful push off of the foot while jumping and the stability on pointe; working eccentrically it helps to provide a soft landing in the plié.

times the body weight – but it is only minimally elastic.

The muscar "sling" of the hindfoot: As if in a hammock, the foot hangs in a sling of muscles which attaches on both sides of the hindfoot. Along the outer side of the fibula the **long** and **short peroneal muscles** attach. Both cross around the back of the lateral malleolus; the short peroneal muscle continuing as far as the fifth metatarsal bone and the long peroneal muscle passing underneath the sole of the foot to its insertion on the medial cuneiform and the first metatarsal on the inner side of the foot. Their task

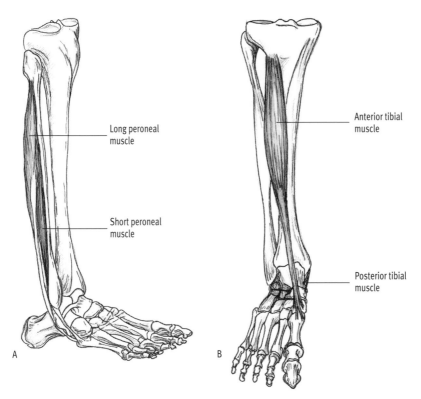

Long peroneal muscle

Short peroneal muscle

Anterior tibial muscle

Posterior tibial muscle

A

B

Figure 6.9 The muscular "sling" of the hindfoot:
A) outside, B) inside.

Foot Shapes

Depending on the footprint, one can differentiate various shapes of feet. A healthy foot with a functional longitudinal arch shows a typical recess on the inside of the weight-bearing surface. Ideally the width of the footprint at its narrowest point, at the isthmus, is about one-third of the entire width of the forefoot. The various foot forms are defined depending on this width.

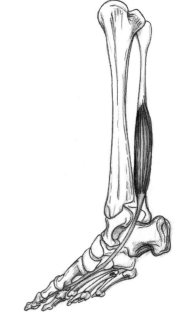

Figure 6.10 The flexor hallucis longus muscle.

Table 6.1 The movements in the ankle and foot and the primary muscles involved

Movement in the ankle	Primary muscles
Plantar flexion ("Point")	Calf muscle: • Gastrocnemius • Soleus *In addition:* Posterior tibial muscle Flexor hallucis longus muscle Long flexor muscle of the toes Long and short peroneal muscles
Dorsiflexion ("Flex")	Anterior tibial muscle Long extensor muscle of the toes
Movement in the foot	**Primary muscles**
Pronation (Rotation inwards)	Long peroneal muscle
Supination (Rotation outwards)	Anterior tibial muscle Posterior tibial muscle

If the footprint is wider than usual, we speak of a **fallen arch**: the longitudinal arch decreases. If the logitudinal arch is entirely lost the isthmus may possibly be even broader than the forefoot, which is then called **flat foot**. Whether a decrease or a total loss of the longitudinal arch, the foot lacks its natural elasticity, which may lead to wear in the tarsal joints. Care should be taken, however, in assessing the footprint of people of African origin. Under a completely functionally longitudinal arch they often show a cushion of fatty tissue which pads out the sole of their feet. Their footprint gives the impression of a flat foot although the bony structure is completely unremarkable.

If the weight-bearing area at the isthmus is smaller than one-third of the forefoot, or if it is completely absent, we speak of an abnormally **high-arched foot** (*pes cavus*). The longitudinal arch is excessively high and the spiral of the foot is increased. It is important to distinguish between the resilient dancer's foot with a high arch and a medically problematic, abnormally-contracted,

high-arched foot. An abnormally-contracted high-arched foot will progressively lose flexibility and elasticity; in the long run, its rigidity makes dancing almost impossible (see p. 142).

The most common malalignment of the foot – found especially in young dancers – is the **hyperpronated foot**. If it is assessed only by the footprint it can imitate a flat foot on the one hand or hide a high-arched foot on the other. The footprint alone is of no use here. "Un-spiralling" of the foot leads to hyperpronation of the hindfoot. The reversal of the foot spiral counteracts the wedge principle. The hindfoot tilts inwards, thus allowing the talus to slide down on the calcaneus towards the inner side of the foot; the tarsus sinks towards the floor. The muscles on the inside of the foot are overstretched and weaken; the long peroneal muscle on the outside loses its functionality. The hyperpronated foot can best be assessed from behind, standing with the feet parallel: the calcaneus tilts inwards showing a kink in the Achilles tendon (see Figure 6.12.)

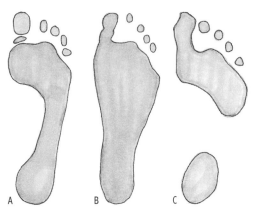

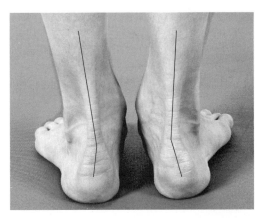

Figure 6.11 Different foot shapes and their classification based on the footprint: A) normal foot, B) flat foot, C) high-arched foot.

Figure 6.12 The hyperpronated foot can best be assessed from behind: the heel bone tilts inwards showing a kink in the Achilles tendon.

In dance a **"sickling" foot** refers to a foot that is sickled, or curved, inwards when pointed. This malalignment is frequently seen in beginners, as through the diagonal axis of the upper ankle joint the calf muscle automatically pulls the foot inwards if the long and short peroneal muscles do not work against it. The sickling foot in dancers should be clearly distinguished from the medical pes adductus, which is a structural congenital malalignment in which the forefoot deviates towards the inner side of the foot. Here the inside of the foot, from the heel to the big toe, is shortened compared to the outside, with the big toe pointing inwards.

Dance in Focus: Load and Overload

Feet pointed to the maximum, dancing in pointe shoes, high heels or barefoot – some dancers' feet show the strain they deal with on a daily basis. For many dancers, pain or even injury to the feet is part of everyday life. The list of complaints extends from calluses to weals and blisters, not to mention the deformations of the forefoot. Who else spends hours of their working day on demi-pointe in thin slippers or barefoot?

Load

Every day a dancer will stand on demi-pointe, will land in demi-plié, and will point the foot to the maximum. This places strain on the dancer's foot, training its resilience on the one side, but also leading to overload on the other.

The relevé

Anatomically speaking, demi-pointe means standing on the metatarsal heads. The foot is in maximal plantar flexion of the upper ankle joint and the tarsal joints. The metatarsophalangeal joints, on the other hand, are dorsiflexed to the maximum. The determining factor here is the flexibility of the metatarsophalangeal joint of the big toe: 90° of passive dorsiflexion in the MTP 1 are necessary for a high relevé. Ideally the line of gravity runs between the first and second metatarsal. This distributes the load between these two bones and the foot is

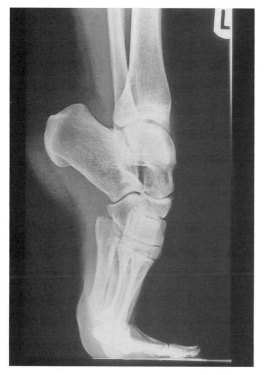

Figure 6.13 Position of the bones on half point in X-ray: the foot stands on the metatarsal heads.

the prerequisites for a high arch in the dancer's foot. A high arch is especially important when dancing on pointe: tibia, talus, midfoot and forefoot should all be aligned in a vertical line, the optimal line of gravity. This allows the load to be axially applied to the bones of the foot that, biomechanically, provides the greatest stability.

The plié

The correct performance of the plié is not only helpful for dance technique; it also prevents injuries. Anatomically speaking, during a plié the ankle mortise formed by the tibia and fibula slides forwards on the talus. Because of the oblique axis of movement in the upper ankle joint the gliding forwards is combined with a mild sliding inwards – against which the dancer has to work actively. If the foot is weak, it will tilt onto the inner side moving the knee inwards. What follows is an unwanted rotation within the knee joint. In the deep plié the heel bone plays a key role. Through the traction of the calf muscle, the rear section of the calcaneus is slightly pulled upwards. This leads to a pre-stretch of all structures on the sole of the foot positioning them to give the optimal impulse for a powerful jump.

vertically aligned in extension of the lower leg. The toes are relaxed and as many toes as possible are in contact with the floor. In order to enlarge the standing area, the metatarsal heads spread out, the ligaments and the intrinsic foot muscles get stretched and the transverse arch flattens. The danger is obvious: frequent stretching of the transverse arch will reduce its elasticity. Through active training of the intrinsic foot muscles this can be prevented. (see p. 149).

The high arch

In dance a high arch, also referred to as high instep, indicates the ideal line of the pointed foot in extension of the aesthetic leg axis. In medicine, the term "instep" is the name for the highest point of the longitudinal arch, the area between the navicular and the medial cuneiform. High flexibility in the upper ankle joint, sufficient mobility in the tarsal region and slightly arched metatarsals are

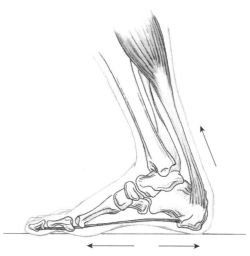

Figure 6.14 The biomechanics of pliés: the ankle mortise formed by the tibia and fibula slides forward on the talus. The rear part of the heel bone is pulled upwards, the structures on the sole of the foot are stretched.

Overload

Everyone agrees that dancing places strain on the feet. However, it is often ignored that by increasing intensity too fast, using inaccurate dance technique, wearing poor shoes, dancing on hard floors or simply having too-short rest periods can add unnecessary strain to the foot. There are many reasons for overload and injuries to the dancer's feet; usually they are due to more than one factor. It is striking that chronic overload is highest on the list of problems; acute foot injuries are much less common.

Chronic overload of the forefoot

Splayfoot: The most common problem in dance is the splayfoot. By spreading out the metatarsal heads in order to increase the standing area in the relevé, the ligaments and intrinsic foot muscles are stretched. If after this stretching the active counteracting of the muscles is missing, the transverse arch will slowly become flattened over time. The ligaments and foot muscles get weaker and lose their elasticity; the metatarsal heads spread out and the transverse arch breaks down. This mechanism also frequently occurs in non-dancers, as high-heeled shoes have a similar effect to standing on demi-pointe.

Metatarsalgia: If the transverse arch has been overloaded and has lost its natural elasticity, the metatarsal heads 2 to 4 in particular are subjected to excessive strain. Then, even when walking normally, contact with the ground is considerably harder. In relevé the strain increases even more. Through the maximal dorsiflexion of the toes the joint capsules get stretched. It is precisely these stretched joint capsules which are placed under the most pressure if elasticity is lacking in the transverse arch. Inflammation of the joint capsules or even in the metatarsal heads can result.

Hallux valgus: The deviation of the big toe towards the second toe, usually combined with a prominent enlargement of the ball of the foot, is known as hallux valgus (bunion). Genetic predisposition plays a major role, but to a considerable extent, the function of the foot is also involved in its development. Hallux valgus is often the result of a combination of hyperpronated foot and splayfoot. If the first metatarsal is deviating towards the inside, the muscles will pull the big toe in the opposite direction, outwards. Evolution plays a trick here, as the mobility of the first metatarsal at its connection with the tarsus can be very mobile – like in the thumb. If the transverse arch does not firmly support the forefoot, the first metatarsal loses its stability and slides down- and inwards. Often the "un-spiralling" of the entire inner foot is to be seen: the navicular and the first metatarsal supinate while the big toe turns in the opposite direction pronating – and the nail of the big toe "squints" inwards.

Many dance styles encourage the formation of a splayfoot and this in turn increases the risk of a hallux valgus. "Rolling in", weak foot muscles and

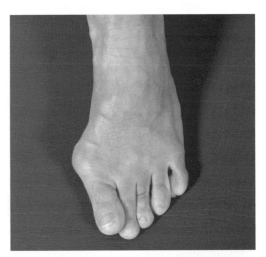

Figure 6.15 Hallux valgus, the typical lateral deviation of the big toe, with the big toe nail "squinting" inwards.

starting with point work at too early an age, also seem to add to this risk. If the malalignment increases, both dance shoes and "street" shoes squeeze on the joint of the big toe, leading to an inflammation of the ball of the foot, the characteristic irritation of the synovial bursa. Advanced hallux valgus changes the statics of the entire foot. Osteoarthritis in the joint of the big toe, combined with reduction of mobility, may follow. If a prominent hallux valgus is present already in childhood, a professional dance career is not recommended.

If there is a tendency to hallux valgus, a specific training for the intrinsic muscles of the foot can help to support the transverse arch (see p. 149). The aim is to avoid further flattening of the transverse arch, to align the big toe on its axis and to restore the architecture of the three-dimensional foot structure. A tape bandage for supporting the transverse arch or massages for releasing the pressure in the big toe joint are passive methods which, however, cannot replace strong musculature.

Hallux rigidus (Latin: *rigidus* = hard, firm): In the strictly medical sense we speak of hallux rigidus, a stiff big toe, only when movement in the big toe joint is restricted to an angle of 30° dorsiflexion. In dance a hallux rigidus is diagnosed much earlier.

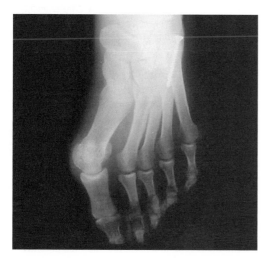

Figure 6.16 Hallux valgus on X-ray. Showing the medial deviation of the first metatarsal, and the big toe drawn to the outside by muscle activity.

Already a dorsiflexion in the MTP 1 below 80° is referred to as a hallux rigidus, as high demi-pointe ideally requires a mobility of 90°. If this high flexibility is missing, by way of compensation there may be increased movement in the interphalangeal joint of the big toe, or – as the mobility of the big toe joint is used to the utmost – microtraumas may occur, which result in wear of the joint structures. Osteoarthritis of the MTP 1 will follow leading to even further restriction of mobility. For dancers, who suffer from a hallux rigidus, it is difficult to perform a high relevé without "sickling" the foot.

Sesamoiditis: The two little sesamoid bones lie directly beneath the metatarsophalangeal joint of the big toe. Their task is to guide the tendon of the flexor hallucis longus muscle (FHL) on its way to the distal phalanx of the big toe. Besides, they distribute the pressure on the MTP 1 joint. With each relevé most of the weight of the body is placed on these two little bones. Weak foot muscles, a flattening of the transverse arch, poor weight distribution on demi-pointe or the notorious "rolling in" can lead to excessive strain on these structures. Also traumas caused by jumping on a hard floor or long rehearsals on high heels can cause inflammation of the sesamoid bones, a sesamoiditis.

The "over-long" second toe: The diagnosis of an "over-long" second toe can be made by a quick external assessment. However, there are two possible causes for the "over-long" second toe which can lead to completely different problems. If it is the second toe itself that is longer than the big toe, problems will arise, above all, in dancing on pointe, especially when the second toe is forced to curl in the pointe shoe because of its length. The problems are more far-reaching if it is not the toe itself but the second metatarsal that is considerably longer than the other metatarsals. Because of its length, it has to bear a disproportionate amount of weight when standing on demi-pointe. It is then virtually impossible to distribute the weight evenly across the entire forefoot and the balance in the high relevé is even more difficult.

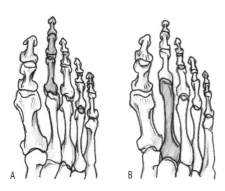

Figure 6.17 The "over-long" second toe:
A) the three phalanges are too long,
B) in relation to the neighbouring metatarsals the second metatarsal is too long.

Claw toes: Not only unattractive and the cause of many a blister, claw toes are also a sign of weak intrinsic foot muscles. If, when pointing the foot, the long flexor muscles of the toes running to the distal phalanges, are the most engaged ones, the toes will become flexed in all their joints, resulting in the typical deformation of the claw toes. Training the intrinsic toe flexors provides help (see p. 149).

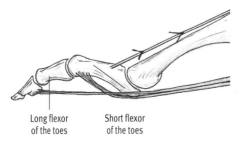

Long flexor   Short flexor
of the toes   of the toes

Figure 6.18 Claw toes are often caused by muscle imbalance.

Blisters and corns: These are everyday problems for virtually all dancers. They can mostly be found where there is excess pressure and friction. They can cause problems if they become infected, which happens particularly if they are manipulated

with sharp, non-sterile objects. Tears under the ball of the foot can arise either if the skin is very calloused or after dancing barefoot.

Chronic overload of the midfoot and hindfoot

Stress fractures: Stress fractures, a slowly developing fracture of the bone, do not arise as a result of an acute trauma but following increasing stress with constant pressure and torsion at susceptible locations of the bone. The second and third metatarsals are particularly affected since on demi-pointe or full pointe they carry most of the body weight. If the bone is unable to withstand the constant stress, anything from a tiny fissure to a real fracture may occur. This can be caused by weak foot muscles, an "over-long" second metatarsal, hard floors, extreme stress during sensitive growth periods or "thin" bones as a result of malnutrition and low body weight. Usually, the pain begins insidiously, slowly becoming more intense. An early diagnosis is often difficult and treatment is protracted. Quite often stress fractures force the dancer to stop their dancing career.

Dancer's tendinitis: The inflammation of the tendon of the flexor hallucis longus muscle, the FHL, is a typical dancer's problem. Pain can occur at the transition between the muscle belly and the tendon somewhat above the medial malleolus, along the length of the tendon sheath behind the medial malleolus or on the inside of the foot. When inflamed, the tendon swells, getting thicker and losing its sliding ability. There is virtually no space left in the tendon sheath and every attempt to slide smoothly causes pain. Muscle imbalance is a common cause: if the short flexor muscles of the toes are too weak, the FHL takes on the work. There are many reasons for an overload on the FHL, like curling the big toe when the foot is pointed or while dancing on point, a one-sided transfer of the body weight onto the big toe joint on demi-point or "rolling in" causing excess stress on the inner side of the foot. If the toes are curled – for example, in slippers that are too short, or on relevé – the long flexor muscle of the toes contract.

During its course this muscle crosses above the tendon of the FHL. If its tension is increased it pinches on the tendon of the FHL, thus leading to inflammation of the tendon. The detailed anatomy of the FHL is of great importance; a combination of a relatively short tendon and a long muscle belly has severe disadvantages. In deep demi-plié or grand plié the muscle belly may then be pulled into the tendon sheath: the tissue rubs and the tendon sheath gets inflamed. Because of its location, pain in the flexor hallucis longus muscle is often misinterpreted as pain in the Achilles tendon.

Chronic overload of the ankle joint

Impingement: Impingement in general describes the squeezing of bone or tissue at the end of a movement. In the ankle joint we distinguish between posterior and anterior impingement. In the *posterior* impingement, maximal plantar flexion of the foot can lead to a stabbing pain in the back area of the ankle joint. The cause of the posterior impingement is often a prominent lump of the talus or a small additional bone, known as the *os trigonum*. An enlarged synovial bursa can also cause pain. When the foot is plantar flexed to the maximum, the tissue between the talus and the tibia is squeezed; repeated impingement leads to local irritation and inflammation. About 10 per cent of the population show an os trigonum, meaning that every fifth dancer carries this additional bone. But not every os trigonum causes pain, and dancers may not experience symptoms for years, until excessive strain, a change in dance technique or new shoes suddenly cause problems.

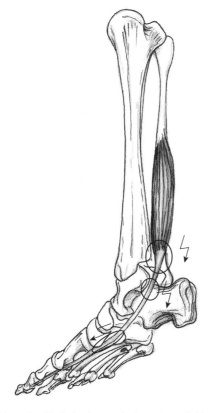

Figure 6.19 Typical pain areas in dancer's tendinitis: junction between tendon and muscle belly, course of the tendon sheath, and inside of the foot.

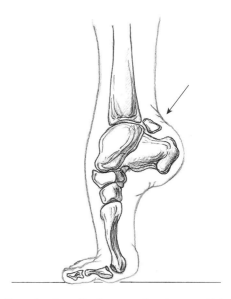

Figure 6.20 Dorsal impingement. On pointe or on high relevé, tissue or bone is pinched in the back area of the ankle joint.

Improving the sliding mechanism in the upper ankle joint and working on the fine coordination of the muscles are helpful approaches for treatment.

We speak of an *anterior* impingement if bone hits bone in the frontal region of the ankle joint during plié. If the talus and the front edge of the tibia receive bony contact, this will not only lead to pain and restrict movement. The constant jarring will provoke a reaction in the bones: jagged edges of bone form along both the talus and the tibia; movement is restricted even further. Dancers with a high arch or an exceptionally deep plié will be affected most often.

Achilles tendonitis: Jumping on hard floors, not putting the heel on the ground when landing, tense calf muscles, "rolling in" and even mechanical rubbing of shoe ribbons can lead to inflammation of the Achilles tendon. Typically, there will be local swelling as well as pain when stretching and moving. Repetitive microtraumas can weaken the tendon to such an extent that it eventually tears. Therefore special care should be taken to ensure both elasticity of the calf muscles and good dance technique.

Chronic overload of the lower leg

Shin splints: The main symptom of shin splints is pain along the front and inner side of the tibia. Causes for this may be a hardening of the muscle, an inflammation of the periosteum or poor blood supply to the muscles. Often, dance technique plays an important role – for example, when the weight is too far back, the knees are hyperextended or the heels are not touching the floor when landing. But inadequate warm-up and cool-down, muscle imbalance or hard dance floors can also lead to shin splints.

Stress fracture: It is important to distinguish between shin splints and a tibial stress fracture. Local heat, swelling and pain when pressure is applied, are serious symptoms which require medical examination and treatment.

Acute injuries

Supination trauma: A twisted ankle is the most common acute injury in dance. It typically happens when landing from a jump or simply when losing balance. If the muscles do not counteract quickly enough, the joint capsule and the lateral ligaments of the upper ankle joint get overstretched or even rupture. The anterior talofibular ligament is taut during maximal plantar flexion – whether on pointe, on demi-pointe or when wearing high heels. If the foot is twisted outwards, the tension in the pre-stretched ligament increases, thus overstretching or tearing the ligament. Depending on the mechanism of the accident one or more ligaments are affected; treatment and the required rest period from training will vary accordingly. Ligament injuries always affect the receptors within the ligaments; the proprioception of the joint and thus the fine coordination necessary for balance will be disturbed. Treatment must be aimed at restoring both as soon as possible.

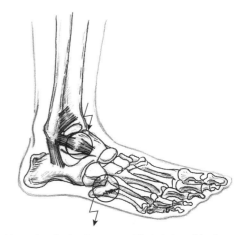

Figure 6.21 Supination trauma. The twisting of the foot can lead to various injuries: a tear of one or more lateral ligaments, or spiral fracture of the fifth metatarsal.

Dancer's fracture: When twisting the ankle, the outer edge of the midfoot may hit the floor so hard that the fifth metatarsal fractures. Spiral fractures in the distal third of the fifth metatarsal occur frequently in dance and are therefore also known as "dancer's fracture".

Cuboid blockage: The high flexibility of a dancer's foot requires good mobility of the cuboid bone. When plantar flexion reaches its maximum, the cuboid slides to the dorsum of the foot; whereas in dorsiflexion it sinks down towards the sole. This mobility is essential for a healthy foot. But the high range of motion has its dangers, as a hypermobile joint can easily lock. If the cuboid sinks down towards the sole of the foot, it can get caught in this position. The sliding mechanism is disrupted and the cuboid is blocked. Then pointing the foot is limited and painful. Typical for a cuboid blockage are pain on the outer side of the foot and weakness when jumping.

Pitfalls in Dance

"Stretch your feet", "Don't roll onto the inner side of your foot" – which dancer has not heard these corrections time and time again? High flexibility and optimal load distribution are essential for a healthy dancer's feet. But a number of technical mistakes can make this impossible.

Rolling In – the Functional Hyperpronated Foot

A widespread postural fault is "rolling" onto the inner side of the foot, known as "rolling in". Forcing the turnout is a common cause for this. Performing a large turnout in spite of a small external hip rotation twists the knee, the ankle joint and especially the foot. The optimal spiral of the foot gets lost. Instead of putting the weight on the outer side of the heel, the heel tips inwards thus turning in the same direction as the forefoot; now the first metatarsal has to bear the most weight. The wedging of the cuneiforms is released and the talus slides forwards–inwards–downwards. The arches of the foot collapse, which makes it even more difficult to point the foot and encourages the formation of a bunion (hallux valgus). Overly turning out the foot in itself is also common in dancers, when trying to achieve a bigger turnout. The forefoot is turned out even further than the foot axis, putting an additional strain on the inner side of the foot. This results in the typical, functional hyperpronated foot. Even outside the dance studio dancers tend to maintain this foot position. The feet "get used" to this disadvantageous position losing their dynamic spiral even when walking normally. Walking turned out in everyday situations encourages the "un-spiralling" of the foot still further.

How to recognize: A short test allows the dancer to assess the cause of the hyperpronated foot. Does it lie in the foot itself or in the forced external

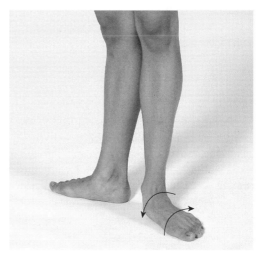

Figure 6.22 "Rolling in" leads to a functional hyperpronated foot. The heel tips inwards, the pronation of the forefoot becomes lost.

rotation? Stand upright, with the feet parallel, slightly apart directly under the hip joints. Simultaneously increase the contact of the big toe joint and the outer side of the heel with the floor, in order to spiral the foot optimally. Is it possible to straighten up the heel into the vertical position without losing the contact of the big toe joint on the floor? If so, the foot is sufficiently mobile; however, it lacks the muscle strength to hold the spiral of the foot in the turnout position. If the big toe joint lifts off the floor when the heel is straightened up into the vertical position, the foot lacks its most important mobility, the ability to pronate sufficiently. In this case, the cause of the "rolling in" lies in the foot itself.

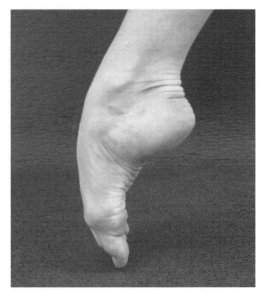

Figure 6.23 The ideal line of the pointed foot.

What you can do:
- The legs should only be turned out as far as the muscles in the hip joint can actively hold the external rotation (see Chapter 4, p. 83).
- The awareness of anchoring the ball of the big toe and the outer side of the heel into the floor, helps to improve the stability of the foot.
- Walking outside the dance studio with the feet turned out places unnecessary strain on the foot. When walking parallel one can perfectly train the 3D spiral of the foot, thereby strengthening the foot for its tasks in dancing.

Point and Relevé – the Great Range of Motion in the Foot

Sufficient mobility in the ankle joint, the tarsus and the MTP joint of the big toe are essential for a biomechanically ideal position both in point and on relevé. If mobility is absent in one of these joints, compensation strategies may be trained and these are often more of a hindrance than a help: limited mobility in the MTP 1 joint (hallux rigidus) may tempt dancers to sickle while performing the relevé. They sacrifice the ideal

What you can do:
- When rising onto the relevé, and rolling back down again, the centre of gravity should always lie between the first and second metatarsal. It is better to aim for a relevé that is not as high but well balanced.
- When standing with feet flat on the floor, it is helpful to actively engage the transverse arch from time to time. Especially after balancing on demi-pointe for a long time, this will strengthen the intrinsic foot muscles and reduce the strain on the forefoot.
- When the foot is pointed one should be able to draw a straight line from the tibia across the middle of the ankle joint to the gap between the big and second toe.
- Always avoid curling your toes! Curled toes *do not* improve plantar flexion; on the contrary, they reduce mobility in the ankle joint and even reduce the arch of the foot.

weight distribution within the foot to the attempt to achieve a higher demi-pointe. The result is excessive strain in the ankle joint, on the outer edge of the foot and in the forefoot region. If movement is restricted within the ankle joint or in the tarsal region, the foot is often sickling inwards in order to increase the pointing. When stretching the foot, the toes are frequently curled, a sign of maximum muscle engagement.

How to recognize: The flexibility of the foot should always be examined in detail in the individual joints (see p. 144). That is the only way to recognize potential compensation strategies in advance and specifically work against them.

The Deep Plié – too much Tension is Harmful

For many dancers, a deep plié is synonymous with suppleness and flexibility. Achieving a deep plié is therefore a goal that is often pursued with great determination. This is unfortunate, because high muscle tension prohibits just what is essential for a deep plié: a relaxed ankle joint in which the talus can slide unimpeded in the mortise of the tibia and fibula. Typically, many dancers try to force themselves into the plié using muscle strength, or struggle frantically to prevent their feet from "rolling in". This involves the anterior tibial muscle in particular. Its efforts can be clearly seen in the tension of its tendon at the front of the ankle joint. If this tendon can be seen prominently during the plié, the pressure in the upper ankle joint increases. The dancer thus restricts mobility and achieves the opposite of the desired effect: the plié becomes smaller.

How to recognize: Protrusion of the tendon of the anterior tibial muscle during the plié is a sign of excessive muscle tension. Possible causes include placing the body weight too far back, so that the anterior tibial muscle has to keep the balance. Relaxing during the plié would lead to a loss of balance. Also, bony restrictions to the movement in the upper ankle joint or increased muscle tension in the calf muscles can tempt dancers to overly engage the anterior tibial muscle. Instead

of working from the top via the deep external rotator muscles of the hip, some dancers attempt to compensate for the "rolling in" of the foot locally by actively pulling the inner side of the foot upwards. Here too, the anterior tibial muscle is engaged, making a relaxed plié impossible.

> ***What you can do:***
> - Be aware of the tensing and relaxing of the muscle: stand with the feet parallel, hip-width apart. Use the tendon of the anterior tibial muscle to test the activity of the muscle. It is often easier to feel the relaxation with your eyes closed. Do a second run-through in first position.
> - To facilitate the relaxation of the upper ankle joint, it might be helpful to imagine the bony movement within the joint – especially the mortise of the tibia and fibula sliding forwards on the talus (see Figure 6.14, p. 133).

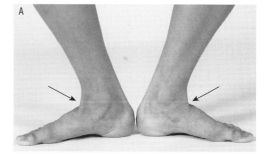
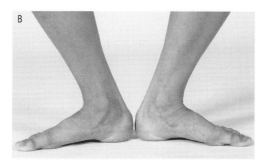

Figure 6.24 A) By engaging the anterior tibial muscle the dancer tries to deepen the plié. B) As the muscle relaxes, the pressure in the ankle decreases.

Pes cavus – a High Arch with Problems

It is not only for aesthetic reasons that a high arch is important in dance. The vertical alignment of tibia, talus, midfoot and forefoot in the optimal line of gravity allows axial loading of the foot bones, which ensures maximum stability, from a biomechanical point of view. But be careful: the desire for this "high arch" leads to dancers being selected who have the very type of foot which will not be able to live up to the enormous demands made on it: the pes cavus or abnormally high-arched foot. Over time a pes cavus will lose its flexibility; it will become hard and rigid and its ability to bear loads will drastically decrease. The lack of flexibility reduces the shock absorption in the foot and thus can lead to sprained ankles and even to stress fractures of the metatarsals. Furthermore, pes cavus reduces mobility even in the upper ankle joint; a deep plié becomes progressively more difficult. Thus, it is of upper-most importance to distinguish between the "high arch" which is a desirable characteristic in dance and a rigid pes cavus.

How to recognize: There is an easy method for distinguishing between a high arch and a pes cavus. For this you will need to make a footprint.

Step 1: To print his own footprint the dancer wets the foot with water or rubs it with oil and stand son a sheet of paper in a fully weight-bearing position.

- If the footprint is divided into two sections with no connection between the forefoot and the heel, this might indicate a pes cavus. (The assessment continues with Step 2.)
- If there is a clear connection between the forefoot and the heel, a pes cavus can be excluded. The dancer has a high arch but the foot demonstrates sufficient flexibility.

Step 2: The static footprint is repeated as described above, but this time with the heel aligned vertically. The new footprint is checked once more to see if there is a connection between the forefoot and the heel.

- If the footprint is now "normal", this indicates a high arch in combination with a hyper-pronated foot. In this case it is important to improve the alignment of the heel in order to counteract the tilting in of the calcaneus. There is no higher risk of the typical early rigidity of the pes cavus.
- If there is still no connection, this indicates a pes cavus and should be examined by a doctor specializing in dance medicine.

A) **Step 1**: static footprint. Is there any connection between forefoot and heel?

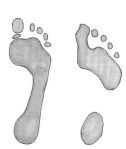

B) **Step 2**: static footprint with heel upright. Any connection between forefoot and heel?

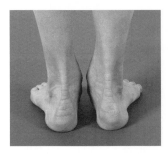
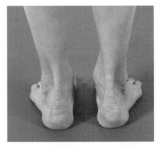
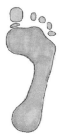
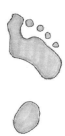

Figure 6.25 Differentiation of high arch and pes cavus.

What you can do:

- In order to improve their foot arch visually, dancers often force their feet into narrow, short slippers. This is not a good idea, as the foot elongates when weight bearing, a sign of its elasticity. If the shoe prohibits this elongation, the flexibility of the foot will be reduced in the long term. It is important to note that narrow slippers are fine, but too-short ones are not!
- The selection criterion for a dancer's foot should not only be the high foot arch, but above all a stable yet flexible foot. An assessment of a dancer's feet should always include the testing of muscle strength – especially of the intrinsic foot muscles – and of the mobility of midfoot and tarsus.

On Pointe, but When?

For years this question tortured dance teachers, young dance students, parents and doctors alike. For a long time, the magic age was 12 years old, but today's recommendations are based primarily on a functional assessment. Unfortunately, it is not helpful to wait until growth in the foot is completed, as this occurs in girls between the ages of 13 and 16, which is too late – at least for professional classical dancers.

Minimum requirements for starting point work:

- Good stability and optimal alignment of leg and foot when performing a turned-out relevé (a straight line running from the hip joint, knee, shinbone and the centre of the upper ankle joint down to the space between the big toe and second toe)
- Sufficient strength in the feet (see p. 145)
- Core Stability

Thus responsibility for assessing and deciding when is the right time to begin dancing on pointe goes back to the dance teacher. As a guideline, we can generally assume serious classical dance training twice a week for a period of at least three years before the conditions listed above are fulfilled. The guideline "from age twelve" would therefore seem to have a certain justification for most dance students. It is also helpful to consider a comment by George Balanchine, who when asked for his opinion on starting to dance on pointe at an early age answered: "Why should children get on pointe, if they don't know what to do up there?"

A Closer Look – Self-analysis

Good mobility, optimal function and strength are the main parameters for a stable and resilient dancer's foot. Self-analysis can help to identify weak spots and by individual foot training increase its resilience.

Form and Mobility

To a large extent, the mobility and shape of the foot are genetically predetermined, but nevertheless, with optimal training from an early age on both can improve to a considerable amount. The box below shows the degree of mobility necessary in the individual joints of the foot.

Classical dance technique requires a great deal of flexibility in the following foot joints:
- **Upper ankle joint:**
  Dorsiflexion at least 25°
  Plantar flexion at least 70°
- **Tarsus:**
  Plantar flexion 10° to 20°
  Pronation of the forefoot 15°
- **MTP joint of the big toe:**
  Dorsiflexion at least 80°

A **pronation** of the forefoot of 15° is a basic requirement for optimal foot function. This shows an easy way to evaluate the pronation ability: hold your foot with both hands, one at the heel and the other one at the dorsum of the foot, at the attachment point of the anterior tibial tendon. Rotate the foot with both hands in opposite directions; the entire foot is "wrung out" like a wet cloth. The correct directions of the spiral are important: the forefoot rotates inwards towards the floor and the heel is held outwards. During the spiralling movement the foot should kept lengthened in its longitudinal axis, the movement can be felt in the tarsus. Optimally, there is a soft and elastic stop to be felt at the end of the movement, a sign of good mobility in the tarsus (see Figure 6.31, p. 147).

The **arch** is easiest to test actively in relevé or on pointe: the dancer should be able to stabilize the foot in straight alignment to the lower leg. This

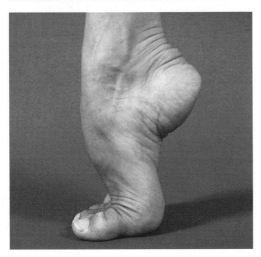

Figure 6.26 On demi-pointe maximum mobility in the ankle joint, the tarsus and the big toe joint is required.

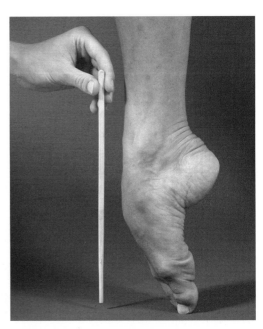

Figure 6.27 Assessment of the instep with a pen: one should be able to stabilize the foot in straight extension of the lower leg.

requires sufficient mobility in the upper ankle joint and in the tarsal region. The greater the mobility of the upper ankle joint, the less mobility is necessary in the tarsal region. This reduces the strain on the small joints. By positioning a stick along the front side of the tibia you can evaluate the arch quickly and easily: ideally the pointed foot forms the direct elongation of the front side of the tibia. Any deviations to the side – whether "sickling in" or "winging out" – should be avoided.

Function

In order to assess the **longitudinal** and **transverse arch** the following points are tested either standing with feet parallel or sitting. For some tests the assistance of a partner is recommended.

Standing with feet parallel, evaluating the weight-bearing foot:

- Is the heelbone vertically aligned when viewed from the back?
- Is the inner ankle well integrated into the course of the inner leg or does it tilt inwards?
- Do all the toes lie relaxed on the floor without curling up?

Sitting, evaluating the non-weight-bearing foot:

- Do the metatarsal heads form a harmonious arch during plantar flexion of the metatarsophalangeal joints?
- Can one find a longitudinal groove on the sole of the foot between the ball of the big toe and the little toe?

Strength and Stability

In order to provide the foot with strength and stability, the extrinsic and intrinsic foot muscles have to work together harmoniously. The more actively the intrinsic foot muscles are engaged, the more relaxed and dynamically the long foot muscles will be able to act.

Intrinsic foot muscles:

- The strength of the **small flexor** and **extensor muscles of the toes** can be tested while sitting. The foot and toes are relaxed without any tension or curling. Using your hand, press the extended toes alternately into plantar flexion and dorsiflexion. The foot muscles resist the pushing, trying to keep the toes in their position, with the toes remaining stretched. Take care: do not allow any movement in the upper ankle joint. If the small flexor and extensor muscles of the toes are strong, you will not be able to push the toes out of their starting position with your hand.
- The strength of the **transverse arch** can also be tested while sitting. Put your foot on the floor in a relaxed position. Firmly anchor the metatarsal of the big toe and little toe on the ground, actively raising the transverse arch. Slightly raise the middle three metatarsophalangeal joints off the floor, ensuring that the toes remain relaxed.

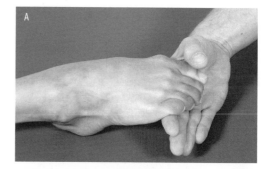

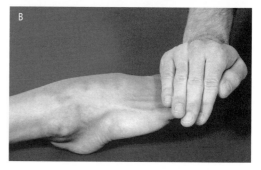

Figure 6.28 Strength test of the small flexor and extensor muscles of the toes: with the hand push the toes alternately in A) dorsiflexion and, B) plantar flexion.

Then exert counter-pressure with your hand in the middle of the transverse arch, pushing the metatarsal heads back onto the floor. When activated the transverse arch should be able to withstand this pressure.

Extrinsic foot muscles:
- The strength of the extrinsic foot muscles **in total** can be easily assessed when standing. Stand with your feet parallel, hip- width apart, both hands on the barre. Perform as many relevés on one leg until the calf muscles starts to hurt. Be carful about the correct foot alignment. A strong dancer's foot should be able to carry out 25 relevés without the muscles becoming too tired.
- The strength test for the **peroneal muscles** should be carried out seated, with a partner. Point the foot at your maximum with the toes extended, not curling up. Now your partner makes contact with the outside of your midfoot and pushes the midfoot towards the inside. A strong dancer's foot has to withstand this pressure remaining stable in its starting position, without extending or flexing the toes.

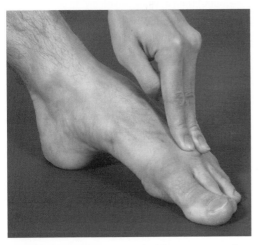

Figure 6.29 Testing the strength of the transverse arch.

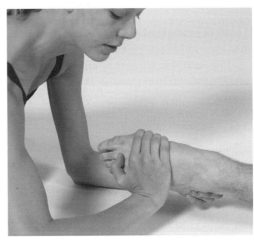

Figure 6.30 Testing the power of the peroneal muscles.

Tips and Tricks for Prevention

Problems in the foot area can have many causes and not all of them can be influenced by the dancer himself. Nonetheless, appropriate training and precaution can help to prevent injuries and overload.

In Everyday Life

Walking is ideal training for the feet. The constant alternation between load and unload strengthens the foot automatically; an opportunity of which dancers particularly should take advantage. The ideal weight bearing of the foot, from the outside of the heel to the ball of the big toe, leads to the foot's spiralling movement. While taking on weight, the foot lengthens and the arches get flatter; the heelbone remains vertical. Shortly before the push off, the weight is placed on the ball of the foot; the structures are stretched like a spring which rapidly pulls together when released. The transverse arch tenses and the toes press against the floor: optimal movement quality for walking. During the course of their careers, some dancers adopt the typical dancer's "waddle" – either out of habit, because they hope to train their turnout in everyday life, or in order to draw attention to themselves. The fact is that feet are not designed to be turned outwards, and the opportunity to give the foot some ideal "training" through walking will be lost.

Tips:

- Watch out when walking – and especially when jogging – to put down your feet as parallel as possible and push off from the transverse arch.
- Let your feet have a rest sometimes. A footbath in the evening will relax the foot muscles. Massage the painful spots and pay particular attention to the inner side and the sole as well as to the insertion of the Achilles tendon.

- Take your time when buying shoes. All of your shoes should fit properly, not only dance ones. Especially after long training days, your walking shoes should not put additional strain on your feet.

Specific Exercises

Mobilization

 Mobilizing the tarsus

Starting position: Seated. Pull one foot towards you. With one hand take hold of the instep at the attachment point of the anterior tibial muscle. Hold the heel with the other hand.

Action: Spiral the foot in opposite directions. The front hand rotates the tarsus inwards towards the floor, the back hand rotates the heel in the opposite direction thereby being aware of lengthening the foot in its longitudinal axis; you can feel the movement in the tarsus. Repeat the mobilization several times rhythmically, each time increasing the range of motion. Then mobilize the other foot.

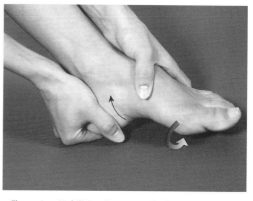

Figure 6.31 Mobilizing the tarsus: the front hand rotates the tarsus inwards towards the floor, the rear hand turns the heel against it.

Awareness

 **Awareness of the 3D spiral
of the foot**

Equipment: Pen or rolled Thera-Band

Starting position: Seated with one foot placed on the floor.

Action: Firmly anchor the ball of the big toe and the outer side of the heel to the floor, building up the arches of the foot like a bow. As a support under the foot you can use a pen or a rolled Thera-Band – but take care not to roll it up too thickly. Now place the foot so that the pen runs from the inner side of the heel to the small toe. The ball of the big toe and the outer side of the heel curve over the pen like a bridge. After a few minutes, remove the pen and compare the arching feeling of the exercised foot with the other side.

Training the proprioception of the ankle joint

Equipment: Towel folded several times or cushion

Starting position: Stand upright with the feet parallel. Place the standing leg on the towel or cushion.

Action: Raise the working leg off the floor; the standing leg should be slightly bent. Now close your eyes and try to keep your balance. In order to stabilize the joint, the receptors in the ankle joint will have to work hard. In order to increase the difficulty you can also perform the exercise in turnout or even on demi-pointe.

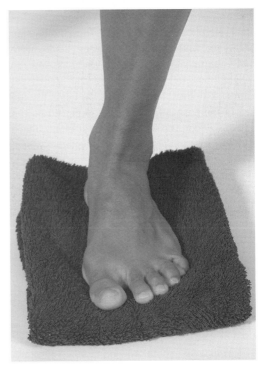

Figure 6.33 Training the proprioception of the ankle joint.

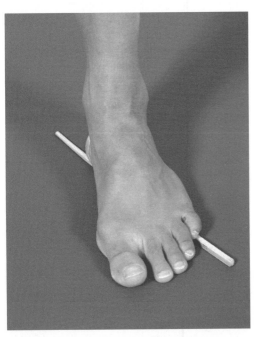

Figure 6.32 Awareness of the 3D spiral of the foot.

Strengthening

E **Strengthening the transverse arch, respectively the intrinsic foot muscles**

Starting position: Seated with one foot parallel on the floor.

Action: Anchor the metatarsal of the big toe and the little toe firmly to the ground. Now try to raise the three middle metatarsophalangeal joints slightly from the floor. Imagining rolling in the first and fifth metatarsal along their axes may help. Make sure that the toes remain extended! This exercise can also be used as a "one-second workout" which you can incorporate into your everyday life.

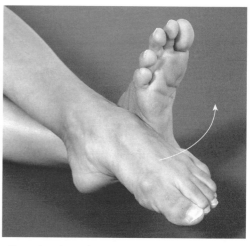

Figure 6.35 Strengthening of the long peroneal muscle I: press the upper foot outwards against the one beneath so that the peroneal muscles engage.

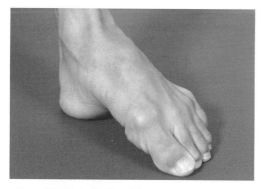

Figure 6.34 Strengthening of the transverse arch and the intrinsic foot muscles: the toes remain straight.

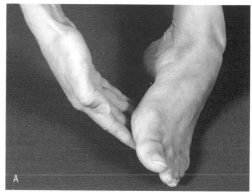

E **Strengthening the long peroneal muscle I**

Starting position: Seated with legs crossed. Flex the lower foot – this will later provide resistance – and point the upper one.

Action: Press the upper foot outwards against the lower one; the long peroneal muscles will contract. Repeat the exercise with the foot stretched to different degrees until you feel a slight burning sensation on the outer side of the lower leg. You should be able to perform 25 repetitions without the muscle showing signs of fatigue.

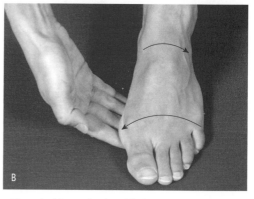

Figure 6.36 Strengthening of the long peroneal muscle II: A) starting position, B) the active rotation against resistance at the ball of the big toe strengthens the muscles.

E **Strengthening the long peroneal muscle II**

Starting position: Seated with one foot parallel on the floor, knee in line with your toes. Place the foot on the outer side, with the heel firmly anchored to the floor. Place the index and middle finger of the opposite hand under the ball of the big toe.

Action: Against the resistance of the fingers, rotate the forefoot towards the floor, until the ball of the big toe makes firm contact with the ground. Make sure that the pressure of the outer side of the heel remains constant. At the end of the movement, the ball of the big toe and the outer edge of the heel will be evenly anchored on the floor. You should be able to perform 25 repetitions without the muscle showing signs of fatigue.

Relaxation

E **Stretching of the peroneal muscles**

Starting position: Stand upright with the feet parallel, hip-width apart.

Action: Tilt onto the outside of both feet and slowly roll down the upper body, starting from the head, until you can feel the stretching of the muscles on the outside of the lower leg. Remain in the stretched position and intensify the stretch by breathing out deeply.

E **Contract-relax stretching of the calf muscles**

Starting position: Stand upright with the feet parallel, hip-width apart. Position the balls of both feet on a stairstep; hold on tightly.

Action: To stretch the gastrocnemius muscle, bring the heels down with the knees stretched. The outer side of the heel should drop even

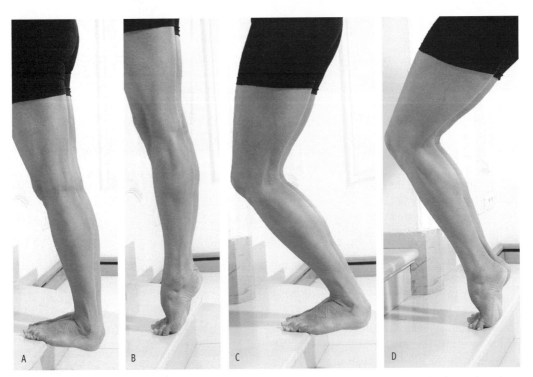

Figure 6.37 Contract-relax stretching of the calf muscles. 1. Stretching of the gastrocnemius muscle: A) stretch, and B) engage with the knee extended. 2. Stretching of the soleus muscle: C) stretch and D) engage with the knee bent.

lower than the inside. Remain in this position for eight seconds, then rise up on demi-pointe for eight seconds. Repeat the whole exercise five times, finishing with the stretching position. For the soleus muscle repeat the whole exercise five times with bent knees. Here too, finish the exercise with the stretching position.

The Timing for Pointing the Foot

The timing of the muscle work when pointing the foot is of decisive importance for increasing the arch. It can enable you to achieve up to 10° more plantar flexion. When the plantar flexion of the foot is at its maximum the talus is positioned backwards–upwards–outwards compared to the other bones of the tarsus. This increases the arch of the foot. The goal of the coordinated pointing of the foot is therefore first to allow the talus to slide backwards–upwards–outwards on the calcaneus, before it moves forward in the ankle mortise for the plantar flexion of the foot. How can this be achieved? Six flexor muscles are involved in pointing the foot (the long and short peroneal muscles, the posterior tibial muscle, the long flexor muscle of the toes, the flexor hallucis longus muscle and the calf muscle). The order in which these muscles engage

Training for muscle timing when pointing the foot:

1. Sitting. Flex the foot, hold the heel firmly in position with one hand. Tighten the large calf muscle without moving the heel. The muscle activity can easily be felt.

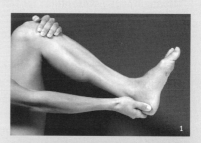

2. From the same position, now point the foot, *without* engaging the calf muscle. The movement starts from the highest point of the longitudinal arch, from the navicular bone. The posterior tibial muscle initiates the movement. This movement sequence takes time! Don't give up, even if it doesn't work first time.

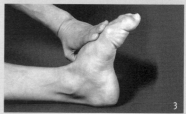

3. With the foot flexed, extend only the toes downwards, without moving the foot in the ankle joint. Now the long flexor muscle of the toes assists in bringing the talus into the desired position.

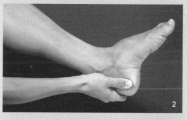

4. Stretch the foot to its maximum and use your hand to put pressure on the instep of the foot. Resist the pressure of your hand in trying to flex the foot but without moving the ankle joint. Repeat this isometric exercise five times.

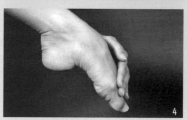

5. Once again repeat the pointing of the foot using the posterior tibial muscle as described under step 2. The pointing is usually already much easier the second time.

is important for the positioning of the talus: in order to move the talus in the desired direction, it helps to first initiate the plantar flexion with the muscles attaching further to the front, in other words to point *without* using the calf muscle. Unfortunately, the combined strength of all of these muscles together is considerably less than that of the calf muscle on its own – roughly in the ratio 1:4 – so that, initially, it may be difficult to be aware of their activity at all.

In Training

- The "honest" turnout is one of the most important injury preventions for the foot. In turnout, the foot can only make use of its dynamic spiral if the external rotation in the hip is sufficiently stabilized.
- Imagining the connection between the ball of the big toe and the outer side of the heel helps to initiate the three-dimensional foot spiral in all positions, whether with the foot flat on the floor, on demi-pointe or on pointe.
- Additional training of the intrinsic foot muscles helps to keep the transverse arch active and to strengthen its function as a shock absorber. A tip: add a short activation of the transverse arch to the regularly performed préparation of each dance exercise at the barre.
- It is best to start every tendu by engaging the transverse arch. It will take practice but the effect is enormous.
- When jumping, make a point of using your transverse arch. The powerful push-off from the forefoot will enable you to jump both more easily and higher.
- During every relevé, pay attention to the optimal weight distribution in the foot. The main load should lie between the first and second metatarsals. Especially if the mobility of the MTP joint of the big toe is limited, do not compensate this lacking range of motion by "sickling" the foot when rising up to relevé.

- To deepen the demi-plié it can be helpful to imagine the sliding movement of the ankle mortise: the further it slides forward on the talus, the deeper the plié. The tendon of the anterior tibial muscle should remain relaxed.
- Do not train in slippers that are too short. The foot lengthens during weight bearing. Short slippers might appear to increase the arch, but they are not supportive for the foot. Ribbons and elastics should not be fastened too tight. The foot needs adequate circulation while working. Frequent muscle cramps in the sole of the foot may be a sign of insufficient blood circulation.
- From time to time train without shoes. Training in socks exercises the intrinsic foot muscles. But be careful not to slip when turning or jumping!

Check your dance technique:

Don't:
- Am I forcing the turnout from the feet upwards?
- Do I often stand on the inner or outer side of my feet?
- Do I curl my toes?
- Do I put weight on my big toe in the tendu?

Do:
- Can I relax my toes in the relevé?
- In the relevé does my axis lie between the first and second toe?
- Can I start the tendu with the conscious engaging of the transverse arch?
- Do I put my heel down when landing?
- Can I relax my anterior tibial muscle in the demi-plié?
- Can I feel the 3D spiral of the foot in all positions?

7. Shoulders and Arms: Stability Despite Mobility

Shoulder blades smoothly resting against the back; arms allowing the movements of the body to harmoniously continue down into the hands – in many types of dance, shoulders and arms constitute an essential element of style. Different movement qualities are required here: they range from the powerful arm movements in flamenco to the supple lyrical movements of classical ballet and the muscular support in breakdancing.

Good coordination of shoulder and arm movements is important, not only for the aesthetics but also for stability and balance. In recent years, the strain on shoulders and arms in dance has increased dramatically. Lifting has become more acrobatic – nowadays it is by no means only the men who show complicated lifts

on stage – and the increasing amount of floor work requires dancers to support a large part of their body weight with their arms. Nonetheless, shoulders and arms are seldom given the attention they need during dance classes.

The remarkable mobility of the shoulders, the fact that people can reach almost all the surrounding space with their hands, permits a wide variety of movements. But this mobility also causes problems: the flexible shoulder girdle, the shoulder joint, which can be moved in all directions, and the complex system of muscles that stabilizes the joint, make the shoulder region susceptible to injury. Even minor imbalances can disturb the sensitive equilibrium between mobility and stability.

3D Anatomy

Shoulder girdle, shoulder joint and arms form a functional unit. Their task is to ensure maximum stability in weight bearing and mobility in movement.

Structure

It seems logical to compare the anatomy of the arm and the leg, since from an evolutionary point of view the arm, freed from weight bearing, is the more mobile and lightweight version of the leg. The bony structure of the shoulder girdle, arm and hand in many ways resemble the structure of pelvis, leg and foot (see Table 7.1).

Table 7.1 Comparison of the anatomical structure of arm and leg

Arm	Leg
Shoulder girdle	Pelvic girdle
Shoulder joint – Ball-and-socket joint	Hip joint – Ball-and-socket joint
One bone in the upper arm *humerus*	One bone in the upper thigh *femur*
Two bones in the forearm: *radius, ulna*	Two bones in the lower leg: *tibia, fibula*
Carpals	Tarsals
Five metacarpals	Five metatarsals
Five fingers	Five toes

The Shoulder

The **shoulder girdle** consists of the two shoulder blades (*scapula*), the collarbones (*clavicula*) and the breastbone (*sternum*). Like a girdle it lies on top of the ribcage. In contrast to the pelvis the shoulder girdle lacks bony stability. The connection at the back between the shoulder blades and the spine is stabilized by muscles only. At the side, the outer extension of the shoulder blade forms the acromion, which is linked to the lateral end of the collarbone via a small articulation. The only bony attachment of the entire shoulder girdle to the torso is the *sternoclavicular joint*, the articulation between the inner end of the collarbone and the breastbone.

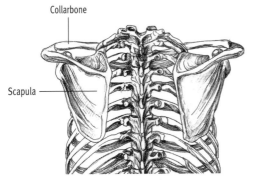

Collarbone

Scapula

Figure 7.1 The shoulder girdle is formed by the two shoulder blades (*scapula*), the collarbones (*clavicula*) and the breastbone (*sternum*). View from behind.

The **shoulder blade** (*scapula*) is a large, triangular-shaped flat bone with a concave inner surface that lies on top of the ribcage. Both surfaces – the inside of the shoulder blade and the outside of the ribcage – are covered with muscles. The sliding ability of the layers of these muscles, allow the shoulder blade to glide freely across the ribcage. Across the back of the shoulder blade runs the prominent spine of the scapula (*spina scapulae*), which, at its lateral side, forms the acromion. On the outside of the shoulder blade lies the shoulder joint socket.

In the course of evolution the position of the shoulder blades changed radically. The erection of mankind to an upright stance allowed them to slowly move from the lateral position typical for quadrupeds towards the back of the ribcage. The degree to which this migration has taken place varies from individual to individual. One thing is certain: the further the shoulder blades are anchored at the back, the more the shoulder joint socket is angled towards the side. This increases the action radius of the arms.

The **collarbone,** or clavicle, shows an S-shaped form that is slightly spiralled. Its shape determines the position of the shoulders: the more extended and horizontal the collarbones are, the more likely the shoulder blades are to be positioned towards the back and not to the side. But the function also influences the form. As the ossification of the

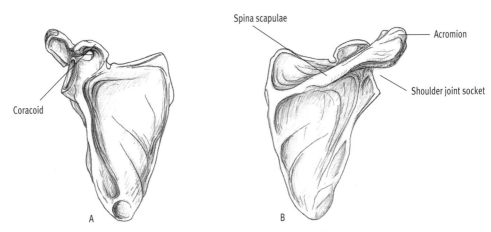

Spina scapulae

Acromion

Shoulder joint socket

Coracoid

A

B

Figure 7.2 The shoulder blade: A) front view, B) rear view.

collarbones is completed at a late stage, their shape can be modified even into adulthood. So it is not only genetic predisposition, but also the shoulder placement and movement patterns during youth that forms the collarbones – whether in a positive or negative way.

Arm and hand

The **humerus** is the smaller version of the thigh bone (see Chapter 5, p. 101). However, there is an important difference: while the head of the femur turns forwards in the horizontal plane thus forming the anteversion angle which is so important for the rotation ability of the hip joint (see Chapter 4, p. 76), the head of the humerus directs backwards. The angle of retroversion amounts to about 40°.

Ulna and **radius** together form the forearm. They are linked to each other by a membrane of connective tissue. The ulna is fairly straight. At its top end one finds a prominent, hook-shaped bony extension, which can be regarded as the equivalent of the kneecap. However, this extension is not mobile like the kneecap, but firmly connected to the ulna. The radius is considerably wider at its lower end. There it forms the socket for the wrist.

Analogous to the anatomical structure of the foot, the skeleton of the hand consists of the **carpals**, five **metacarpals** and the **finger bones**. All fingers consist of three phalanges and it is only the thumb that is "special", like the big toe (see Chapter 6, p. 123): it consists of only two phalanges.

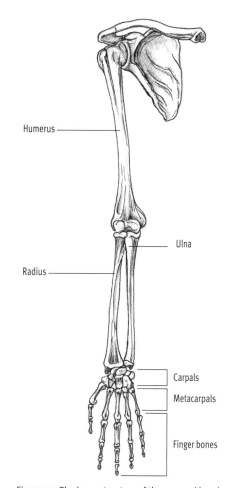

Figure 7.3 The bony structure of the arm and hand.

The Joints

The shoulder joint

The shoulder joint socket lies at the top lateral angle of the shoulder blade. Together with the head of the humerus, it forms the shoulder joint, a ball and socket joint that is mobile in all directions. The socket is small and fairly flat. In spite of a fibrocartilaginous ring (*labrum*) that surrounds the socket, just as it does in the hip joint (see Chapter 4, p. 76), the contact area between the head of the humerus and the shoulder socket is quite small: no more than one-third of the head of the humerus is in contact with the socket. This permits a large degree of joint mobility but makes stability considerably harder to achieve. Despite its lightweight construction an intelligent structural trick relieves the shoulder joint of pressure. The collarbone, the spine of the scapula and the humerus together form the three sides of a pyramid with the shoulder joint building the top. A sophisticated system of muscles and ligaments brings all parts of this pyramid together. Thus pressure in the joint is transformed into traction on the ligaments, and the load is evenly distributed throughout the whole joint. This helps to take the pressure off the individual structures.

The elbow joint

At the elbow, the humerus joins with the two bones of the forearm: the radius and ulna. Its movements include flexing and extending as well as rotation of the forearm both when bent and with the elbow joint extended. The joint between humerus and ulna is responsible for flexing and extending; rotation – both, supination and pronation – is the task of the joint between ulna and radius. In supination, the two bones of the forearm are parallel. In pronation, by contrast, the radius rotates around the ulna: in the elbow joint it turns around itself, while in the wrist it rotates around the ulna. This spiralling of radius and ulna increases the stability of the forearm.

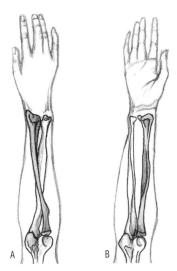

Figure 7.4 Rotation of the right forearm: A) in pronation the radius crosses the ulna, B) in supination radius and ulna are parallel.

3D Function

The stability of the shoulder blade is crucial for all arm movements. Its placement on the ribcage backwards–downwards–outwards gives the shoulder girdle its necessary stability. The shoulder blade is optimally positioned on the posterior ribcage and the shoulder muscles are in balance. Directing to the side, the shoulder joint

is placed in an ideal starting position for providing the arm and hand with the greatest possible range of motion.

Analogous to the legs, the rotational directions of the arms are of decisive importance. In the hip joint, it is the external rotation that is predominant (see Chapter 4, p. 78). This is different in the shoulder joint. Here the internal rotation appears to be more important: the internal rotator muscles dominate as regards both number and strength. The opposing orientation continues: the lower leg bends backwards at the knee, while the forearm bends forwards at the elbow.

Raising the hand to the mouth and weight bearing: these are mankind's archaic movements, which played an important role in evolution. Their movement patterns are reflected in the three-dimensional use of the arms. The head of the humerus and the hand form the opposite poles that lead the movement. When bending the arm,

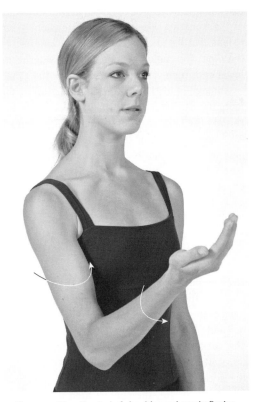

Figure 7.5 The 3D spiral of shoulder and arm in flexion.

the shoulder blade is positioned to the back- down-outside. The head of the humerus rotates inwards in the joint socket and simultaneously slides backwards and downwards. In order to move the hand towards the mouth, the forearm turns outwards (supination). This spirals the entire arm.

When supporting the body weight, the rotational directions are exactly opposite; only the position of the shoulder blade stays the same. Analogous to the spiralling of the leg (see Chapter 5, p. 103), when bearing weight, the upper arm turns outwards whereas the forearm rotates in the opposite direction, inwards (pronation). With the pronation of the forearm, ulna and radius twist round each other like a spiral; this increases stability. The spiralling of upper arm and forearm has further advantages: it aligns the axis of the arm in the direction of the strain, thus increasing the stability of the whole arm.

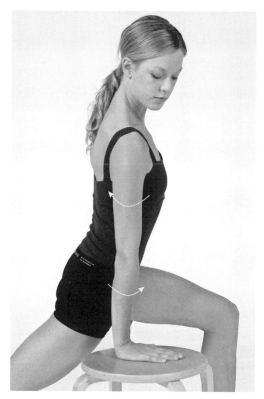

Figure 7.6 The 3D spiral of shoulder and arm when weight bearing.

Movements of Shoulder and Arm

The shoulder joint

The shoulder joint is the most mobile joint of the body. As a rough guideline, the degree of movement amounts to almost 90° in all directions – except for raising to the back where the mobility is considerably less. If the movement exceeds the mobility of the shoulder joint itself, first the shoulder girdle and second the thoracic spine will participate. See Table 7.2 for the movements that can be made by the shoulder joint.

Table 7.2 Possible movements in the shoulder joint

Axis	Movement	Range of motion
Horizontal axis	Raising arm forwards (*Flexion*)	70°
	Raising arm backwards (*Extension*)	50°
Sagittal axis	Raising arm sideways (*Abduction*)	80°
Vertical axis	External rotation	80°
	Internal rotation	110°

The movements within the shoulder joint are always the result of a combined motion, whereby the head of the humerus rotates and simultaneously slides in its socket. When the arm is raised forwards, the head of the humerus slides backwards and downwards in the socket while turning around its horizontal axis. The head of the humerus creates space for itself: through the sliding movement, the gap between the head of the humerus and the acromion increases so that painful "trapping" of the structures passing below the acromion is avoided. The combination of sliding and turning centres the head of the humerus in the joint socket throughout the whole movement: this ensures the necessary joint stability.

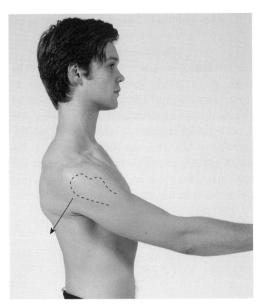

Figure 7.7 When lifting the arm to the front, the humeral head slides backwards and downwards in its socket.

long before the end of motion is reached in the shoulder joint the shoulder blade starts to move. The shoulder blade rotates around its sagittal axis, moving the socket of the shoulder joint upwards. This allows over 150° of abduction for the arm, although the mobility of the shoulder joint itself is limited to about 80°.

Musculature

Together, the muscles of the shoulder and arm form a complex system. Over 50 muscles are involved in the movements of the arms. In an effort to simplify this system only those muscles which are functionally most important are shown below.

Shoulder muscles

On all sides muscles connect the shoulder blades to the torso. Every edge, angle and protrusion is used as an attachment point for the muscles. The arrangement of these muscles can best be explained by three loops: one horizontal muscle loop and two diagonal ones. As if in a sling, the shoulder blade is embedded in these muscle loops. Thus, the coordinated interplay both within and between the various muscle loops is decisive for the stability and mobility of the shoulder blade.

The shoulder blade

In moving the arm, the motion seldom takes place only in the shoulder joint. The shoulder girdle is involved in virtually every movement of the shoulder. The shoulder blade turns and slides across the ribs. Via the collarbone the movement continues to the sternoclavicular joint, which links the collarbone to the breastbone. The shoulder blade can turn in all three dimensions, and at the same time it slides on the ribcage up and down and towards the side. It is the combination of these sliding and rotation movements that leads to its tremendous mobility.

The movements of the shoulder blade and shoulder joint are closely linked. Usually the movement starts in the shoulder joint and continues further into the shoulder blade. If the shoulder blade is easily movable across the ribs, the position of the shoulder joint socket can always be adapted as required, thereby almost doubling the mobility of the shoulder. This can clearly be seen when raising the arm to the side (abduction). Here the movement impulse starts in the shoulder joint, but already at about 30° of abduction, in other words,

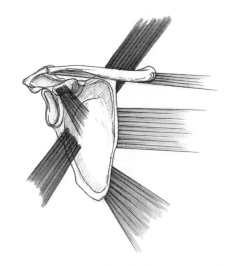

Figure 7.8 The muscles of the shoulder blade: two oblique and one horizontal system.

Table 7.3. The muscle loops of the shoulder blade

System	Primary muscles
Lower diagonal system	Pectoralis minor muscle Lower trapezius muscle
Upper diagonal system	Serratus anterior muscle Upper trapezius muscle
Horizontal system	Subclavius muscle Middle trapezius muscle

The **pectoralis minor muscle** plays an important role in positioning the shoulder blade. It runs from the upper ribs to a prominent protuberance on the front of the shoulder blade, the coracoid process. If the pectoralis minor muscle is shortened, it pulls the entire shoulder blade forwards–inwards–downwards, which is an unfavourable position for coordinated shoulder movements.

Arm muscles
The shoulder joint is a "muscle-dependent-joint" as both its stability and mobility depends on the surrounding muscles. Four muscles enclose the head of the humerus like a cylinder. Together they form what is known as the **rotator cuff**. With their tendons actually merging into the capsule of the shoulder joint, they stabilize the head of the humerus in the socket. When engaged, they centre the head in the socket and are responsible for the inner and outer rotation of the humerus.

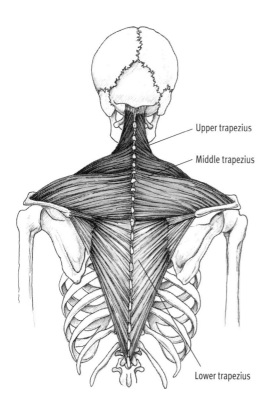

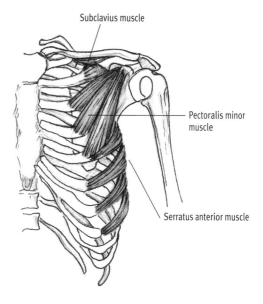

Figure 7.9 The main muscles of the scapula:
A) rear view: the trapezius with its three parts,
B) front view.

Two large muscles run from the torso to the upper arm: the **pectoralis major muscle** at the front and the **latissimus dorsi muscle** at the back. Both contribute to the internal rotation of the arm.

The two-headed muscle of the upper arm, better known as the **biceps muscle,** consists of a long and a short head. With its tendon, the short biceps head originates at the front of the shoulder blade, at the coracoid process. The tendon of the long biceps head runs from the upper rim of the shoulder joint socket through a narrow gap between the acromion and the head of the humerus. Together, the two muscle heads pass along the humerus attaching at the front side of the forearm. The long head of the biceps has a special task in the shoulder joint. When the muscle is engaged, the tension in the tendon increases, thus pushing the head of the humerus backwards and downwards at the same time. This creates the space under the acromion. The common "impingement problem" when raising the arm to the side is solved in an intelligent manner.

The 3D spiralling of the arm is coordinated by the two **guiding muscles**: the biceps and the triceps. When flexing the shoulder and elbow joints the biceps dictates the direction of movement. The long biceps tendon pushes the head of the humerus backwards and downwards; at the same time it supports the internal rotation of the upper arm. The forearm rotates outwards turning the palm of the hand up. By contrast, when supporting the body's weight, the movement is coordinated by the triceps muscle, which lies on the back of the humerus acting as an antagonist to the biceps. It guides the upper arm in an external rotation. Together with the internal rotation of the lower arm this stabilizes the arm while weight bearing.

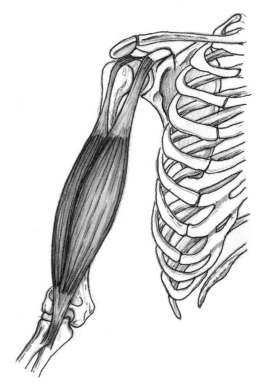

Figure 7.10 The best-known muscle of the upper arm: the biceps, with its long and short muscle head.

Dance in Focus: Load and Overload

The fact that shoulders and arms lie well down on the list of dance injuries is not due to their good training state, but rather to the fact that they are subject to less load. Although floor and partner work are increasing in many dance styles, the stress to shoulders and arms is usually much less than the demands made on hips and legs. But fewer demands also mean less training, and that is the crux, because lack of coordination, lack of stability and weak muscles are the main causes of strain and overload on shoulders and arms in dance.

Load

High flexibility, strength and stability when supporting and lifting: these requirements can be met, and injuries can be avoided by shoulders and arms which are optimally coordinated.

The port de bras – mobility of shoulders and arms

The high degree of mobility in the shoulder joint permits an almost unlimited range of movement variations, but the anatomical structures provide clear guidelines. The basic principles of well-coordinated arms are the same in all styles of dance.

The basic position of the arms in classical dance, the bras bas, takes up the ideal anatomical spiral of the arms. The arms are held down slightly away from the body; the elbows are slightly bent with the hands extending the line of the forearm. The palms of the hands face upwards leaving a small gap between the fingertips. Anatomically this action involves the following movements: the shoulder blades are positioned on the back of the ribcage; they are stabilized backwards–downwards–outwards by the muscle loops. The upper arms rotate inwards at the shoulder joint thereby sliding the head of the humerus slightly backwards and downwards thus centring it in the joint socket. The elbows are slightly bent and direct sideways. As a counter-movement to the internal rotation of the upper arm, the forearm

rotates outwards; it supinates. The palms of the hands are facing upwards, and the back of the hands including the middle finger continue the line of the forearm thereby slightly bending the wrist. The 3D spiral is also kept during movement. Thus, for example, in the classical second position of the arms it supports the way they are held to the side. When lifting, a partner the principle is the same: shoulder blades are in a stable position backwards–downwards–outwards, the upper arm is turned inwards and forearm is turned outwards.

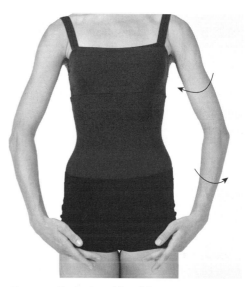

Figure 7.11 The basic position of the arms in classical dance: the bras bas shows the ideal spiral of the arms.

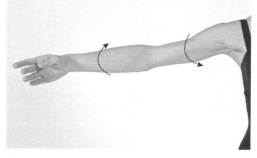

Figure 7.12 The second arm position: the three-dimensional spiral supports the arms when held to the side.

The internal rotation of the upper arm in the shoulder joint is an important key for the coordinated movement of the shoulder girdle and the arms. In abduction, one can retain the internal rotation until the arms are raised to an angle of about 90°. Further abduction reverses the directions of movement – the head of the humerus turns outwards in the shoulder socket. Independent to the position of the upper arm the forearm can supinate and pronate. To a large degree, the form and aesthetics of the entire arm are dependent on the position of the elbow and the forearm, as well as on the placement of the wrist and the fingers.

Weight bearing – stability of shoulders and arms

When providing support, the spiral looks different. Here the rotational movements within the arms are reversed: the head of the humerus turns outwards in the shoulder joint, while the forearm counteracts in rotating to the inner side; it pronates. Through the pronation, the radius spirals around the ulna, the weight-bearing axis of the arm is directed in a straight line and the arm supports itself by its bony structure (see Figure 7.6, p. 157).

Overload

Overload in the shoulder and arm region is becoming increasingly frequent in dance. Acrobatic floor elements and demanding partner work require a stable, well-coordinated shoulder girdle and strong arms. Both are often not adequately trained in dance classes.

Chronic overload

Shoulder-arm pain: Some shoulder pain is not the result of injury to the shoulder itself, but can be attributed to changes in the cervical spine. The shoulder and arm region is supplied by the nerves of the lower cervical spine. Problems in this area can irritate the spinal nerves and thus lead to pain in shoulder and arm. The abdominal inner organs can also be involved. For example, because of their location, the kidneys, liver, stomach or spleen can irritate the diaphragm. This can affect the key nerve of the diaphragm, the phrenic nerve. Via cross connections this irritation can be transferred further onto the nerves of shoulder and arm. The pain is projected into the shoulder, although the cause of the pain is located somewhere completely different.

Instability of the shoulder joint: The relatively large head of the humerus and the small, flat socket make the shoulder joint extremely mobile, thereby reducing its bony guidance. This is why the shoulder joint owes its stability to the well-coordinated interplay of the joint capsular ligaments and the musculature. But this interaction does not always function as it should and leads to instability in the shoulder. The head of the humerus is no longer centred in the joint socket; usually it slips forwards and upwards, placing the joint in a position of subluxation. If the shoulder joint is very loose, those affected can spontaneously subluxate their shoulders themselves – a bad habit which should be avoided at all costs. Genetic disposition or repeated microtraumas are frequent causes for instability in the shoulder joint.

Impingement of the shoulder: Painful irritation or degeneration of tendons and the synovial bursa mainly occur at the functional bottleneck of the shoulder, the space between the head of the humerus and the acromion. Numerous muscles, tendons and ligaments run underneath the acromion. With poor statics of the shoulder girdle or uncoordinated shoulder and arm movements these structures can become trapped between the head of the humerus and the acromion. If this occurs frequently it will lead to inflammation of the impinged tissue. The tissue swells and restricts the space beneath the acromion even further. It is essential to break this vicious circle.

Tennis elbow: Dancers are also familiar with the pain that is felt on the outer side of the elbow, increasing when the hand is raised and the fingers extended. Unusual strain – for example, with increased floor work or intensive lifting – can overload the extensor muscles of hand and fingers at their attachment on the outer side of the elbow. This may lead to micro-tears at the insertion points of the tendons; local pressure and movement are painful and strength is reduced.

Acute injuries

Fracture of the collarbone: Fractures of the collarbone are the second most common fractures in adults. Falling directly on the shoulder or on the outstretched arm are the most common causes. In two-thirds of all clavicular fractures it is the middle section of the collarbone that cannot withstand the sudden strain and breaks.

Shoulder dislocation: Poor leverage or force applied directly to the shoulder are the most common causes for a shoulder dislocation, a luxation of the humeral head out of its socket. In more than 90 per cent of cases we find an anterior shoulder dislocation: the head of the humerus slipping forwards and downwards. Damage to the joint capsule, the supporting ligaments, the labrum of the shoulder socket or the ball of the humerus is typical. In young people in particular there is an increased risk of repetition following a shoulder dislocation. An operative treatment is often necessary.

Pitfalls in Dance

"Don't pull your shoulders up" – corrections like this aim to prevent what is often a sign of great tension and concentration: the visible tensing of shoulders and arms. A tense shoulder and arm region is not desirable in dance, not just for aesthetic reasons. The high degree of muscular tension makes isolated movement between the shoulder blade and the upper arm impossible; the coordination of the joints is disturbed allowing the entire shoulder region to only move en bloc. The muscles do not work together – but against each other. This is detrimental to the resilience of the entire shoulder region.

Raised Shoulders

One of the most common mistakes in dance is the raising of the shoulders, either due to tension, pure habit or simply in order to elevate the arms. Whenever the arms are raised above the horizontal, the shoulder blades move as well, and so they should. If the arm moves to the side, the tip of the shoulder blade turns outwards around the sagittal axis; the shoulder joint socket moves upwards thus enlarging the range of motion of the arm. The trick is to allow the shoulder blade to rotate without raising the shoulders at the same time. Ideally, dancers are able to consciously

isolate the movement in the shoulder. At the beginning, the head of the humerus slides

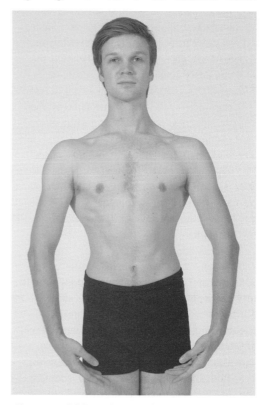

Figure 7.13 Visible tension: raised shoulders are usually a sign of high concentration.

downwards in its socket thereby raising the arm. Only when coming close to the end of the motion of the shoulder joint should the shoulder blade participate in the rotational movement. The serratus anterior muscle and the lower trapezius support the guided rotation of the shoulder blade and prevent the shoulders from being raised.

How to recognize: When elevating the arms, the movement seems to be carried out by the shoulders en bloc. From the beginning the shoulder blades are already raised as well; it is almost impossible to identify an isolated movement in the shoulder joint. Instead of sliding downwards in the socket, the head of the humerus is pushed upwards making it impossible to allow free movement to the joint.

What you can do:
- Always make a point of relaxing your shoulders, allowing both shoulder blades to sink backwards–downwards–outwards. First of all, it is helpful to pull the shoulders forwards–upwards–inwards, which, by contrast, makes it easier to feel the muscles relax afterwards. It might also be helpful to imagine "the neck muscles melting like ice in the sun".
- "Pull your arms down before you raise." Imagining this movement helps to promote awareness of the small initial movement in the shoulder joint – the sliding downwards of the head of the humerus – thus training the fine coordination of the movement.
- Imagining weights on the inside of the shoulder blade can help to address the stabilizing muscles of the shoulder blades. They hold the shoulder blade down during rotation and prevent the shoulders from being lifted.
- Even when lifting, always watch out for the isolated movement in the shoulder joint. The shoulder blade should remain stable and the impulse of the movement should start in the shoulder joint itself.

Pulled Back Shoulder Blades

"Pull your shoulder blades back together." "Make your shoulder blades touch your spine." These corrections aim to prevent a phenomenon that is frequently seen in dancers, especially in young dancers: shoulders which are hunched forwards. There are numerous reasons for this posture, e.g. a rounded ribcage, increased kyphosis of the thoracic spine, rapid growth of the spine, or weak back and shoulder muscles. The shoulder blades slide forwards across the ribs and the arms no longer hang by the sides but in front of the body. This is termed *protraction* of the shoulders. Whether it is cause or effect, one muscle is generally particularly prominent in this: the pectoralis minor muscle. Running from the front of the shoulder blade to the upper ribs, a too-short pectoralis minor muscle will pull the shoulder blade forwards–downwards–inwards. If, in line with the dance correction, the shoulder blade is

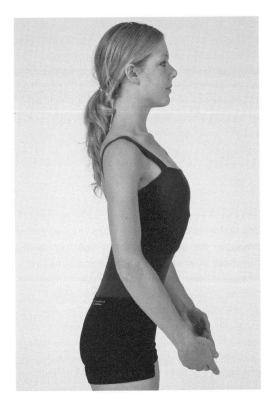

Figure 7.14 "Pull your shoulder blades back together " – a correction that often has undesirable consequences.

pulled backwards towards the spine, not much will have been gained: a short pectoralis minor muscle at the front, and tense shoulder blade fixators at the back. Now the shoulder blade is pressed against the ribs, but neither ideally positioned, nor freely movable. The mobility of the ribs is restricted and the span of the arms reduced. The thoracic spine also suffers. If the shoulder blades are pulled towards the spine, the spine too will become fixed and unable to move. This is not good preparation for dance.

How to recognize: A well-meant correction of shoulders that are hunched forward can lead to a variety of negative consequences: an over-extension of the thoracic spine, a ribcage which opens up to the front, shoulder blades which are pulled back and a high muscular tension.

What you can do:
- In the case of shoulders that are hunched forward the first step is the relaxation and extension of the pectoralis minor muscle (see p. 167).
- When correcting dancers, it is worth remembering that focusing on the lengthening of the pectoralis minor muscle helps to position the shoulder blades optimally on the posterior ribcage.
- Backwards–downwards–outwards is the ideal movement perception for the orientation of the shoulder blades in their basic position. The shoulder girdle becomes wider, the spine remains mobile; and there is no longer anything to interfere with the coordinated movement of shoulders and arms.

A Closer Look – Self-analysis

Form and posture of the shoulder girdle provide a clue as to its function. An open, wide shoulder area and centred shoulder joints are indications of the mobility and stability of shoulders and arms.

- When viewed from the side, is the head of the humerus centred beneath the acromion?
- Is the inside of the elbow rotated roughly 45° to the inside and do the palms of the hands point towards the thighs?

Form and Position

With the help of bony references it is not difficult to assess the coordinated **shoulder and arm position**. The dancer stands with the feet parallel hip-width apart; beside the body the arms hang relaxed without muscle tension. The following is easiest to evaluate with a partner:
- Are the collarbones slightly curved? Do they run more or less horizontally?
- Do the shoulder blades integrate flat on the ribcage and do they lie almost in the frontal plane?
- Do the inner sides of the shoulder blades run parallel to the spine?

Function and Strength

The basis for the resilience of shoulders and arms is their three-dimensional spiral and their coordinated muscle activity.

Flexion of the arm: Feel the right shoulder joint with your left hand. Move the right hand towards the mouth: the elbow bends and the upper and forearms rotate in opposite directions. Can you feel the internal rotation in the shoulder joint during the movement? Can you perceive the head of the humerus sliding backwards and downwards in the socket at the beginning of the movement? (see Figure 7.7, p. 158).

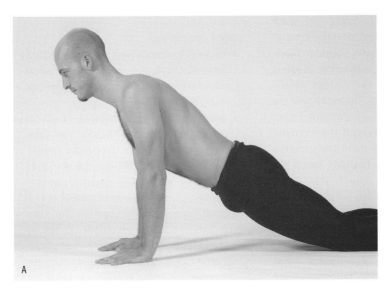

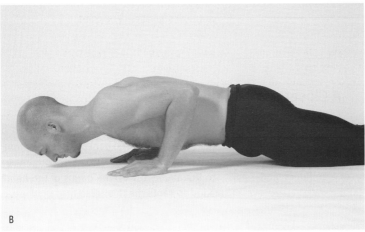

Figure 7.15 Strength when weight bearing: A) starting position, B) slowly bend your elbows backwards until your nose almost touches the floor, then straighten your arms again.

Weight-bearing position: Position yourself on all fours, with knees hip-width apart, hands at the width of your shoulders and fingers pointing forwards. Now transfer your weight alternately onto your right and left arm. What happens when the arm takes your weight? Can you feel the three-dimensional spiral of the arm? The upper arm rotates outwards, the forearm inwards. This gives bony stability to the arm (see Figure 7.6, p. 157).

Strength in weight-bearing position: This is a modified press-up: hands against the floor at the width of your shoulders, with fingers pointing forwards. Slowly bend the elbows backwards towards your knees until your nose almost touches the floor, then push away from the floor to stretch your arms again. Female dancers should be able to complete at least 15 repetitions; male dancers at least 25, without losing the 3D spiral of the arms. NB: keep your weight on the arms during the entire exercise; do not lose the width of the shoulder blades.

Tips and Tricks for Prevention

By means of active posture and focused movement awareness, overloading of the shoulder and arm region can be prevented.

In Everyday Life

In everyday life, our shoulders and arms are constantly moving. From the natural swing of the arms when walking, the coordinated arm rotation when lifting the hand towards the mouth, to the fine coordination when shaking hands: there are plenty of opportunities to train the shoulder and arm region in our daily movements. It is the quality of the movement that determines the efficiency of the training.

A relaxed shoulder girdle and shoulder blades which are positioned backwards–downwards–outwards are the ideal preparations for coordinated shoulder and arm movements. When lifting or carrying, remember: rotate the upper arm inwards and the forearm outwards. This improves mobility and eases the work of the muscles. When using the arm for support the exact opposite occurs: analogous to the leg spiral, the upper arm now rotates outwards and the forearm inwards; the bony stability will increase.

Tips:

- Take advantage of everyday situations to repeatedly check the position of your shoulder blades. Each time you pass through a doorframe, when making phone calls or shaking hands you can, just by the way, allow your shoulder blades to sink backwards–downwards–outwards thereby improving the form and function of your shoulders in the long term.
- When raising your arms, pay attention to the fine coordination in the shoulder joint. The head of the humerus should rotate inwards and simultaneously slide backwards and downwards *before* the arm is raised. This increases the space below the acromion and prevents tendons, muscles and the synovial bursa from being trapped painfully.
- Be aware of the spiral rotation of the arm. Whether lifting, carrying or supporting: the conscious use of the spiral improves mobility and increases stability.

Specific Exercises

Mobilization

 Mobilizing the shoulder blade: relaxation of the pectoralis minor muscle – "spiral staircase"

Equipment: Thera-Band

Starting position: Seated. Sit with the left buttock on one end of the Thera-Band. Pull the band diagonally upwards across the back to the right shoulder, cross the Thera-Band over the shoulder and pull it along the armpit straight down under the right buttock. The band is held in place by the two buttocks; it should be pulled fairly tight.

Action: Against the resistance of the Thera-Band raise the right shoulder blade forwards–upwards–inwards towards your nose. Slowly release the shoulder and allow it to move backwards–downwards–outwards. The traction of the Thera-Band shows the precise direction. The pectoralis minor muscle eccentrically relaxes and stretches; at the end of the movement you can feel the "opening" of your shoulder (see Figure 7.16, p. 168).

 Mobilizing the shoulder joint

Starting position: Seated. The right arm hangs loosely by your side. To feel your right shoulder joint with the left hand your fingers should be placed on the head of the humerus.

Action: Slightly turn your right arm inwards and lift forwards leading with your elbow. The left hand supports the impulse of the humeral

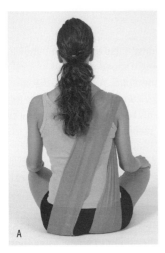
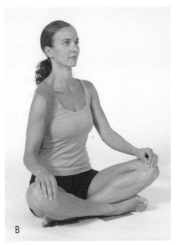
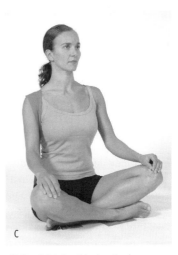

Figure 7.16 Relaxation of the pectoralis minor muscle: A) starting position, B) the right shoulder is raised forwards–upwards–inwards, C) release tension. The Thera-Band supports the shoulder blade in moving backwards–downwards–outwards.

head: it rotates inwards and simultaneously slides backwards and downwards. Repeat the exercise on the other side (see Figure 7.7, p. 158).

Awareness

E **Arms à la seconde – awareness of 3D spiralling I**

Equipment: Thera-Band
Starting position: Seated. Sit with the left buttock on one end of the Thera-Band. Pull the band from behind over the right shoulder, around the upper arm, behind the elbow and along the forearm to the right hand. Hold the Thera-Band firmly with your right hand, stretching it tightly. Place the right arm à la seconde to the side.

Action: The course of the Thera-Band trains your awareness of the three-dimensional spiralling; the shoulder blade is positioned backwards–downwards–outwards, the upper arm rotates inwards and the forearm turns against it to the outside. Repeat the exercise on the other side.

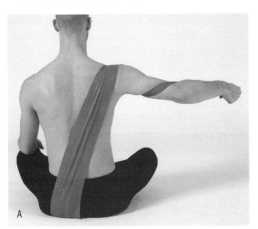
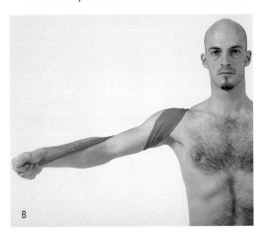

Figure 7.17 Arm in second position – awareness of 3D spiralling I:
A) starting position, B) awareness of the spiralling with the help of a Thera-Band.

Arms à la seconde – awareness of the 3D spiralling II

Equipment: Thera-Band

Starting position: Standing or seated, with Thera-Band placed as shown in Figure 7.17 (A).

Action: With your left hand, take hold of the end of the Thera-Band which was previously held in place by the buttocks and increase the traction on the band as required. In this way you can feel in isolation the spiralling of the shoulder joint in opposite directions – the shoulder blade rotates backwards–downwards–outwards and the upper arm turns inwards. Repeat the exercise on the other side.

Weight-bearing position– awareness of 3D spiralling

Starting position: On all fours with knees hip-width apart, your hands at the width of your shoulders, the fingers pointing forwards.

Action: Stabilize both shoulder blades backwards-downwards-outwards. Turn the upper arms outwards, and rotate the lower arm inwards, in the opposite direction; the arms should be kept straight along the vertical axis. Now reverse the rotary direction of the lower arms: the forearms turn outwards with the fingers pointing sideways. Upper and forearm are now rotating in the same direction; the spiral is lost and the

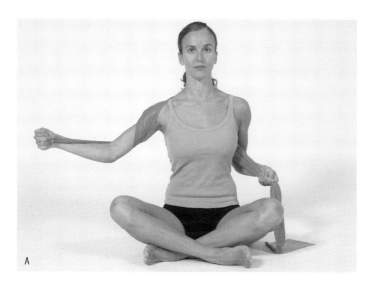

A

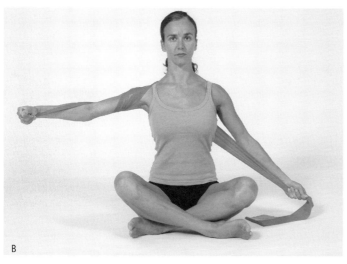

B

Figure 7.18 Arm in second position – awareness of 3D spiralling II: A) starting position, B) the tension of the Thera-Band may be adapted.

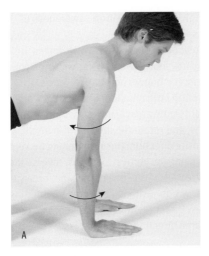

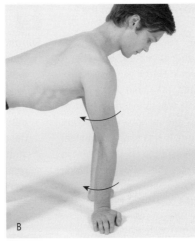

Figure 7.19 Weight bearing – awareness of the 3D spiral.
A) Bony stability: upper arm rotates outward, forearm inwards.
B) The upper and lower arm rotate outwards together, losing stability.

pressure in the elbow joint increases. Return to the starting position of the optimal arm spiral. Notice the release of pressure in the elbow joint and compare the stability in the weight-bearing position.

Strengthening

E **Strengthening the shoulder and arm muscles in movement**

Equipment: Thera-Band, a small massage ball
Starting position: Seated with the back against a wall. Sit with the right buttock on one end of the Thera-Band. Take the band with your right hand pulling it slightly taut. Place the massage ball directly behind the humeral head of the right arm.

Action: With the head of the humerus press the ball against the wall. Now raise the right hand against the resistance of the Thera-Band towards the left shoulder. The elbow is bent and the forearm is turned outwards. The head of the humerus rotates inwards and at the same time slides backwards. Allow the arm to sink down again slowly and release the spiral. NB: During the entire exercise the ball remains trapped between the head of the humerus and the wall. Repeat the exercise on the other side.

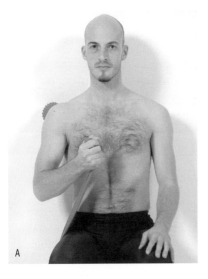

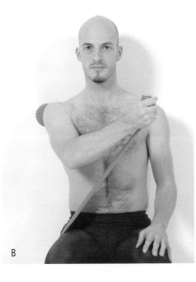

Figure 7.20 Strengthening the shoulder and arm muscles in movement: A) starting position, B) the right hand pulls towards the left shoulder against the resistance of the Thera-Band.

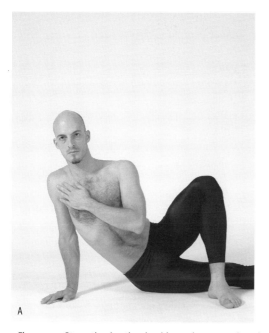 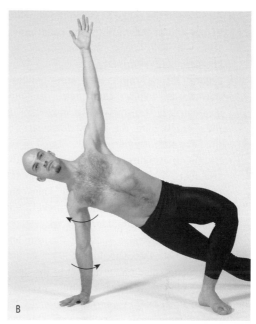

Figure 7.21 Strengthening the shoulder and arm muscles when weight bearing: A) starting position, B) push the pelvis off the floor until the entire body from the head to the right foot is aligned in a straight diagonal.

E Strengthening the shoulder and arm muscles when weight bearing

Starting position: Sit on your right side extending the right leg; the left leg is bent at hip and knee, with the foot parallel on the floor in front of the right knee. The right hand is placed on the floor, acting as support to keep the upper body upright.

Action: Push the pelvis off the floor until the entire body from the head to the right foot is aligned in a straight diagonal. Firmly rotate the shoulder blade of the right arm backwards–downwards–outwards. The upper arm turns outwards and the forearm inwards. Stretch the left arm towards the ceiling in extension of the right arm. Both hands reach away from each other as far as possible. The right shoulder blade remains firmly anchored on the back. Repeat the exercise on the other side.

Relaxation

For the relaxation of the pectoralis minor muscle, see first exercise, 'Mobilizing the shoulder blade: relaxation of the pectoralis minor muscle – "spiral staircase"', p. 167.

In Training

- Relax your shoulders in dance class! The correction "pull your shoulder blades together" should disappear from the dance studio. Let your shoulder blades slide backwards–downwards–outwards. It might help to pull the shoulders firmly upwards in order to become more aware of the relaxation in the muscles afterwards.

- Focusing on the extension of the pectoralis minor muscle helps to position the shoulder blades backwards–downwards–outwards on the posterior ribcage.

- Be aware of the space between the shoulder blades and of the width of the collarbones. This will also assist in positioning the shoulder blades correctly.
- Before lifting, pull the arms slightly downwards. This can help enhance awareness of the small initial movement in the shoulder joint: the sliding downwards of the head of the humerus.
- Imagining weights on the inside of the shoulder blade helps to activate the stabilizing muscles. This will keep the shoulder blade down and thus prevent you from pulling your shoulders up.
- A mobile ribcage also improves the form and mobility of the shoulders. During arm movements, also pay attention to the small movements in the thoracic spine.
- In all arm positions, pay attention to the three-dimensional spiralling of shoulder blade, upper arm and forearm in both the arm weight bearing and non weight bearing.
- A good weight-bearing position requires a stable arm axis: the head of the humerus rotates outwards and the forearm inwards. The arm spirals itself lengthways thus preventing the unwanted hyperextension of the elbow.
- Do not position your arms too far behind your body. Even with good mobility of the spine, ribcage and shoulder blades it will be virtually impossible to centre the shoulder joint in this position. A good tip is to remember that when looking forwards you should be able to still see your hands out of the corner of your eye.

Check your dance technique:

Don't:
- Do I tend to pull up my shoulders when I am stressed?
- Do I pull my shoulder blades together at the back?
- Do my shoulder muscles feel hard and firm?
- Do I often move my shoulder blades and shoulder joints together en bloc?
- Do I tend to form a sway back when I raise my arms?
- Do I hyperextend my elbows when using my arms to support my weight?

Do:
- Can I position my shoulder blades on my back in a relaxed way?
- Can I feel the length and extension in my pectoralis minor muscle?
- Am I aware of the movement of my shoulder blades on my ribcage?
- Can I coordinate the movement of my shoulder blades and arms and use them independently?
- Am I aware of the 3D spiralling of my arms during movement and when weight bearing?

8. Dancing with Heart and Soul

The joy of moving to rhythm and music, creativity, expression through one's body: there are lots of reasons why people dance. Although in dance the body is trained, challenged and strained just as it is in sports, competition is not of prime importance. Comparing dance with gymnastics is frowned upon, as dance embraces more than the purely physical aspect. Most dancers do not consider themselves athletes but artists. The consequence of this is while sportsmen and sportswomen do not need to hide their physical effort – a strained expression on the athlete's face does not reduce the effect of the performance – dance is generally supposed to appear free of physical effort. This is not altered by the fact that in many dance styles technique becomes increasingly more demanding and acrobatic.

The body is the dancer's instrument; it is the base used to perform movements, enriching them with life and emotion. This accounts for the fascination of dance but at the same time harbours dangers. The dancer cannot "hide" behind a musical instrument, and there is no set text to create a distance between the performing body and the person inside. That makes dancers vulnerable, not just physically, but also emotionally. The dividing line between the dancing body as an instrument of art and the personality of the dancer is easily blurred as body and mind cannot be separated, neither on the stage nor in the dance studio.

Demands on the Psyche

Only a small number of dance enthusiasts will make dancing their profession. For most people, the dance studio remains the centre of their dance experience; the dance training will frame their relationship to dance. This makes the atmosphere during dance classes particularly important. It not only influences the enthusiasm for dancing, but also has a considerable impact on the speed and effectiveness of the learning process. This can be explained scientifically: certain areas of the brain judge all events, actions and learning contents for their emotional impressions. Events linked to positive emotions are more deeply embedded in the brain while unpleasant emotional experiences obstruct the memory. Knowledge transmitted in an unpleasant learning atmosphere is usually confined to the short-term memory only. Thus, effective learning cannot take place, whether inside or outside the dance studio.

Impact of the Dance Class

Most people learn dancing in a group. A dance class motivates; it creates opportunities to compare, but also to compete. It is necessary to find your own position: both as part of the group and your space in the dance studio. Dancing together increases the awareness for space. Where do I stand? How much room does the choreography require? This trains the dancers' awareness of closeness and distance, and sensitizes for one's own movements and for those of the other dancers.

Support from and competition with one's fellow dancers, are two sides of the same coin.

No dance teacher can observe all dancers in a studio all of the time; it is impossible to accompany each individual step. Dancers therefore quickly acquire the ability to work on themselves, correcting themselves and training in a disciplined manner even when the teacher's attention is focused on another dancer. Constant self-monitoring, working independently to improve dance technique and a high degree of personal responsibility are important when it comes to dancing. However, too much control can be detrimental, as this leaves little room for spontaneity and relaxation. The quality of movement gets lost, and the dynamic of the dancing decreases. Often, the need for control also finds expression in everyday life. For many dancers is seems difficult to find the ideal balance between challenging themselves and relaxing. Eating disorders are more common in the dance world than among the general population (see Chapter 9, p. 189). There are many reasons for this, and one might be the high rate of self-monitoring.

Different Forms of Dance Correction

Dance training is characterized by corrections, suggestions for improvements, criticism and support by the teacher. The optimal performance of any given movement is of prime importance, and feedback from another person is essential for achieving that. But the way in which feedback is communicated dictates its effect. In dance, the focus tends to be on the aspects of the dance step that is still missing, on the "mistakes". This negative point of view – the look out for mistakes – characterizes the dance class, the dance teacher and, naturally, the dancer, too. Corrections are often given quite directly in front of the entire group. This is a good thing as many suggestions

> **Corrections** are essential for improving one's dance technique. Framing them in a **positive manner** is important for the dancer's psyche.

addressed to individual dancers are also helpful to others. But public criticism can also be hurtful, particularly if it is formulated in a negative way. Small adjustments can make a big difference here. "You can stretch your leg more" rather than "Your leg is not stretched" has a motivating effect and simultaneously shifts the focus to what actually needs to be done. In fact, in addition to being potentially hurtful, the use of negative formulations has another considerable disadvantage: it directs attention away from what is most important, focusing on the problem without offering a solution.

No Dance Studio without a Mirror?

Mirrors are an important prop in virtually all dance studios. Mirrors allow dancers to correct themselves independently, to analyze their movements on their own and compare their perception of the movement with what they see in the mirror. This is helpful. However, dancers must learn how to use the mirror. Both the dancer's technique and, significantly, also his body must withstand his own critical gaze. It can be frustrating

> Selective use of a mirror is helpful to dancers.

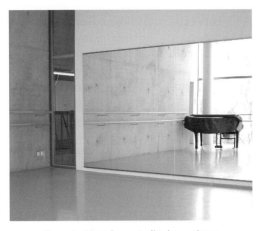

Figure 8.1 Most dance studios have mirrors.

when the reflection in the mirror does not live up to one's own expectations.

The visual fixation on the outer form threatens to sideline the process of perceiving and exploring the movement from within. This impairs movement quality and often saps the dancer's awareness of his body. Too much tension can considerably disrupt the coordination. Constantly looking in the mirror not only harms the dance line, but can also lead to moments of inattention and, as a result, to injury. Furthermore, the performance can suffer from the focus on the mirror. Dancers get often irritated, forget the choreography, or feel insecure simply because the mirror has been covered up or the room direction has been changed. Training from time to time without a mirror can prevent this.

Dancing as a Profession and as a Mission

Professional dancing is more than just a job. Most dancers are absolutely and completely committed to dance, making great sacrifices during their training from a young age onwards, with the aim of becoming professional dancers. Anyone who has experienced the flow of a performance, dancing as though nothing else in the world exists, the intense concentration, the solidarity and that moment when everybody gives their all; this person will understand how you can become addicted to dance, why dancers choose to make dancing the focus of their lives despite financial insecurity, inappropriate working conditions and lack of social recognition. This is wonderful for the art of dance, but this passion often demands a high price from the dancers.

Working Conditions in Dance Schools and Dance Companies

Starting professional dance training often forces dancers to leave their family home at an early age, tearing them away from their familiar environment at a young age. In later years, joining a new dance company is often associated with moving on, losing dear friends and even, in some cases, entering a foreign culture. Dancers have to be geographically flexible. This explains the great role that dance schools and companies play in many dancers' lives. Fellow dancers often serve as substitutes for family and friends, and contact with people from outside the dance world is limited. It is therefore virtually impossible to separate the world of dance from private life, with the consequence that dance-related problems are doubly distressing.

Professional dancers do not only place strain on their bodies, but also on their psyches:

- **Discipline:** In the everyday schedule of training and rehearsals, discipline is a fundamental prerequisite for a career as a professional dancer. Dancers must work with perseverance, purpose and concentration. They are used to accepting, and swiftly reacting to, criticism and taking instructions in a constructive manner.
- **High demands:** The dancers' demands on themselves, as well as the demands placed on them by parents, teachers, choreographers, ballet directors or critics can lead to constant stress and negatively influence the performance.
- **Stage-fright:** Stress is the body's natural response to demands perceived as threat. The adrenal cortex releases adrenaline, a stress hormone that propels the body into a state of alertness thus preparing it to withstand the greatest possible strain. This is a prerequisite for peak performance. But stage-fright can also be a block. Extreme stage-fright can cause palpitations, high blood pressure, blackouts and inappropriate reactions.
- **The pressure of competition:** An authoritarian style of teaching and working, short-term work contracts, mysterious criteria for

examination and assessment and decision-making that is incomprehensible for the dancers increases competition in the group both in the dance school and in the company.

- **Social isolation:** Frequent rehearsals and performances in the evenings and at weekends make social contact outside the theatre virtually impossible. If working in a foreign country, language problems and intercultural differences make it even more difficult for dancers to adapt to their new environment.
- **Financial insecurity:** Short-term work contracts, low pay, frequent changes of work place and a short career span are considerable stress factors in the dancers' lives.

Extreme physical strain over years and decades demands an extraordinary degree of discipline, self-motivation and a strong sense of personal responsibility. On the other hand, working as an artist, developing and interpreting dance on stage, requires openness, sensitivity and dedication. Dancers are highly motivated, often push their own boundaries and even step beyond them. This increases the risk of injury – both physical and emotional.

Maintaining a Healthy Balance

Dancing implies stress, a strain to body and soul. This does not have to be negative as stress comes in different forms: while *distress* (negative stress) is perceived as unpleasant, threatening and overwhelming, *eustress* (positive stress) can increase attentiveness and even increase resilience. In athletes whose negative-stress levels are high, injuries take longer to heal. Conversely, a positive attitude to life can speed up the healing process. Dancers can protect themselves from distress with their own attitude and a good balance between strain and relaxation.

Tips for maintaining a healthy emotional balance:

Be an active member of the group: Take responsibility in your dance school or company. Even if your group is small, nominate a speaker to communicate your common interests and represent them to the management. This will allow you to actively influence your environment.

Multifaceted training: Maintain variety in your training methods. Endurance training is not only a good counterbalance to dance training; it also improves your stamina (see Chapter 12, p. 219).

Openness: Learn the language of the country in which you work, even if you will only be there for a short period of time. Acquaint yourself with the foreign culture. This will help you to feel at home wherever you are.

Distraction: Maintain friendships and contacts outside of your school and company. Distraction is important for getting yourself ready to completely dedicate to dancing again. Thus regular distractions can help to improve your dance.

Contrasts: Make time for hobbies and interests that go beyond dance and theatre. This, too, is a form of relaxation!

Relaxation: Allow yourself to enjoy breaks for recreation and make sure you get sufficient sleep. Relaxation techniques can help to cope with stress. Methods such as Feldenkrais, Qi Gong, Alexander Technique, yoga or autogenic training help to reduce stress.

Chill out: Allow yourself to just do nothing ... and enjoy it!

Life after Dance

Whether due to age, injury or for other personal reasons; whether the decision is made during the professional dance education or after a long active dancing career – it is always difficult to leave the world of dance. When you have to stop dancing, there is a big void. Dance cannot simply be replaced by something else. The fascinating combination of artistic work and physical challenge is lacking in other art forms or in sports.

Leaving the world of dance causes grief. Grief over an all-too-short career as a dancer, over goals not achieved, over all the beautiful things that are now in the past. Unpleasant elements are usually forgotten: the daily physical exertion, the many long hours of often-monotonous rehearsals, working with difficult choreographers or under terrible conditions. Juxtaposing the positive and negative sides can help dancers to reconsider their view of the past, and to differentiate between leaving behind the realities of life as a professional dancer and their dream of dancing. Young dancers will often not be able to make this distinction if they already, during their dance studies, had to give up their dreams of becoming a professional. Frequently, their goals are widely separated from reality. If a dance career ends before it has actually started, that means letting go of a dream. And that is doubly difficult.

Dancers often move on to their second career as early as their 30s, a time when many other people are just establishing themselves professionally. They must reorient, train or retrain, and might find themselves in a completely new environment. Dancers who are aware of the extraordinary skills they have acquired through dance, and realize that they have learned far more than dance steps and choreographies, have already cleared the first hurdle: the fear of the world outside of dance. It is a frequent occurrence that dancers feel they are "failures" once their dance careers have come to an end. They fall into deep depression and seem unable to position themselves in society without dance. They feel as if they cannot do anything but dance. But this is definitely not true!

Dance training: beyond the physical

Does dance develop special personality traits, or do people w ho already have these characteristics do feel particularly drawn into dance? It is impossible to answer this question conclusively. However, one thing is certain: dance nurtures skills that go far beyond the physical.

Dance teaches people how:
- to work in a concentrated and precise manner;
- to pursue accomplishing a task with discipline and perseverance;
- to ignore distractions;
- to work in a goal-oriented way;
- to follow instructions;
- to implement ideas creatively;
- to accept criticism and apply it constructively;
- to react to change with flexibility;
- to work as part of a team;
- to take over team and individual responsibility;
- to perform at a high standard, even under pressure.

For the body, a slow decrease in strain and a step-by-step reduction of the training is of crucial importance (see Chapter 12, p. 237). The psyche, too, benefits from this gradual "phasing-out". It takes time to adjust to no longer being an active dancer, to reorient towards new goals and discover interests beyond the world of dance. Many dancers will have to build up a social network first, one that will support them when they retire from professional dancing. The earlier they start the better.

The end of a professional dance career does not have to indicate the end of dancing. Even after an injury, it is often possible to start dancing again, albeit at a lower intensity and perhaps in a different style of dance.

9. Nutrition: An Important Aspect of Training

Why do we eat? Science has a clear answer to this question. Every second approximately 10^{30} chemical reactions take place in our bodies. Every day, 600 billion cells die, and the same number are renewed, integrating seamlessly back into the system. Physical strain increases the demands made on the metabolism. Intense training leads to micro-injuries of the tissue, releasing toxic substances and radicals. Damaged tissue is repaired, toxins neutralized and discharged from the body through complex biochemical processes. This is only possible with help from the outside: the food we eat supplies us with the necessary building materials, nutrients and sufficient energy to cope with the building and rebuilding processes within our body. But who thinks of the body's metabolic processes when taking a bite of a juicy apple? For most people, pleasure and emotional satisfaction are decisive when it comes to what they eat, how they eat and how much they eat. Many eat out of enjoyment or boredom, to reward themselves or to reduce stress. Seldom do people eat out of the primal human feeling – out of hunger.

Countless nutritionists throughout the world are engaged in a debate on what constitutes a "healthy diet". Advice and trends change rapidly and contradictions are rife. Diet is a highly complex subject. Discussed below are some important facts that can help dancers to improve their health and performance through healthy nutrition. Achieving high performance needs both optimal training *and* a thoughtful diet!

The Components of Nutrition

"Five-a-day" campaigns encourage consumption of at least five portions of fruit and vegetables per day. In this way, government departments and organizations worldwide aim to improve the health of the population. But most people, including a great many dancers, are far removed from eating the suggested 600g of fruit and vegetables every day. However, fruit and vegetables are very important parts of our nutrition, as they contain just about everything we need for a healthy, balanced diet: carbohydrates, protein and fat, dietary fibre, vitamins, minerals, trace elements, phytochemicals and water.

Fruit and vegetables: five a day!
Eat 600g, combining different types and colours, half of them raw.

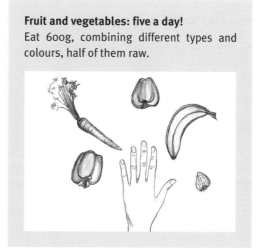

Carbohydrates – the Body's Energy Supply

A lot of food contains carbohydrates, from bread and pasta to fruit and vegetables. Glucose, one of the smallest carbohydrate molecules, is the only nutrition source for the brain. Compared to burning protein or fat the body requires much less oxygen when converting glucose into energy. This makes carbohydrates the most important and most easily accessible energy source for the body.

Carbohydrates exist as single molecules (*monosaccharides*), such as fructose or glucose. In *disaccharides*, two molecules combine, such as with sucrose – our everyday sugar – or lactose – the sugar found in milk. *Polysaccharides* consist of long chains of sugar molecules. In order to make these complex carbohydrates accessible for the body and allowing their transfer to the blood, they first have to be broken down into their smallest molecules. This takes time, and time is what leads to an important difference.

When we eat potatoes or wholegrain foods, before we can digest them, these complex carbohydrates first have to be peeled out of the dietary fibre and then broken down into single sugar molecules. These sugar molecules are released into the blood one at a time, so that the rise of the blood sugar level is slow. With many foods of modern civilization the mechanism is different. As soon as we have eaten sugar or white flour, or had a drink of lemonade, immediately the sugar molecules are released into the blood raising the blood sugar level rapidly. This puts a strain on the body, as one of its primarily goals is to level out the blood sugar. Being swamped with sugar molecules causes large quantities of insulin, which is the key hormone for the regulation of blood sugar, to be released. This has several undesirable consequences. Insulin speeds up the process of storing sugar in fat cells, thereby isolating this glucose from further metabolic utilization. Furthermore, the high concentration of insulin makes the blood sugar drop down rapidly. When blood sugar falls below its initial level, the body reacts in getting hungry again – and so a vicious circle begins.

The **glycaemic index** represents the effect of different foods on blood sugar levels.
- A *high glycaemic index* indicates that the carbohydrates in this food are digested quickly and also quickly released into the blood. This makes blood sugar level and insulin level skyrocket.
- Foods with a *low glycaemic index* are slowly and consistently released into the blood. Blood sugar level and insulin level rise evenly; the body is supplied with energy steadily over a long period of time.

Why carbohydrates are vital for dancers

Carbohydrates are the most important energy source for strenuous activities of relatively short duration – as in dance. The body is able to store carbohydrates in the form of glycogen, but the quantity of the storage is limited. Up to 300g of glycogen can be stored in the musculature, and up to 100g in the liver. The amount of glycogen the body can store is sufficient for about 90 minutes of dance, after which the reserves are exhausted. Clearly, therefore, it would be good to increase this storage capacity. This can be achieved through optimal coordination of training and eating. The normal rate of replenishment for the glycogen stored in the muscles is approximately five per cent per hour. This means that it takes at

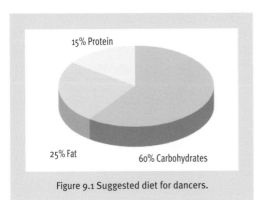

Figure 9.1 Suggested diet for dancers.

Advice for the dancer's diet – carbohydrates:

- By eating high-fibre, complex carbohydrates such as pasta, rice or potatoes, as well as fruit and vegetables you can level out your blood sugar throughout the whole day.
- Never start training when you are hungry! Carbohydrates with a low glycaemic index are slowly metabolized and are therefore an ideal energy source for physical activity. Wholegrain bread, pasta, potatoes, vegetables or muesli, eaten three to four hours before training, supply the body with the required energy.
- Refined sugar as found in energy bars, chocolate and sweets should never replace a balanced, carbohydrate-rich meal before intensive training.
- Abstain from eating food with a high glycaemic index for at least one hour before intensive training! Eating a chocolate bar shortly before training or during rehearsals leads to a rapid rise in blood sugar level to begin with, but the corresponding release of insulin causes the blood sugar to fall just as quickly again. Tiredness, lack of concentration and coordination problems are the undesirable consequences, increasing the risk of injury.
- To replenish muscle energy reserves, eat carbohydrates within the first two hours after training. This increases your glycogen stores. It need not be a fancy pasta dish: even a fruit juice diluted with water contains carbohydrates and therefore contributes to the replenishment of the glycogen store while simultaneously compensating for the electrolytes lost through perspiration.
- Sixty per cent of your total diet should consist of carbohydrates.

least 20 hours for the stores to be replenished. However, eating carbohydrate-rich food within the two hours immediately after training can speed up this process by a factor of five, so that the muscle glycogen store can be filled up to half within just two hours. Furthermore, the rapid supply of carbohydrates leads to overcompensation: the stores are enlarged and their glycogen-storage capacity can be doubled.

Problems begin when the ingested or stored carbohydrates can no longer keep the blood sugar constant. Hypoglycaemia sets in. Concentration drops and the knees become wobbly. Some people break into a sweat, feel dizzy or develop circulatatory problems, increasing the risk of injury. Initially, a simple sugar cube will help to raise the blood sugar level. But beware: large quantities of quickly metabolized glucose – such as dextrose or energy bars – can soon lead to the next blood sugar crash. Complex carbohydrates prevent this from happening.

Fat – Unloved but Necessary

Fat has a bad reputation, and not just among dancers. Fat causes arteriosclerosis (hardening of the arteries), heart attacks and strokes, as well as disfiguring the body in the form of big bottoms and beer bellies. The aesthetic of the slim dancer seems to exclude the presence of fat. And yet fat is vital: the body uses it to build up hormones, cushion the inner organs (see Chapter 1, p. 8), keep cell membranes and the skin supple, protect the nerves, isolate the body against the cold and store fat-soluble vitamins and hormones. The fat consumed as part of one's diet is either burned immediately for energy, or stored in fat deposits to create energy reserves. While just about 400g of carbohydrates can be stored in the body, the storage capacity for fat is almost unlimited. Depending upon one's age, the proportion of bodyfat in women should be between 19 and 27 per cent, and between 11 and 20 per cent in men.

According to their chemical structure, we distinguish between two types of fatty acids: saturated and unsaturated. *Saturated fatty acids,* in other words fatty acids with no double bonds between carbon atoms, are virtually un-reactive because of their chemical structure. They are primarily found in animal products such as egg yolk, butter, uncooked ham and cheese. Although coconut oil and palm oil are vegetable fats, they too consist mainly of saturated fatty acids. These oils are the exception to the rule, as most other vegetable oils are famous specifically for their large content of unsaturated fatty acids. *Unsaturated fatty acids* contain one or more double bonds between carbon atoms, and are much more reactive. Olive oil is a well-known example: it consists of 76 per cent mono-unsaturated oleic acid, which has a considerable protective effect on blood. Polyunsaturated fatty acids cannot be built up by the body itself and therefore have to be consumed with one's diet. These polyunsaturated, *essential fatty acids* are found in nuts and vegetable oils, particularly in soy oil, thistle oil and rapeseed oil, as well as in numerous saltwater fish such as mackerel, salmon and sardines, for example.

The composition of the fats, the ratio of saturated to unsaturated fatty acids, determines their effect on the body and dictates whether they are healthy or unhealthy. The higher the proportion of unsaturated fatty acids, the better they are in terms of health. This is because unsaturated fatty acids lower the blood fat, support the immune system and inhibit inflammatory reactions in the body. They also improve blood flow and thus guard against the dreaded sediments in the walls of the blood vessels.

Why fat is vital for dancers

Fat is the most energy-rich of all food. Without fat, the body's energy metabolism grinds to a halt. When the body works over a long period of time at a lower intensity level, fat is used as the principal source of energy. Long-distance runners are a typical example. Their bodies have learned to increase their fat metabolism thus preserving their glycogen reserves. This allows to remain fit and concentrated even throughout long periods of physical exercise. This intelligent principle is certainly worthy of imitation by dancers. But fat has yet more advantages: unsaturated fat inhibits inflammatory processes in the body and supports the metabolism during regeneration. And it is important to remember that fat is the basic element and storage organ for oestrogen, the female sex hormone, and this in turn is mainly responsible for the bone structure. Only with sufficient body fat can good bone stability and resilience be achieved.

Advice for the dancer's diet – fat:
- Wherever possible, avoid saturated fats and increase your intake of unsaturated fats. Reduce animal fats as these contain large quantities of saturated fatty acids. Choose vegetable fats as they are rich in unsaturated fatty acids.
- Avoid convenience food such as ready-meals, soups and sauces! They can contain a great amount of particularly unhealthy saturated fats.
- Eat fish regularly. Saltwater fish have a large proportion of unsaturated fats and therefore have a positive effect on your health.
- Use cold-pressed oils as the gentle extraction methods do not damage the unsaturated fatty acids.
- Because of its composition rapeseed oil, an essential fatty acid, is particularly highly recommended. It is tasty and easily digested and is also suitable for cooking in a frying pan.
- Fats can make up to 25 per cent of your diet. But beware: not all fats are easily identified. Look out for hidden fats in foods such as nuts, energy bars and chocolate.

Protein – the Body's Building Material

Bones and joints, enzymes and hormones, muscles and blood, the immune system and even serotonin, the "happiness hormone", are all composed of protein. Its importance for the body is even part of its very name: "protein" is Greek and means "that which is most important". The body constantly uses up proteins. During the course of each training session, muscle cells are destroyed; blood cells, enzymes and the immune system work at full speed. Repair and modification processes exact a high price: every day the body loses up to 100g of protein and this protein has to be replaced through food. The normal daily requirement of a dancer is 1–1.4g of protein per kilogram of body weight. This quantity is necessary to ensure replacement of lost cells and rapid regeneration. If the body lacks protein, this will have far-reaching consequences. Body and mind switch down into a "standby" mode; the bones become instable, the muscles weaken, the immune system slows down and even the psyche suffers. Weakness, vulnerability to injury and a bad mood do not create the ideal conditions for dancing.

In addition to quantity, the quality of the protein is also significant for health. Every protein consists of a large number of individual elements known as *amino acids*. Up to several thousand amino acids can be involved in the formation of a single protein molecule; the composition determines its value to the body. Thereby it is of great importance how readily the body can build up its own material from the protein consumed. Twenty different amino acids are used in the construction of human proteins. Some of these can be produced by the body itself, but ten of them have to be consumed within the food. These are known as *essential amino acids*. They determine the quality of the protein.

Protein is classed as complete or of high biological value, if it is rich in essential amino acids. Animal protein – such as meat, fish, eggs, milk or milk products – contains all of the essential amino acids and is therefore considered to be particularly nutritious. Vegetable protein –

contained in pulses such as soy beans, beans and peas, in nuts and sprouts, but also in grains, potatoes and rice – does not contain all of the essential amino acids. While it is possible to consume all of the important amino acids with an entirely animal-product-free diet, it does require careful planning. The safest way to ensure the supply of complete proteins is through a mixed diet, in other words one that includes animal and vegetable protein. Clever combinations allow us to further improve the efficacy of the proteins we consume. Potatoes with egg, wheat with beans or the popular combination of muesli with milk provide the body with an ideal cocktail of essential amino acids.

Why protein is vital for dancers

Proteins act as building materials for the body and are therefore of great importance for rapid regeneration and for optimizing the metabolism. In contrast to carbohydrates, which are responsible for the supply of energy before and during physical exercise, proteins are particularly important after intense training. A dancer weighing 52kg should eat at least 52g of protein a day. To give an idea of this: 10g of protein are contained in 0.3l of milk, 50g of mozzarella, 50g of veal fillet or 50g of beans. In contrast to carbohydrates and fat, protein cannot be stored in the body long term, making a daily supply even more important.

Proteins act as transport vehicles, taking on important courier services in the body: the protein haemoglobin is responsible for the transportation of oxygen in the blood, while the protein transferrin carries iron. Physical exercise is not possible without these transport systems. An adequate supply of protein during periods of intense training or when injured is therefore essential.

Vitamins, Minerals etc.

Vitamins, phytochemicals, minerals and trace elements are what are called vital nutrients: although they do not supply the body with energy, they are of central importance for cell growth, regenerative and healing processes. A sufficient

Advice for the dancer's diet – protein:

- As a dancer, you require more protein than the average person! Always remember: it is impossible to dance without sufficient protein.
- After an exhausting training session sufficient protein intake is essential for rapid regeneration.
- The body cannot make use of too much protein consumed in one go. Eat small quantities several times a day. Buttermilk, kefir, cottage cheese or yoghurt with fruit, a piece of poultry or fish will replenish your protein store.
- Mix different types of protein into your daily menu. Combinations always provide more benefits than their individual components.
- Drink plenty of liquid so that the waste products of the protein metabolism can be flushed out thoroughly.
- Be sure to get an adequate protein supply during periods of intense training and when suffering from chronic inflammation.
- Fifteen per cent of your total diet should consist of protein.

protein structures and can cause considerable damage if not kept in check: free radicals cause degenerative processes in the body's cells – oxidation processes that can destroy cell particles and entire body cells. Every cell is exposed to around 100,000 attacks by free radicals per day. But natural antioxidants like Vitamin A, C and E can bind free radicals, neutralize and remove them.

There are two categories of vitamins, based on their solubility: those that are soluble in water and those that are soluble in fat. Water-soluble vitamins – such as Vitamin B and C and folic acid – can be absorbed easily by the body, and any excess is expelled through the kidneys. Fat-soluble vitamins include Vitamin E, D, K and A. These can be stored in the body. This can lead to overdoses, especially through haphazard intake of vitamin supplements. In most cases, a balanced diet can meet the body's vitamin requirements without additional supplements. However, through exposure to light, or by long periods of storage or by cooking, the vitamin content of fruit and vegetables is greatly reduced. Fruit that has been frozen with care immediately after being harvested can therefore be healthier than "fresh" fruit that has been stored for long periods or transported long distances.

quantity of these vital nutrients is necessary to ensure that we are fit, wide awake and able to concentrate, have a stable immune system, shiny hair, healthy teeth and nice skin.

Vitamins and phytochemicals

Vitamins and phytochemicals are produced by micro-organisms and plants. For humans, the main sources of these are fruit and vegetables. Scientists have identified 13 vitamins, most of which have to be taken in with food. In addition to their role in metabolism, the immune system and cell division, vitamins are responsible for protecting the body against free radicals. Free radicals attack the body's immune cells and

Minerals and trace elements

Minerals and trace elements are involved in the formation of teeth and bones; they are to be found in proteins and hormones, play a role in metabolism and energy production and support the functioning of nerves and muscles. Through daily nutrition the body has to be supplied with 23 different minerals. Depending on the quantities needed by the body, we refer to these either as minerals, of which the body needs a few grams, or as trace elements, of which only the tiniest amounts are required. The body constantly loses minerals and trace elements through digestion, urination and sweating. This loss has to be compensated for through diet.

Advice for the dancer's diet – vitamins, minerals, trace elements:

- Buy the freshest fruit and vegetables available and use them while still fresh. Long storage periods reduce vitamin and nutrient content considerably.
- Short transportation routes and careful storage retain the vitamin content of fruit and vegetables. Therefore choose local products whenever possible.
- Trimmed and chopped vegetables such as peppers, carrots and kohlrabi make for appetizing little snacks between meals.
- Cook vegetables gently, for example, by braising them with only a small amount of fat.
- A glass of fruit or vegetable juice is tasty and supplies valuable nutrients.

Sodium, chloride and **potassium** are responsible for the electrical excitability of muscle cells. Increased loss of these elements during long and intensive training sessions can lead to disruptions in muscle contraction, from muscle weakness to muscle cramps. The loss of salt (NaCl) through sweating is particularly high. Up to three grams of salt per litre of sweat can be lost! This must be compensated. Dancers who sweat a lot can need up to 20g of salt a day to replace their loss, roughly four times as much as non-athletes. Potassium loss can be balanced by eating the famously potassium-rich banana.

As an activator of a variety of enzyme systems, **magnesium** plays an important role in metabolism and is also of central importance for the electric stimulation within the nervous systems. Magnesium deficiency can lead to muscle cramps and muscle ache. Pulses, seeds, vegetables and fruits are natural magnesium suppliers.

Iron is important for blood production. If iron levels drops, as can happen as a result of exhausting physical activity, blood production is reduced. This, in turn, reduces physical performance. Compensating for this by way of an iron-rich diet, for example meat or white beans, is important.

Calcium and **phosphorus** are needed to build up bone. Calcium deficiency results in a loss of bone mass, known as osteoporosis (see Chapter 11, p. 209).

Drinking – the Body's Source of Water

Water is the most important elixir of life for humans. Without water, there will be no blood circulation, no metabolism, no regulation of body temperature – no life. Water constitutes the largest part of our human body. Depending on age, gender and state of training, it consists of up to 80 per cent water. A healthy fluid balance is vitally important, and not just when it comes to training. Loss of water – and thus also of minerals – not only decreases the body's ability to regulate its temperature; it also strains the circulation and leads to rapid exhaustion with all that this implies. The body loses water via a variety of channels: we eliminate approximately 0.5l of urine a day through the kidneys, and the same amount of water is lost through breathing and metabolism. Sweat production during and outside of training add to this total.

One can counteract the process of dehydration by drinking sensibly. This reduces physical stress, maintains performance potential and accelerates regeneration – advantages that dancers should certainly make use of.

Perspiration – an intelligent cooling system for the body

Muscles heat up during training: almost two-thirds of the energy expended on muscle performance is lost in the form of heat. In order not to let the body overheat, an intelligent cooling system is required: sweating. Water is transported from the centre of the body to the warm muscles and from there to the skin's small blood vessels. Together with minerals and waste products, it is released through the skin in the form of sweat. On the surface of the skin it evaporates thus achieving the desired cooling effect; the body's temperature decreases. A fine layer of minerals remains behind, which is responsible for the salty taste of sweaty skin.

It is not possible to prevent the body from sweating. On the contrary: the better one's physical condition, the better the discharge of heat from inside the body to the surface of the skin. The cooling process through sweating starts earlier and the sweat rate is increased. People who do not train on a regular base can produce approximately 0.8l of sweat per hour, whereas those who are well trained can sweat as much as 3l per hour! Concentration, amount and composition of sweat are also dependent on the temperature of one's surroundings, the humidity and the diet, and of course on the length of the training session.

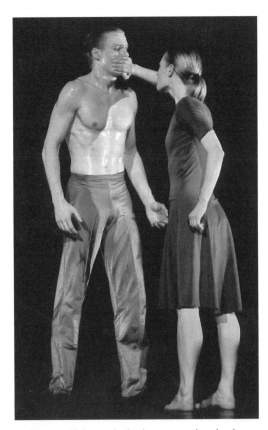

Figure 9.2 High perspiration is common when dancing.

Dehydration is Unhealthy

If the body is dehydrated, this has consequences for the amount and composition of the blood. Water deficiency thickens the blood thus decreasing circulation in the small and smallest blood vessels. The important transport of oxygen and nutrients to the muscles and organs gets delayed, and the elimination of waste and metabolic products slows down. Muscle cramps, circulation problems, lack of concentration, trouble with coordination, headaches, dizziness and even vomiting are possible consequences. Already a water deficiency of as little as 1–2 per cent of body weight can reduce mental performance. The brain reacts particularly sensitively: concentration problems and a reduced reaction speed are the first symptoms of dehydration. Energy metabolism in bodily cells, too, is impaired. This results in an early onset of metabolic acidosis and exhaustion of the muscles. A water deficiency of about 6 per cent or more leads to a strong feeling of thirst, irritability, weakness and exhaustion. Motor coordination is affected. Through perspiration, the body loses not only fluid, but precious minerals as well. Typical symptoms of mineral deficiencies such as muscle weakness and muscle cramps develop.

What and When to Drink

A healthy water balance before you start is a prerequisite for any dance-related activity. This means you should never start training while you feel thirsty!

When training for less than 60 minutes, it is fine to wait until the end to compensate for the lost fluid. If training lasts longer, one should start drinking during the training session. This is necessary in order to maintain concentration, physical performance and coordination throughout the entire dance class.

Isotonic drinks (drinks that feature a particle concentration similar to that found in blood, e.g. isotonic sports drinks) and *hypotonic* drinks (drinks that have a slightly lower particle concentration than blood, e.g. juice diluted with water) are suitable for the rapid replenishment of fluids. *Hypertonic* drinks (drinks that have a slightly higher particle concentration than blood), on the other hand, are not recommended.

How much liquid do you need?

A simple weight method can be used to calculate one's personal fluid-intake requirement during training: weigh yourself *before* and *after* physical activity, always wearing dry clothes and with an empty bladder.

Fluid-intake requirement during physical activity		weight before training		weight after training
	=		−	

What you drink during training should:

- compensate for the loss of fluid due to perspiration;
- replace the minerals and trace elements lost through sweating;
- supply energy in the form of carbohydrates for periods of activity longer than 60 minutes;
- be quickly re-absorbable;
- taste good and refreshing.

Table 9.1 Properties of various drinks

Drink	Fluid replacement	Energy replacement	Electrolyte replacement
Juice diluted with water	+	+	+
Fruit tea or herbal tea	+	−	+
Mineral water	+	−	+
Lemonade/coke	−	+	−
Milk	−	+	+
Undiluted fruit juice/vegetable juice	−	+	+

Advice on fluid-intake

- Thirst is a bad indicator when training. It develops only when fluid is already lacking. So drink before you feel thirsty!
- Small quantities of liquid consumed frequently throughout the day or during training are better than few large ones. Every training session should start with a healthy fluid balance!
- Slightly hypotonic drinks are best for the quick compensation of water and energy loss during training. The well-known mixture of water and juice (three to five parts water to one part juice) is easy and inexpensive. It provides adequate fluid replacement and quick-release energy, minerals and trace elements.
- No fizzy drinks before or during training! Carbon dioxide expands the stomach slightly, which can be undesirable during training. In addition, fizzy drinks are only absorbed with delay.
- Slightly chilled drinks (5–10°) have a stimulating effect on fluid absorption. In low temperatures, warm drinks like fruit teas and herbal teas are highly recommended.
- Drink liquids rich in carbohydrates (for example, juice diluted with water) as soon as possible after training. This will replenish your glycogen stores.

- Undiluted fruit juices, sugary coke drinks, "energy drinks" and lemonades delay fluid absorption. They are unsuitable as sports drinks. Coffee and alcohol, too, are inappropriate for the replenishment of fluids.

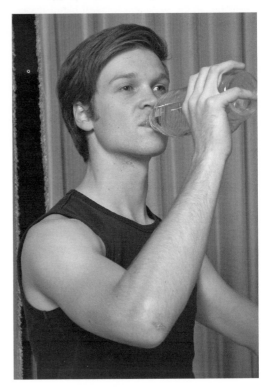

Figure 9.3 Drinking is important.

Eating Disorders – it's all about Weight

Dancers are slim, very slim. The idealized image of the well-proportioned, elf-like dancer is anchored in the minds of many people. In order to live up to this ideal, young women in particular often set out on a wide variety of diets, up to and including going without food. Whether it is due to external pressures or a personal ambition to "look like a dancer", the result is the same. In order to achieve their "ideal" weight, many resort to unhealthy methods. The consequence is the very opposite of the desired: they do not become successful dancers with dream figures, but extremely skinny women, weak, tired and frequently injured.

The figures are frightening: up to 35 per cent of all professional dance students and dancers suffer from eating disorders, with women making up the majority. One-third have a body mass index below 17 kg/m², and more than half of all female dancers do not menstruate regularly; 13 per cent make repeated use of laxatives and two-thirds worry about their weight. The relationship to food is a cause for concern in the world of dance. This has to change.

Supply and Demand – Energy Balance Determines Body Weight

The daily energy requirement, for everyone, is the sum of two factors: the basal metabolic rate and the active metabolic rate. The *basal metabolic rate* refers to the energy needed every day for vital bodily functions, excluding any physical exertion. In addition, there is the *active metabolic rate*, which is the extra energy that is needed for physical activity. Depending on the intensity and the dancer's age, gender and physical condition, one hour of dance burns between 250 and 600kcal. If the quantity of energy consumed by one's diet corresponds to the energy required, body weight will remain constant: input and output are balanced.

Body Mass Index (BMI) serves as a measure for assessing body weight. In general it does not take account of age, gender or body composition, so it should only be used as a rough guide. A person with a BMI lower than 18 is considered to be underweight while somebody with a BMI above 24 is considered overweight.

$$BMI = \frac{\text{body weight in kg}}{(\text{body height in m})^2}$$

Types of Eating Disorders

Anorexia nervosa (or "anorexia") and *bulimia nervosa* (or "bulimia") are typical eating disorders that are particularly prevalent among girls and young women. As psychosomatic disorders they must be taken seriously and require psychological treatment. Advice on nutrition alone is certainly not sufficient. The difficulties experienced by those affected are not the result of insufficient

---

Warning signals that might indicate an eating disorder:

- Body Mass Index ≤ 17.5 kg/m²;
- Self-induced weight-loss beyond the target weight;
- Unhealthily distorted self-awareness (perceiving one's body shape to be "too fat" despite being extremely slim);
- Absence of menstruation ;
- Excessive physical activity;
- Withdrawal from social contact ;
- Weighing frequently;
- Eating secretly and/or feeling guilty while eating;
- Concentration on "feeding" others;
- Almost everything revolves around the subject of food;
- Repeated vomiting after eating;
- Regular use of laxatives.

knowledge about the basics of nutrition, but are mainly rooted in their attitude to their own body weight and to their own bodies in general.

Anorexia athletica is a special form of eating disorder that arises in the worlds of dance and sports. In contrast to "common" anorexia and bulimia, it is not categorized as a psychosomatic disorder. Weight-loss is managed – at least at the beginning – in a controlled manner and with the sole aim of improving one's performance and increasing one's odds on the dance market. Physical performance can remain unaffected for a long time despite very low body weight. But be careful: anorexia athletica can easily tip over into a defined eating disorder at any time!

Physiological Consequences

In addition to mental and emotional changes, a lack of adequate nutrient supply for energy and repair puts a great strain on the body. All metabolic processes are reduced to a minimum – switching to katabolic metabolism, which involves removing material instead of building it up – effectively, the body shuts down and energy levels sink close to zero. Even after successful treatment, the physiological consequences remain visible for years to come.

The reduced supply of nutrients leads to a decrease in the quality of bone composition. In order to cover the body's needs, minerals are even drawn out of the bone. The bones become "thin" and susceptible to stress fractures, while the risk of osteoporosis increases (see Chapter 11, p. 209). Extreme weight-loss leads to a lack of oestrogen,

Consequences for dancers:
Dance alone is not responsible for the fact that eating disorders are more common among dancers than in the general population. And yet some practices in the world of dance should be scrutinized when considering the prevention of eating disorders:
- Dancers weighing themselves daily at home or – worse still – being weighed in front of the group;
- Weight reduction through excessive sweating with insufficient fluid intake, including the use of "sauna trousers" or plastic wrap;
- Going to the sauna without compensating for the fluid lost through perspiration;
- Sanctions if a dancer's weight increases (for example, losing a dance role);
- Commenting on one's body and weight in front of others;
- "Hushing up" the eating disorder.

reflected in irregular or totally absent menstruation. The oestrogen deficiency increases the risk of osteoporosis yet further. Heartbeat and breathing rhythm become slower and blood pressure drops. Sufferers frequently feel cold, dizzy, sick and may even experience a circulatory collapse. The consequences of the imbalance in body minerals are muscle injuries and cardiac arrhythmias, this just being a small selection of the possible physiological consequences.

10. Dance and Growth

Dancing is popular among children and teenagers. Television dance shows are responsible for fully booked jazz and street dance classes; school dance programmes familiarize children with artistic dance; and hip hop lures even cool guys into the dance studio. All dance styles have one thing in common: they train children in multifaceted variations and make use of their natural urge to move. This is of great value, especially in times of increasing immobility.

The fact that somebody is a good dancer does not automatically make him or her a responsible dance teacher. Adapting training to the various needs of the individual age groups and adjusting dance techniques that are often developed not for children's but for adults' bodies, requires more than just pedagogical skills. It also calls for well-founded knowledge about the developmental stages of childhood, about the changes that every one has to go through on their journey from baby to adult.

> "The child is not a smaller version of the adult." (*Josef Huwyler*)

Compared to adults, children are subject to quite different constraints, from the physical to the mental and the physiological. The bodily changes are clearly visible. They demand a great deal from children in everyday life, and even more so when it comes to dancing: as the body develops and the proportions change, skills that have been acquired do not simply persist but have to be continuously rediscovered.

The Basics of Growth

Basic knowledge about the psycho-physical characteristics of growth helps dance teachers to understand children's development, and to adapt dance training to the requirements of the individual age groups.

Growth Takes Place in the Bones

Most bones of the human body are formed through *endochondral ossification*: hyaline cartilage is converted into bone tissue, and the parts of the skeleton initially formed by cartilage are replaced by bone substance. The infant's soft, flexible framework of cartilage is transformed into the stable and resilient bone skeleton of an adult.

Growth is primarily the result of a lengthening of the long bones. At the ends of the long bones, at the contact between epiphysis and diaphysis (see Chapter 1, p. 10), one can find the epiphyseal plates. This is where growth takes place. When the body is growing, cell division occurs at an increased rate within the epiphyseal plates, which thereby becomes thicker. The more active the cell division, the thicker the epiphyseal plate, and the more sensitively it reacts to shearing forces and torsion. Strain and overload can deeply damage the epiphyseal plate, thus hindering further growth. Therefore, particularly during periods of rapid growth great care must be taken to avoid any damages to the epiphyseal plates. Application of external pressure, whether by the dance teacher or by a friend who attempts to "bend something into place", is particularly dangerous. Lengthening has been completed when the epiphyseal plates are closed. This usually occurs between the ages of 18 and 21, and generally happens earlier in girls than in boys.

The **thickening** of the bone takes place at the diaphysis. Bone substance is stored directly underneath the periosteum, while the bone tissue inside the medullary cavity is eroded; the diameter of the diaphysis increases.

Growth Happens in Spurts

From birth to adulthood children grow slowly and continuously, with decreasing speed; but there are two exceptions: the two growth spurts. The first growth spurt takes place at the age of about six to eight years, and the second during puberty. In its development from a baby to an adult, the human body goes through considerable changes in size: while the circumference of the head doubles, the length of the torso triples and the legs even become five times as long. This changes the proportions and influences balance; both have an impact on dance.

The timing of the growth within the individual body parts varies considerably, but follows this general rule:

> **Growth of the body as a whole:**
> The body grows from the outside in – from the periphery to the centre.

- First, the hands and feet begin to grow. Most people are familiar with the image of the small boy with enormous feet. Pointing the feet or placing the hands in optimal alignment with the lower arm becomes increasingly difficult for young dancers during growth spurts.
- The growth of the arms and legs follows. Hands and feet become more and more distant from the centre of the body. This influences coordination: rapid foot and leg movement are particularly difficult at this time.

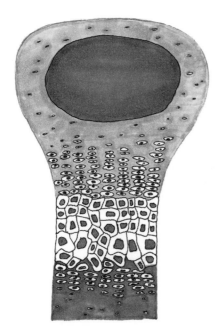

Figure 10.1 Lengthening takes place in the epiphyseal plate.

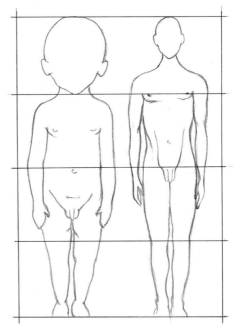

Figure 10.2 Development from newborn to adult: change of proportions.

- Changes to the pelvis are next. In boys, this is accompanied by a broadening of the chest and shoulder girdle.
- The lengthening of the spine marks the final stage of growth.

Young dancers are usually divided into dance classes according to age. This corresponds to the children's psychological development and range of experience, although calendar age does not actually reflect the maturity of the body. *Biological age* is crucial to performance development and to the capacity to deal with stress when it comes to dancing. It can greatly diverge from chronological age. Through X-ray examination of the carpal bones in the hand, biological age can be determined to within one month. Research shows, that there can be a difference of up to five years from the biologically youngest to the biologically oldest of the same chronological age. This is one cause for the major differences in performance within a given age group. Be aware that body size alone does not indicate the biological age.

Table 10.1 The developmental stages relevant to dancing

Developmental stage	Calendar age (in years)
Preschool age	3 – 6/7
Young school-age	6/7 – 10
Older school-age	10 – beginning of puberty girls: 11/12, boys: 12/13
Puberty Pubescence (first pubertal phase)	girls 11/12 – 13/14 boys 12/13 – 14/15
Adolescence (second pubertal phase)	girls 13/14 – 17/18 boys 14/15 – 18/19
Adulthood	beyond the ages of 17/18 respectively 18/19

Every Age is Different

The classification of the five developmental stages is a helpful reference for dance teachers; it is not a rigid set of rules. The transition between the individual developmental stages is fluid and subject to considerable variation.

Preschool age
Preschool age covers the period between age three and the start of the first school year at the age of around six or seven. This age group is characterized by a great urge for movement and play, by curiosity about everything unfamiliar, by powerful imagination and a strong willingness to learn. The driving forces in the brain outweigh the inhibition, which can easily be seen by the lack of concentration ability within this age group. Towards the end of the preschool age the first growth spurt takes place. The increase in length gradually alters the infant proportions.

Consequences for dance training:
Interest in and joy of exploring are the primary characteristics of this phase. Movement stories and space to independently solve movement tasks support motor skills and body creativity and encourage self-awareness, as well as expanding the range of movement.

Young school-age
The first years of school up to age 10 represent an excellent time for the learning of new skills. This is due to children's increased ability to concentrate, the refinement of their motor skills and coordination, and their greater understanding of movement instructions and correction. New movement sequences are learned quickly, but cannot yet be reproduced in a reliable manner.

Consequences for dance training:
Training focuses on the improvement of coordination skills and the expansion of the movement repertoire. A multifaceted movement routine allows the dancing child to learn the basic skills and selectively refine them. Frequent repetition is important, thus firmly integrating newly learned skills into the movement repertoire.

Older school-age

The period between the age of ten and the onset of puberty is also referred to as the "golden age of learning". Physical proportions become optimized. While height and weight increase only marginally children become progressively stronger, which can lead to exceptional body control. By the age of around ten, the sense of equilibrium and the body's proprioceptive system are almost fully mature. With a high level of motivation and a continued love of physical activity, this is a key phase for learning movement.

Consequences for dance training:
Age-appropriate training and specific dance technique training should be combined. Now it is of special importance to avoid the automatization of "incorrect" movement patterns as their correction at a later age gets more and more difficult.

Pubescence (First Pubertal Phase)

Pubescence, the second growth spurt, starts from the age of 11 to 12 in girls, and the age of 12 to 13 in boys. It is the time of great changes, both physical and mental. This is when the most height is gained. Increases in height of up to 10cm and weight gain of up to 9kg a year are not unusual. In boys, muscle diameter expands. The young dancers' proportions – and, as a result, their coordination, too – are thoroughly shaken up. This interferes with the harmony of movement, and fine coordination is lost. Complex movement sequences that appeared to be securely learned become shaky, and steps that make high demands on coordination skills become difficult to learn.

Consequences for dance training:
To help the young dancers to keep their enthusiasm for dance, support and individual coaching is now especially important. Adding new, unfamiliar dance styles can help to maintain their love for dancing, and to improve their body awareness, not to mention expanding their horizons as dancers.

Adolescence (Second Pubertal Phase)

Adolescence constitutes the end of the development from childhood to adulthood. The annual increase in height slows down and the body becomes more solid. The sexual hormones induce the epiphyseal plates to close up. The proportions are harmonized as the body converts into a typical adult's shape. This improves coordination skills. The increase in strength and the brain's high storage capacity for movement patterns create the ideal conditions for the further improvement as a dancer. Stamina and coordination are equally receptive to training. Following the phase of older school-age children, adolescence is the second period that allows great improvement of performance.

Consequences for dance training:
Balanced physical proportions, stabilization of the personality and improved observation skills make this phase the second "golden age of learning". A high degree of psycho-physical stamina combined with a still great plasticity of the nervous system allow for comprehensive and intensive exercise. Even the most difficult of movements are learned quickly and retained easily.

Specialities in Growth

During growth metabolism plays an important role. The adolescent body needs sufficient vitamins, minerals and nutrients for the intensive growth processes; the body's basal metabolic rate increases. If, due to comprehensive and intensive training energy metabolism increases too, things can get tight. If the necessary nutrients are missing, growth processes are shelved. The discrepancy between food supply and nutritional demands not only reduces physical stamina, and increases the risk of a stress fracture. It can also considerably disturb a child's entire physical development. A balanced diet (see Chapter 9, p. 179) and sufficient rest periods (see Chapter 12, p. 234) are therefore essential to the health of young dancers.

Compared to adults, the percentage of fluid in total body weight is higher in children's bodies. Therefore, they are much more vulnerable to dehydration. Even a small degree of dehydration can cause loss of concentration, headaches, muscle cramps and a general reduction in physical performance. Sufficient drinking before and during the dance class is therefore an important element of healthy training especially for young dancers.

Particular care must be taken with:

Bones: The resilience of bones to being bent and torn is low until approximately ten years of age. Bone fractures are therefore not rare in children. Compared to the bone itself the periosteum is flexible and elastic, just like the green bark of a young tree. When the bone breaks, this can lead to a particular kind of infantile bone fracture, the so called "greenstick fracture": the bone itself is broken, while the surrounding periosteum remains intact.

Cartilage: In young children, joint cartilage can regenerate to a small degree. This ability is lost with puberty. Then, overload to the joints can lead to lasting cartilage damage.

Ligament system: During growth spurt the ligamental system around the joints and the epiphyseal plates is elongated and loosened up. Forced movements, such as uncoordinated strength training using weights or an exaggerated turnout, can result in considerable damage. For boys, partner work often starts in the middle of their second growth spurt. This can cause back problems. Therefore do not work on lifts until the trunk is sufficiently stable!

All in Good Time – What Can be Trained, and When?

Dance is more than the playfully energetic movement enjoyed by children. The complex movement sequences of dance, both demand and train the physical fitness components of flexibility, coordination, strength and stamina to varying degrees, depending on the type of dance.

Flexibility

The younger the dancer, the greater their flexibility. General flexibility is already reduced by the first few years of primary school; the increasing stiffness of the capsular ligaments constitutes a natural limitation to movement. While this protects the joints, it simultaneously reduces the range of motion and, particularly during growth spurts, can lead to muscular imbalances. Therefore, one aim of dance training during growth is to preserve flexibility and the earlier the better. There is a wide range of different methods (see Chapter 12, p. 215), but as a general rule: the younger the dancer, the more care should be taken in partner exercises. Children's enthusiasm can easily lead to overstretching and, as a result, to injury. During the second growth spurt the reduction in flexibility is particularly noticeable. The reason is to be found in the timing of growth. Bone and muscle usually grow at different speeds: bone first, followed by the surrounding muscle tissue. The relative muscle shortening has unpleasant consequences: flexibility is reduced and stretching exercises that used to be easy become tortuous.

Growth of body parts in detail:
The body grows from the inside out: first bone, then muscle.

Flexibility training during growth:
- Until the age of approximately ten, favour active stretching methods.
- In order to preserve the range of motion, specific flexibility training should be introduced starting with the older school-age children.
- To avoid local instability, do not go for exaggerated flexibility training.

Coordination

Coordination in dance not only refers to the optimization of movement sequences and the economization of muscle use; dancing also improves the coordinated reaction to acoustical, optical and tactile stimuli, as well as increasing spatial awareness, balance and sense of rhythm. Until young school-age the systems of body awareness are not fully developed. Movements are imprecise, and spatial and temporal execution cannot be reliably reproduced. New movement patterns are easily blurred and therefore have to be repeated frequently. Older school-age is considered the period of maturation of the motor skills. Coordination abilities rapidly increase and muscle work becomes more economical. The second growth spurt often leads to a slump in coordination. Balances and pirouettes, for example, can become extremely challenging due to the change in body proportions and growth-related muscle imbalances. But there is at least a thin silver lining: simple sequences of movements that have been practised regularly and are firmly entrenched remain, even during this period of change.

Coordination training during growth:

- It is never too early to train coordination skills. Appropriate, child-friendly practice is essential: the younger the dancer, the simpler the movement repertoire!
- Coordination can be trained particularly successfully in the older school-age children.
- Good coordination also helps growth. The more economical the use of their muscles, the better prepared the young dancers are for the physical changes that occur during puberty.
- Coordination means flexibility of the brain. Therefore dance combinations should always be started from both sides, once from the right, once from the left. For advanced dancers: show the exercise on one side, and let it perform on the other.

Strength

Increased strength is a "by-product" of dancing: increased coordination and improved intramuscular and intermuscular work makes young dancers become stronger. This is not the result of an increase in muscle mass as this is not possible before puberty, before the production of testosterone, the male sexual hormone. Muscle circumference cannot increase until a sufficient concentration of testosterone is present. This applies to boys more than it does to girls, although female dancers also gain muscle during puberty. Hormone concentration, and metabolism too, makes specific strength training pointless in children. Any form of strength training, any maximum or sub-maximum strain on the muscle increases the concentration of lactic acid. In children, high levels of lactic acid increase the level of adrenaline in the body. During strength training, up to ten times as much adrenaline is released into the child's blood than would be present in that of an adult. This is stressful for the child, showing all the well-known stress symptoms.

Strength training during growth:

- Accentuated strength training during childhood is not only ineffective, but actually harmful. Strength training should only be carried out in combination with coordination. This is precisely what happens while dancing!
- Strength training outside the dance studio to increase muscle mass should only start at the end of pubescence.

Endurance

Children can romp around for a long time and with great stamina. Their metabolism is geared towards endurance: the aerobic system – the system that produces energy with the help of oxygen (see Chapter 12, p. 220) – works much more effectively in children than it does in adults. One advantage of this system is that almost no toxins are produced. This kind of energy production is effective and makes the best possible use of energy sources. The produced toxins are removed quickly, and tissue regenerates rapidly. Starting endurance training at an early age allows us to maintain these advantages into adulthood. Conventional endurance training is often boring and dull. If packed into dance, rhythm and music act as motivators. But care must be taken during puberty: some girls experience circulatory problems or even collapse as a result of excessively intensive endurance activities.

Endurance training during growth:

- Even young children's endurance metabolism can be strengthened by specific movement games. In young school children, it is the musculoskeletal system rather than the cardiovascular system that defines the limits of endurance.
- Regular endurance training should start by the age of 13 for girls, and by the age of 14 for boys.

Advice on Training During Growth

- Unnecessary stress on the epiphyseal plates and on tendon and muscle insertions is damaging to development. Children's skeletons are very flexible and therefore particularly susceptible to injury. Flexibility and range of motion should therefore not be forced by external pull or pressure.
- Joints should always be trained in all directions. One-sided training causes muscular imbalance, which can lead to excessive strain, injuries and signs of wear in the short and long term.
- Early onset of core-stability training prepares children for growth: a stable core improves the coordination of the extremities.
- In themselves, many dance styles do not constitute adequate endurance training. Additional fitness training in the form of games or prolonged choreographies is therefore essential.

Growth and Dance have an Impact on Each Other

In dance, as in sports, the course for the future career is usually set during puberty. Various factors determine whether dance will develop into a professional career, a hobby or whether all enthusiasm will fade. Physical development influences boys and girls in entirely different ways. While in boys, dance generally benefits from puberty (as their bodies become more "masculine" and their strength increases), in young female dancers the physical changes they undergo is often not seen in such a positive light. The development of breasts, the broadening of the pelvis, and the increased storage of body fat "disturbs" the image of the graceful dancer. In addition, the changed body proportions and an increase in body weight make partner work more difficult. Puberty is therefore a particularly sensitive time for many women dancers. This is when the fundamentals for their own body-image are set: whether they can accept and approve their own physical development, and use their body in a responsible way or whether they start to fight against natural changes and try to "overcome" their body. Dance teachers and schools can be central to the development of a positive body-image during this sensitive period.

Growth Can Help Young Dancers

During growth, the body undergoes a number of changes that are beneficial to dance and which facilitate the correct performance of dance technique.

Position of the pelvis

Children with a forward-tilted pelvis are often subject to correction (see Chapter 3, p. 59). It is the young dancer's biological age which helps teachers to differentiate whether the pelvis will straighten up by itself or whether incorrect dance technique might be the cause of this posture. The natural position of the pelvis changes from infancy to adulthood. In young children, the pelvis is tilted forwards, resulting in the typical sway back position. As the abdominal muscles are still weak, they allow the inner organs to protrude to the front. This visually increases the sway back posture, which is entirely age-appropriate for young children. During growth the pelvis slowly straightens up, the organs "slide back into the abdomen" and the spine elongates. Older school-age children already tend to show the pelvic position usually seen in adults. Specific correction, with the purpose to increase awareness of the pelvic position, can already be used in young children. This supports the natural development of the body.

Turnout

The external rotation of the leg increases naturally as the bones grow. The bone structure of the leg, which has a considerable impact on turnout, changes in not one but two advantageous ways: tibial torsion increases, and the anteversion angle decreases. Together, these changes improve the external rotation of the leg.

The tibia is turned inwards by about 10° at birth (see Chapter 5, p. 101). Change begins as early as the first year of life. The tibia turns gradually outwards and by the age of ten reaches its genetically determined torsion, ranging from as little as 0° to as much as 40°.

The anteversion angle (see Chapter 4, p.76) decreases as growth progresses. In infants and small children, anteversion is large, at up to 50°. Maximum inward rotation of the hip joint is not a problem at this age. Anteversion is gradually reduced during development, until during the second growth spurt it reaches its genetically determined angle. Whether and to what degree the anteversion angle can be affected by early and intensive training has not yet been conclusively shown. There are, however, recommendations for improving individual turnout in classical dance. Children between the ages of 11 to 14 should train for at least six hours a week as bone plasticity is particularly high during this time.

Challenges for Young Dancers

As beneficial as dance can be to children's development, positive aspects of dance training are often lost as a result of the dance teacher's lack of basic knowledge of children's development, of unprofessional instruction or exaggerated technical demands. Bad dance classes can harm the body as it grows and can interfere with the child's physical development. The hyperpronated foot with fallen arches is a typical example.

Most young children show hyperpronated feet with fallen arches up to a certain age. This is no cause for concern, as the development of the foot is still in progress. Only in young school-age children will the heel straighten up and the longitudinal arch form. Forced turnout at an early age can have negative consequences on the feet. Only few children are actually able to stabilize the external rotation of the legs through engaging their hip muscles. And so the feet are pushed outwards, the heels tip inwards and the whole weight is transferred to the inner side of the feet. This not only harms the feet and hinders the normal straightening of the heels; the knee, also suffers as a result of the rotation of the leg.

Despite careful dance training, slow and gradual increase of intensity, and despite ideal training conditions, there are diseases of the skeleton that force young dancers to limit their training schedule, to take breaks from training, or even to give up dancing entirely. The following diseases are especially problematic during childhood and adolescence. They are discussed in greater detail in the relevant chapters:

- Spondylolysis and spondylolisthesis (see Chapter 2, p. 40)
- Scheuermann's disease (see Chapter 2, p. 40)
- Scoliosis (see Chapter 2, p. 45)
- Hip dysplasia (see Chapter 4, p. 89)
- Osgood-Schlatter disease (see Chapter 5, p. 110)
- Patella dislocation (see Chapter 5, p. 110)

11. Help and Self-help: Dealing with Injuries

For many dancers physical complaints are part of everyday life. But only one-third will actually lead to a break from dance training; the rest is tolerated, ignored, or just considered to be a normal part of the dancer's life: dance and pain often seem to be closely linked. However, acute injuries are relatively rare in dance. Approximately two-thirds of all dance injuries result from chronic overuse: pain with a slow onset that increases gradually. Chronic overuse is not only uncomfortable and often showing prolonged healing, but it also increases the risk of acute injuries. In this chapter, you will find an overview of the most important types of injuries in dance, as well as advice on self-help.

Inflammation and Healing – the Natural Course of Injuries

Whether it is a chronic overuse syndrome or an acute injury, the body starts an entire cascade of repair mechanisms, the first of which is inflammation. Most people consider inflammation as something undesirable that must be avoided at all costs. But the inflammatory response is actually a natural mechanism for protection and defence. It is the immune system's reaction to an attack on the body by bacteria, viruses or by the waste products of injured tissue. Therefore in case of an injury, a primary, localized inflammation is a very beneficial thing.

Inflammation

Redness, heat, swelling, pain and *loss of function* are considered to be the typical signs of inflammation. At first, an acute injury leads to a shock reaction of the small blood vessels. They constrict, thus decreasing circulation. This lasts only for a few minutes before, as counteraction, the blood vessels dilate. This increases blood circulation and the injured area becomes red and warm. Inflammatory substances increase the permeability of the cell walls. Thus, fluid streams into the tissue, increasing the pressure and causing swelling of the area. The pressure within the tissue, the inflammatory mediator molecules – the best-known of which is prostaglandin – and the localized acidosis of the tissue stimulate the pain receptors. Swelling and pain impair function.

The Healing Process

The localized inflammation acts as a signal to the immune system. Immune cells invade the injured area and counteract the effects of damaging substances. Macrophages remove waste products, and the area is cleaned up in preparation for the repair work. This is when the healing process begins.

Ideally, restoration of the tissue takes place by cell regeneration: undamaged cells divide and replace the destroyed tissue. By the end of the healing process, the entire tissue is back to its full function, as the healing process has been carried out *ad integrum* (= to completion). This is why skin injuries are often invisible after complete healing; old and new tissues are identical both in form and function.

But the healing process can also take another course: in addition to or instead of the division of the tissue cells themselves, connective tissue cells can invade the damaged area. They produce connective tissue, which replaces a large part of the original tissue. The formed scar tissue is quite thick, firm and inflexible. Although the healing process has been completed and the damaged structure has been replaced, the inelastic scar tissue impedes function. How disturbing this is depends on the nature of the damaged tissue. It is not uncommon for a scar tissue to "adhere" to the surrounding tissue. Unfortunately, healing by scar tissue is particularly common in muscles. This explains why even small muscle injuries can lead to a long-term, bothersome restriction of flexibility.

The type of tissue that is damaged is not the only factor determining the healing process. Good circulation allows for adequate transportation of building materials and waste products, it improves the metabolism of the affected area, influences the quality of the newly-formed tissue and shortens the healing period. The small and smallest blood vessels in particular are responsible for microcirculation within the tissue. In smokers, these smallest blood vessels are the ones primarily constricted, which creates less-than-ideal conditions for a rapid and complete healing process.

Sufficient rest is crucial to the healing process. If the damaged area is placed under strain too quickly, and if the tissue is stretched too early, the newly-formed connections within the tissue will break down. The body then has to start the process of rebuilding all over again. This not only slows down the healing process, but also leads to increased formation of scar tissue.

First aid in the Dance Studio

An acute injury of the muscles, tendons, ligaments or joints often damages the related blood vessels. The speed at which blood leaks into the surrounding tissue depends on the size of the wounded blood vessel. Pressure inside the tissue increases, which in turn compromises those blood vessels which remained intact. Blood circulation decreases, slowing down the local metabolism. Swelling and pain soon set in. The increased pressure within the tissue slows down the healing process, although this effect only becomes apparent after a few days.

Quick and competent first aid has a considerable impact on the healing process following acute injuries. Restricting the bleeding in the tissue is of primary concern. The "RICE" method covers all aspects of first aid for injuries to soft tissue:

RICE method:

R **Rest** = Immobilize the injured body part.

I **Ice** = Cool it using towels soaked in cold water, or an ice pack, for approx. 20 minutes. Caution: do not place ice directly on the skin!

C **Compression** = Use a compression bandage to prevent blood and interstitial fluid from dispersing into the surrounding tissue. Caution: do not wrap the bandage too tightly.

E **Elevation** = Elevate the injured body part above heart level.

Following a successful first aid intervention, the HARM rule helps further in dealing with the injury. Within the first 24 hours after injury, the following should be avoided:

HARM Rule:
H **H**eat
A **A**lcohol
R **R**unning
M **M**assaging the injured area

Caution: Nicotine constricts the blood vessels. This reduces the metabolism in the injured area, slowing down the healing process: no cigarettes for at least 24 hours after an acute injury!

While they are certainly not acute injuries, **blisters** are among the most common problems for dancers. During their career, most dancers develop a highly individualized form of blister-management. Some advice for treating blisters:

- Sterilize a pin, ideally using boiling water or a flame. Allow it to cool. Carefully prick the blister at two spots. Press a paper tissue against the skin to expel the fluid. This puts an end to the painful pressure. Be careful not to remove the top layer of the skin, in order to avoid infection.

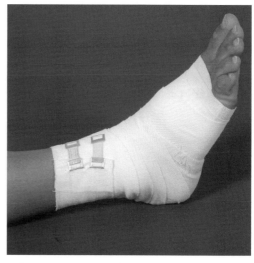

Figure 11.1 Compression bandage after an ankle injury.

- Leave the blister uncovered as often as possible, thus allowing the fluid to dry out completely.
- Cover the empty blister before it is exposed to strain, friction or pressure. Special blister plasters with a hydrocolloid layer are particularly handy, and are available from all pharmacies.

Muscle Injuries

From muscle ache to ruptures of the muscle fibre: muscle injuries are common in dance. A quarter of all dance injuries are related to muscles. Self-help can be particularly effective in promoting rapid healing.

sore muscles do not cause permanent damage. On the contrary, muscles get often stronger and more resilient afterwards, provided that they continue to be trained.

Muscle injuries can be caused by:
- Insufficient circulation within the muscle
- Insufficient fitness
- Muscle imbalances
- Insufficient warm-up and cool-down
- Localized or general fatigue
- Infections
- External factors (e.g. low temperatures)

Muscle soreness can be caused by:
- Physical activity following a long break
- Unfamiliar movement, particularly eccentric movement (this also applies to fit dancers)
- Particularly intense physical or psychological strain, e.g. examinations and competitions (this also applies to fit dancers)

Sore Muscles

At the earliest, muscles soreness can be felt within a couple of hours after unusual or particularly intense training. The muscles swell, become stiff, hard, sensitive to pressure, and sometimes even feel weak. The pain reaches its climax after between one and three days, and can last for up to a week, depending on the intensity. The cause of muscle soreness can be seen under the microscope: tiny micro-injuries of the muscle fibre, tears to the Z-lines (see Chapter 1, p. 14). Fast-twitch type 2 muscle fibres and muscles performing eccentric contractions are particularly susceptible. A high degree of intra-muscular coordination is needed for eccentric work, during which the muscle contracts while simultaneously being stretched. If intramuscular coordination is missing, or if the stress on the muscle becomes too great, the individual sarcomeres within the muscle fibre are put under stress. Weak sarcomeres are highly stretched and eventually can tear. The micro-injury happens while the muscle is working, but pain onset is delayed. The pain receptors are not activated until the pressure in the tissue has considerably increased. Poor local circulation and pain-related tension can worsen the pain. But there is no need to worry,

---

The development of muscle soreness:

Intense or unfamiliar strain on muscles
↓
Tears to the Z-lines
↓
Accumulation of fluid, swelling, pain
↓
Decreased circulation
↓
Reflectory muscular tension

What you can do: The following methods can help to reduce the pain within the sore muscle. However, they cannot reduce the time needed for the healing process.
- It is said that the best way to avoid muscle soreness is to have had sore muscles recently. This is because for several weeks a similar stress cannot provoke new muscle soreness at the same region. One should take this with a pinch of salt, however. There is no doubt that a constant build-up in training schedule, with a slow increase of activity, is the best way to strengthen muscles and avoid sore muscles.

- Enhancing circulation following the training helps to minimize the reactions to the micro-tears. Cool-down, careful stretching, alternating between a hot and cold shower, a hot bath, going to the sauna or putting arnica on the affected area are helpful methods. Deep massages are not to be recommended as they can even increase the mechanical damage.
- Gentle dynamic work improves circulation, decreases muscle tension and thus speeds up repair. Hence, one should also train "the day after", albeit with reduced intensity.

Muscle Cramp

An uncontrolled, painful contraction of a stressed muscle is referred to as muscle cramp. A magnesium deficiency is often considered to be the cause. It is true that low levels of magnesium reduce the threshold level for nerve irritation and increase nerve conduction velocity. Both can result in an overstimulation of the muscle. However, other minerals, too, are involved in muscle contraction. Disturbed sodium, potassium or calcium balances can also impede ideal muscle work. Any liquid deficiency or reduced circulation to the muscle – which can be caused by constricting leggings, for example – and any imbalance in mineral levels can lead to muscle cramp. Fatigue, is also a factor, albeit this is more generally in the brain, or more locally in the muscle.

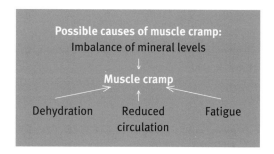

Possible causes of muscle cramp:
Imbalance of mineral levels
↓
Muscle cramp
↑
Dehydration   Reduced   Fatigue
circulation

What you can do:

- Stop training immediately. A muscle cramp is the muscle's cry for help, and one should pay attention to it.
- As first aid, passively stretch the muscle for 30 to 40 seconds, until the cramp has abated. Drink plenty of water. Relax the muscle using massage techniques. Rubbing the area with ice can also help.
- Tight clothing such as leotards with constricting edges should be avoided. They reduce circulation in the muscle and can therefore increase muscle cramps.
- Always drink plenty of fluids. If the training session lasts longer than 60 minutes, you should be drinking fluids during the session as well as afterwards (see Chapter 9, p. 186).

Muscle Spasm and Myogelosis

If muscle tonus is abnormally high, this is known as muscle spasm. Even in rest, the muscle belly remains sensitive to pressure and causes pain. Muscle strength is often reduced, while the high tension in the muscle can be easily felt when touching. Local hardening of the muscle is described as myogelosis. This is often found at muscle attachments, where the muscle belly meets the tendon. The increased muscle tonus is caused by problems of the muscular metabolism. In the long term, the delayed removal of waste products can even lead to changes of the muscle tissue with the muscle becoming "scarred".

What you can do:

- Use deep warmth, e.g. in the form of a mudpack or warming patches (Caution: test skin tolerance first!)
- Careful stretching. The contract-relax stretching is particularly effective (see Chapter 12, p. 217).
- Myogelosis can often be relieved by local massage and pressure: for 90 seconds press your thumb firmly to the most painful area. You will feel your thumb literally sink into the tissue; the muscle relaxes.
- Muscle spasm can be treated with a "warm wrap": apply damp linen to the affected muscle, and cover it with sandwich wrap/ cling film. Wrap a towel around and leave it for 20 minutes.

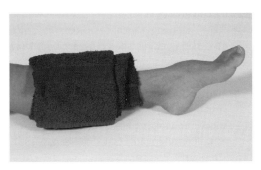

Figure 11.2 A "warm wrap" helps in the treatment of muscle spasm.

Pulled Muscles and Muscle Fibre Tears

Pulled muscles are the most common muscle injuries in dance. The hamstrings (see Chapter 5, p. 106) and inner thigh muscles (see Chapter 4, p. 80) are particularly susceptible. Poor co-ordination within the working muscle is thought to be the cause: while stretching the muscle some fibres are stretched more than others, causing a "shift" between the individual muscle fibres. There is no indication of discontinuity within the muscle fibre.

Pulled muscles and muscle fibre tears can be caused by:

- General fatigue. This increases careless behaviour and often leads to over-estimation of one's abilities.
- Insufficient warm-up and low temperatures reduce muscle circulation and increase the risk of injury.
- Poor communication from skin, joint and muscle receptors impede the functional cooperation of muscles (see Chapter 12, p. 225).
- Previous injuries with extensive scar tissue increase the risk of injury and result in a reduced elasticity of the scar tissue.
- Dancers who tend to suffer from muscle hardening are particularly at risk for pulled muscles and muscle fibre tears.

A muscle fibre tear is a more profound injury. Muscle cells tear, resulting in bleeding within the tissue. Here as well as in a pulled muscle insufficient muscle coordination is a well-known cause both between agonist and antagonist (*intermuscular*) and within the muscle itself (*intramuscular*). Muscle fatigue, poor metabolism and miscommunication between nerves and the muscle are also possible causes. Depending on the location we speak of peripheral or central muscle fibre tears. The former often looks more dramatic because of its often large superficial bruising. Still it usually heals more quickly since the pressure in the tissue can be released outwards, thus not disturbing the metabolism in the rest of the muscle. Depending on the size and location of the muscle fibre tear the healing can take between 14 days to eight weeks. Both pulled muscles and muscle fibre tears are characterized by immediate stabbing pain that can usually be accurately located. A larger muscle fibre tear can be felt as an indentation in the muscle belly.

What you can do: painful movements should be avoided for both pulled muscles and muscle fibre tears. Pain is the main indicator of the extent to which the dancer may use the affected muscle.

For pulled muscles:

- Ice massages several times a day: using an ice cube, carefully massage along the entire painful area. Caution: avoid freezing the skin!

- Be careful when stretching: no passive stretching on a pulled muscle for two to three weeks. Active movement that does not cause pain is allowed.

For muscle fibre tears:

- Use the RICE method, and follow the HARM rule for first aid.
- To avoid contraction of the scar tissue start to stretch carefully after ten days. Caution: stay in the pain-free range of motion.

Tendon Injuries

Tendons are very strong, but almost non-stretchy (see Chapter 1, p. 15). To allow for optimal muscle work, they have to smoothly glide within their surrounding tissue. This makes a direct blood supply via blood vessels impossible. Tendons are primarily nourished by diffusion, by absorbing nutrients from the surrounding tissue. This slows down their metabolism, which explains why it takes them a long time to adjust and regenerate. Adaptation time for tendons is approximately three times longer as for muscle tissue. This makes tendons the weakest part in the tendon–muscle–bone system.

Tendon Insertion Problems

At their insertion point into the bone, tendons have to withstand strong tensile and shearing forces. Repetitive non-axial pull or tense muscles can lead to inflammation, which in turn causes typical symptoms like pain at the area of the tendon insertion, weakness of the affected muscle or tension in the synergists (see Chapter 1, p. 17). Problems at tendon insertions always affect the entire muscle, and this is where treatment starts.

What you can do:

- Ice massage at the area of the tendon insertion.
- Relaxing the affected muscle. Softening the muscle belly reduces the pull on the tendon and the tendon insertion. Heat, a soft, relaxing massage and contract-relax stretches (see Chapter 12, p. 217) can smoothen the muscle.
- Detailed analysis of dance technique is important. Poor dance technique and poor postural habits in everyday life are the main causes of stress to the tendon insertion.
- Check your footwear! Problems at the tendon insertion of foot and knee are often caused by wearing inappropriate shoes.

Tendinitis and Tenosynovitis

Inflammation of the tendon (*tendinitis*) or of the tendon sheath (*tenosynovitis*) causes localized pain, overheating and swelling. Movement is often accompanied by a feeling of friction of the tendon and even a crackling sound. Excessive strain on the muscle, poor posture and localized pressure are common causes. For example, poorly fitting dance or street shoes can irritate the Achilles tendon. Tendon inflammation is an alarm signal for all dancers, as they can lead to chronic complaints if not treated appropriately.

What you can do:
- First step: rest and release any strain from the affected area.
- Massage the area with ice cubes.
- Bandage the area using ointment, and also use a tape bandage for support if necessary.
- Detailed analysis of dance technique; checking of footwear and clothing. Local pressure is often a trigger for tendinitis and tenosynovitis.

Bone Injuries

Injuries of the bone affect both the bone structure itself, as well as the surrounding sheath, known as the periosteum. There are many possible causes. Taking the appropriate steps at an early stage can help to prevent both bone fractures and periostitis.

Periostitis

Periostitis, an inflammation of the periosteum, can be caused by a hit or knock directly to the bone, by increased muscle tonus or by inflammation of the tendon insertion. When a muscle is under considerable strain, its pull on the bone increases. The periosteum at the muscle insertion point responds with irritation and swelling, starting a localized inflammatory reaction. The insertion of the anterior tibial muscle at the front of the tibia (see Chapter 5, p. 104) is an area most affected by periostitis. The front of the tibia becomes swollen, sensitive and painful. Flexing the foot is particularly uncomfortable. As a reflex, the calf muscles become tight. The top priority in the treatment of periostitis is to relax the affected muscles.

What you can do:
- Massage the inflamed area using ice cubes.
- Apply a cold compress to relax the muscles.
- Alternate between hot and cold showers to increase circulation in the muscles.
- Avoid any painful exercises.
- Try to find possible causes: disadvantageous posture and poor dance technique can increase the tension of the muscle and eventually lead to periostitis.

Bone Fractures

Depending on the cause, we distinguish between *acute bone fractures* and *stress fractures*.

No matter how healthy a person may be, adequate trauma can break any bone. Luckily, serious **bone fractures** are not common in dance. Depending on the location of the fracture, it takes a period of three to 12 weeks of rest to fully repair the bone. However, the area of the fracture can remain sensitive for a much longer period of time, for example, it may ache when the weather changes. This does not affect the bone's stability.

Stress fractures are more common among dancers than among the general population. The balance between stress and recovery is out of kilter and the bone gives in slowly, with no indentifiable trauma. It breaks imperceptibly, bit by bit. Depending on the extent of the stress fracture this can lead up to a complete fracture of the affected bone. One distinguishes between two forms of stress fractures, according to their causes:
- **Fractures caused by fatigue:** Constantly repeated micro-traumas lead to an excessive strain on a particular area of the healthy bone. Like a wire that is constantly bent backwards and forwards, the bone eventually breaks.

- **Fractures caused by low bone density and poor bone structure:** the bone's resilience is reduced as a result of changes to the bone's structure. Osteoporosis is the most common cause among female dancers in particular.

Typical locations of stress fractures in dancers:
- Metatarsals 2 and 3
- Sesamoid bones, below the big toe joint
- Tibia
- Lumbar spine (spondylolysis)

Stress fractures show typical signs of inflammation: localized redness, heat, swelling, pain and reduced functionality. As general X-rays often do not show this type of fracture, the diagnosis is difficult, especially at the beginning. Time is of the essence, however, as the length of time needed for the healing equates to the period of time between the first onset of symptoms and the start of treatment. Therefore, rapid diagnosis is of great importance.

Osteoporosis – A Cause of Stress Fractures

Commonly known as a problem affecting older women, in fact, osteoporosis is also a significant problem among young female dancers. By the loss of bone mass, altered microarchitecture and reduced bone mineralization the bone loses its density and stability; the bone quality reduces. Bones affected by osteoporosis can break even under negligible strain. Approximately three million people suffer from osteoporosis in the UK today, and over 10 million in the US. Most of those affected are women, as oestrogen plays an important role in bone metabolism.

To a large extent, osteoporosis is genetic. However, there are well-known factors that also influence bone structure and that, ideally, ensure a balance between bone resorption and bone formation. Exercise, hormonal balance and a healthy diet generally lead to good bone density. Extreme physical activity can damage the bone, however. Intense training is often accompanied by extremely low body weight in female dancers, which often disturbs hormonal balances. Menstruation can become irregular or can even cease, which can be a sign of insufficient oestrogen levels. In combination with an unbalanced diet – calcium is the most important mineral for bones – and too little sunlight – Vitamin D is essential for the uptake of calcium into the bone, and with the help of sunlight can be generated by the body itself – this can reduce bone formation or even increase bone resorption.

Maximum bone density, or "peak bone mass", is reached by the age of approximately 25. Already by the age of 30, bone resorption exceeds bone formation, and thus reduces bone mass. The higher the "peak bone mass", the better equipped one is for old age. Childhood and adolescence are therefore particularly important in the prevention of osteoporosis. This is when the base is laid for adult bone stability.

Prevention is the best treatment
Despite the fact that osteoporosis is largely inherited, there are effective preventive measures that can be taken.

Smoking is harmful to the bones. Nicotine has a negative effect on bone metabolism, and can increase osteoporosis. This is yet another good reason not to smoke.

Vitamin D is essential to the uptake of calcium into the bone. Sunlight allows the skin to produce Vitamin D by itself. As little as 20 minutes a day spent outdoors increases bone mineralization.

Oestrogen is a key hormone in bone regeneration. Late menarche, and irregular or missed menstruation is a warning sign for low oestrogen levels, and should be checked by a gynaecologist.

Maintaining **ideal body weight** reduces the risk of osteoporosis. If the body mass index (see Chapter 9, p. 189) is below 18 in women dancers, they should take particular care of a balanced and calcium-rich diet. Incorporating more calories into the diet would also help.

A **calcium-rich diet** helps to fight osteoporosis. calcium increases bone density and reduces bone resorption. The recommended daily amount of calcium (Ca) is 1200mg.

The following nutrition tips can help to ensure sufficient calcium levels:
- Choose fruit juices and fruit-juice drinks with added calcium, as calcium uptake is improved by the presence of Vitamin C.
- Regularly eat milk products such as buttermilk, soured milk, kefir, yoghurt or cheese. This is a solid base for your calcium level.
- The following vegetables are particularly rich in calcium: kale (212mg Ca in 100g), fennel (109mg Ca in 100g), broccoli (105mg Ca in 100g) and chard (103mg Ca in 100g). Take care to cook the vegetables in as little water as possible as calcium is water-soluble and would otherwise be poured down the drain along with the water.
- Calcium-rich meals late in the day are particularly effective. A yoghurt in the late evening can reduce the bone resorption that takes place at night.
- Drink calcium-rich mineral water, which contains at least 150mg calcium/l or dilute with juices. Use this mineral water for food preparation, too.
- Avoid typical calcium-sapping foods such as phosphate-rich soft drinks (e.g. coke) and curry sausage.

Each Injury has Consequences

Dance injuries seldom happen without warning. Anatomical predisposition, poor dance technique, typical compensation mechanisms, fatigue, nervousness and pressure to perform, low stamina, an inadequate diet, dehydration or simply over-training can lead to an injury-related break. The body is overtaxed. A sufficiently long break and appropriate treatment are the first essential steps on the way back to the dance studio. However, a detailed analysis of the possible causes is equally important both for preventing further injury and for stopping the problem from becoming chronic.

What you can do:
* Undertaking a detailed analysis of the dancer's technique should be the priority following an injury.
* Check all possible causes and create an accurate assessment of the situation.

* Allow injuries to heal properly! Problems can become chronic if, following an injury-related break, activity is increased too quickly.
* Be attentive to potential compensations both in posture and movements. Whether they are used consciously or adopted unconsciously, they might negatively influence dance technique and even lead to acute injuries.
* Take pain seriously. Find a doctor or therapist who is familiar with the problems of your particular dance style, and whom you can contact in case of emergency.
* Regular use of anti-inflammatory medication is not a good solution! Even the short-term use of medication bypasses the important control mechanism provided by pain.
* A regular dance-medical check-up can help to review your dance technique, assess overuse at an early stage, and thus initiate preventative strategies to avoid further injuries. After all, prevention is always the best form of treatment.

12. Dancing the Smart Way: How to Plan Training

Dance techniques and dance styles are not created at the drawing board. New dance steps develop from practice, by trial and error, by testing and discarding. Dance training developed in just the same way. The structure of dance classes is based on practical experience, on what the dance instructors themselves have learned as students, on knowledge that has a long tradition, and which is sometimes actually outdated. The "classic barre" is a good example: its structure, the order of the exercises, has hardly changed from its inception to the present day. What has changed, by contrast, are the choreographies performed by the dancers following their training at the barre. They must push themselves higher, further, faster: the strain on the body has increased considerably. Does the traditional dance training at the barre still offer the best form of preparation?

The science of training, as a subcategory of sports science, has investigated the basic principles of training for many years. How can training be planned most effectively? What are the effects of different training methods? Many of these findings have become firmly entrenched in the world of sports, but until now dance has only benefited to a limited degree from these insights. Most dancers consider themselves artists. There is a new awareness, slowly gaining a foothold in dance studios, that dancers also are professional athletes and that findings in the science of training can support their performance.

In training science we have identified five areas of physical fitness: *flexibility*, *coordination*, *speed*, *strength* and *endurance*. Dancers are particularly notable – in both the positive and the negative sense – in three of these categories: while coordination and flexibility are greatly improved

through dance, many dancers have surprisingly low scores when it comes to endurance. Low stamina, however, leads to early fatigue and fatigue is one of the main causes of injury!

Many aspects of training theory are already optimally incorporated into dance training. The science of training can indeed learn from dance, but this also works vice versa. Old myths and traditions continue to haunt dance studios. Many training methods are rooted in historical explanations, and some are more detrimental than helpful to dancers and their ability to perform. One-sided training, the creation of muscle imbalances and localized hyper-flexibility are typical examples of practices that should be examined more closely. Rhythmic gymnasts

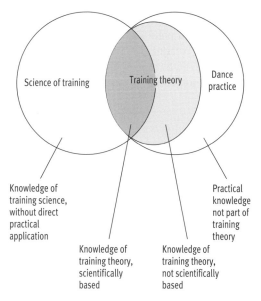

Figure 12.1 The interplay of training science, training theory and dance practice.

jog, footballers practise Pilates: a glance at the world of sports shows that full athletic potential can only be achieved through comprehensive training in all areas. Applied to dance, this means that sometimes it is important to get out of the dance studio to develop fitness in those areas that are neglected in dance.

In what follows, important aspects of dance training and the planning of training are discussed. This is not to supplant the practical knowledge of dance training, but rather to use the science of training to help the dancer perform on their highest capacity in good health and for as long as possible.

Flexibility – Stretching is a Part of Dance

Dance demands an exceptionally high degree of flexibility in the entire body. *General flexibility* refers to a constitutional disposition for basic flexibility. It is genetically determined, although, to a limited degree, it can improve through training. *Specific flexibility* focuses on flexibility in particular joints. Depending on the dance style, the focus is on different body parts. While in classical dance a high relevé is not possible without maximum flexibility in the big toe joint, in Oriental dance the flexibility of the pelvis and of the lower back are most important.

If general, flexibility, or the flexibility of particular joints, is considerably above average, this is called **hypermobility**. Over-flexible joints are exposed to great strain and are therefore at risk of early wearing out. Hypermobility leads to instability of both the joint itself and of the entire body. Balance becomes more difficult and it is

virtually impossible to remain centred. Localized hypermobility is often the result of limited movement in the adjacent joints. This is seen particularly often within the spine. The reduced mobility (**hypomobility**) of the thoracic spine is one of the most common causes for hypermobility of the lumbar spine. The spine has no alternative: if the mobility of the middle part of the back is limited the main movement will take place within the lower back. The segments of the lumbar spine

Flexibility depends on:
- the bony structure of the joints;
- the length and elasticity of the ligaments, tendons and the articular capsule;
- the length and elasticity of the muscles;
- the elasticity and gliding of the nerves.

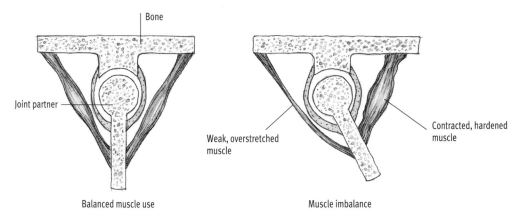

Figure 12.2 In muscle imbalance even in the resting position the joint is not centred.

are strained to the maximum, which might force them into hypermobilty.

Hypomobility, reduced flexibility, is often attributed to a shortening of the muscles. Strictly speaking, however, this does not exist: the structural length of a muscle always remains the same. The shortening of a muscle should better be equated with reduced flexibility or elasticity of the muscle. This is often found in muscle imbalances: a functionally "shortened" muscle opposes a weakened antagonist. These *muscle imbalances* influence flexibility and, in the long term, affect the functioning of the joints. The mobility of the joint is impaired; even in its resting position the joint is no longer centred. The asymmetry overtaxes the structures, from cartilage and articular capsules to ligaments and muscles. Over-stretching and weakening on the one hand and contraction and hardening on the other: joint functioning and muscle coordination are out of balance.

This is frequently seen in the hip joints: one-sided training of only external rotation reduces the ability to rotate inwards. The rotator muscles tighten up, thus preferring external rotation even during everyday movements. The imbalance in the joint can lead to early degeneration.

Advice on flexibility:
- Dancers should be flexible, but not hypermobile. In case of a general or localized hypermobility, flexibility should not be further increased by training. It is more important to work on stabilization.
- Coordination helps to stabilize and balance. Coordination training improves the muscle interplay and simultaneously increases range of motion.
- One-sided training can lead to muscle imbalance. Use specific exercises to equalize the joint play. Don't forget to train the opposite direction, too!

Stretching – the Many Methods

Before, during and after training: stretching is part of every dancer's daily routine. There is hardly any dancer who does not spend time lying in stretching positions on the floor, trying to improve his flexibility through stretching. Stretching has been a hotly debated subject for years, and the "ideal" method of stretching changes depending on the fashion. One thing is certain, and all dancers will have experienced this by themselves: stretching increases flexibility. It can also reduce muscle tonus, support muscle regeneration and allow the muscle fasciae to glide smoothly. Therefore, stretching is an inextricable part of dance. The only question is when and how stretching is most effective.

What you need to know about flexibility:
- Women are generally more flexible than men.
- Flexibility improves as the temperature of the muscle increases. Warming-up and warm outside temperatures soften the muscles.
- Flexibility generally increases over the course of the day.
- Stress and emotional strain decrease flexibility.
- Fatigue leads to increased muscle tonus and thus reduces flexibility.

A wide variety of methods are available for stretching. Generally, they can be divided into active and passive stretching, depending on the ways in which they are performed.

In **active stretching** the muscle is stretched by active muscle work. Usually, by contracting, the agonist stretches its partner muscle (= agonist-contract stretching). This is what is mostly seen in dance: there is no high extension of the leg without stretching the hamstrings; no flexing of the foot without elongation of the calf muscles.

Passive stretching is very popular among dancers. Passively, the muscle is brought into a stretch position, where it is held in place either by its own or by external weight. Numerous dance steps perform passive stretches to the muscles. Every demi-plié stretches the calf muscles and every battement devant stretches the hamstrings, just as every rolling down elongates the back muscles.

Many people, not just dancers, only use passive stretches, whether for warming up, for stretching after the warming-up exercises or for the regeneration after. There are, however, many different methods for relaxing muscles effectively and to increase flexibility (see Table 12.1).

Static stretching

Static stretching is relaxing for both body and soul. It is of only limited use as warm-up or for a long stretching session during training. Holding the stretch position for a long time reduces the elasticity of the tissue, leads to a decrease of velocity in muscle work and even cuts off the blood circulation to the stretched muscle; all of these increase the risk of injury. Intensive static stretching also increases the pull on the Z-lines. If muscle soreness is likely to follow a training session, intensive static stretching after class is not advisable. A specific stretching session, separate from dance training itself, appears to be most effective for training flexibility.

How to do it: Bring the muscle to its maximum stretch position, and remain there for between five and 15 seconds (short stretch) or between 15 and 60 seconds (long stretch). Three to four repetitions are advisable for each muscle. Breathing out while stretching makes it less painful.

Table 12.1 Overview of the most important stretching methods in dance

Active stretching	Passive stretching
Agonist-contract stretching	Static stretching
Eccentric stretching	Dynamic stretching
	Contract-relax stretching

Advantages of static stretching:
- Good control over the stretch.
- Fine-tuning of the amount of stretch.
- "Listening" to the muscle.
- It is particularly suitable for beginners and for dancers returning after an injury.

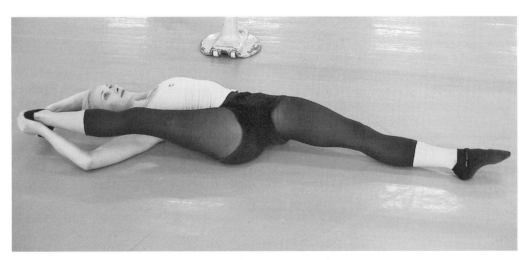

Figure 12.3 Stretching is important for dancers.

Dynamic stretching

Gentle bouncing at the end of one's range of motion improves joint flexibility. Without tugging or tearing, the end position is carefully extended through rhythmic movement. Dynamic stretching is best for warming up, and also for improving flexibility during the training. It requires a good sense of one's physical limits and should therefore only be practised by trained dancers.

How to do it: Bring the muscle to the stretch position. Slightly reduce the amount of stretch, performing five to 15 small bouncing movements. The speed and amplitude of the dynamic stretching can be carefully increased, depending on the dancer's physical condition.

Advantages of dynamic stretching:
- Good preparation for dynamic movements.
- The rhythmic pull on the tissue strengthens the structures.
- In addition to the muscle tissue itself, the muscles' fasciae are also stretched by the bouncing movements.

Contract-relax stretching

In contract-relax stretching (also known as post-isometric stretching), contraction and relaxation of the muscle alternate. This alternating muscle stimulation releases the muscle and reduces the muscle tonus. The effect can be felt immediately: after the isometric contraction the muscle tonus decreases. This allows deepening the stretch without pain.

How to do it: Bring the muscle to the stretch position. In this position, engage the muscle against resistance for three to eight seconds. Relax the muscle, deepen the stretch and keep this position for three to eight seconds. Repeat the cycle of stretching, engaging and readjusting three to five times, ending with the stretch.

Advantages of contract-relax stretching:
- Reduction of muscle tonus and relaxation of the muscles.
- The isometric contraction of the muscle increases circulation and strengthens the muscle.
- Increased awareness of the muscle being stretched by alternation between engaging and relaxing.

Agonist-contract stretching

When a muscle works concentrically, its antagonist is simultaneously stretched. The extent of the stretch depends on one's active flexibility. For example, the higher a dancer can extend the legs by muscle work, the greater the stretch on the muscles at the back of the thighs. This reveals the limits of this form of stretching. Many dancers are not able to actively reach the point where the antagonist's passive limits of flexibility are attained; either because the agonist is not strong enough, or because the antagonist is already very flexible. In such cases, effective stretching of the muscles cannot be achieved by an agonist-contract stretching.

How to do it: Bring the muscle to the stretch position and deepen the stretch by an active contraction of the agonist.

Advantages of agonist-contract stretching:
- It trains the coordination between agonist and antagonist.
- While the antagonist is being stretched the agonist gets strengthened.
- Engaging the agonist increases its blood circulation.
- Agonist-contract stretching is automatically part of all dance training.

Eccentric stretching

When a muscle contracts while being lengthened, this is called eccentric muscle work. This can be used to strengthen and simultaneously stretch muscles. The focus is on the "lengthening" of the muscle. Caution: eccentric muscle contractions can lead to sore muscles.

How to do it: Contract the muscle concentrically. This pulls its two ends closer together, bending the relevant joint. Now slowly extend the joint. This decreases muscle contraction "lengthening" the muscle. Perform the movement continuously until the end of the range of motion. For a few seconds completely relax the muscle tonus in the stretched position. Repeat the entire sequence seven to ten times.

Advantages of eccentric stretching:
- Simultaneous stretching *and* strengthening of the muscle.
- Good awareness of the muscle working and of the course of the muscle.
- Awareness of "muscle lengthening" after the stretching.

Timing is Important – When is Stretching Effective?

How to stretch "properly" is difficult to say. Every stretching method has its own advantages and disadvantages. The time and desired goal of stretching determine the most effective stretching method. Dancers should work out their own stretching programmes according to their individual needs. These can include a combination of the different methods. Table 12.2 provides an overview of the most important stretching methods before, during and after training.

Table 12.2 The most important stretching methods before, during and after training

	Before training	During training	After training
Static stretching	yes (short) no (long)	yes (short) no (long)	yes (short) yes (long)
Dynamic stretching	yes	yes	no
Contract-relax stretching	no	no	yes
Agonist-contract stretching	yes	yes	no
Eccentric stretching	yes	yes	yes

All stretching methods intend to improve flexibility. During training, following the barre or the warm-up training, long static stretching should be avoided. It tires the muscle and thereby increases the risk of injury. Stretching is particularly helpful after training: intense training increases muscle tonus, and the muscle feels hard and short. Stretching relaxes the muscle and releases it to its normal length.

Caution: Stretching is not always the ideal solution. Sometimes it makes more sense to strengthen the antagonist instead of "working hard" to relax a muscle using all available means.

Endurance – the Basis for High Performance

When we think of endurance training, we usually associate it with jogging, cycling, walking or swimming. But there are different forms of endurance, and their various training methods differ accordingly. In general, they are organized by the duration of activity: maximal activity for 45 seconds to two minutes is referred to as *short-term endurance*; an activity lasting two to eight minutes is called *medium-term endurance*; and any activity that goes on for more than eight minutes is referred to as *long-term endurance*. Therefore, the sports mentioned above mainly train long-term endurance, which is also known as "basic endurance" or "physical fitness".

The science of training defines endurance as resilience to fatigue: the slower a dancer tires, the better the stamina. With good stamina, one dances and dances and dances and, ideally, feels little or no exhaustion. A high level of basic endurance is therefore excellent for injury prevention, given that fatigue is considered one of the primary causes of injury in dance.

Unfortunately, dancers do not always score well when it comes to endurance. Studies show that the average dancer's stamina is not at all higher than in people who don't practise any sports at all. This is easy to explain as the focus of dance training is on dance technique and there

usually is no time to incorporate endurance training. Although there is an increasing number of dance pieces and choreographies in which dancers perform for 20 minutes or more, the intensity of the activity is usually too high to work as proper endurance training.

A high level of basic endurance provides dancers with a wide range of advantages. A short discussion of the metabolism of muscle work explains why.

Energy Production – it's All about Oxygen

Every muscle contraction requires energy, which is usually available in the form of **a**denosine **trip**hosphate (ATP). Like a battery, ATP supplies the muscle with the power it needs: by splitting ATP into **a**denosine **dip**hosphate (ADP) and phosphorus, the body generates the energy that it requires for muscle work. But there is not nearly enough ATP in the muscle. The reserves are depleted after just a few seconds and then the pool has to be refilled again. This can be done in one of two ways: either with or without oxygen: aerobically or anaerobically. The mechanism used depends on the intensity and the duration of the activity.

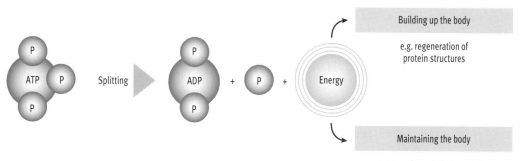

Figure 12.4 Nutrition is transformed into energy: adenosine triphosphate (ATP) is split into adenosine diphosphate (ADP) and phosphorus (P).

Aerobic muscle work

Low-intensity, long-term activity and sufficient oxygen supply are the characteristics of aerobic muscle work. In a slow and laborious process, carbohydrates and – depending on the duration of the activity – fat are metabolized using oxygen. Thereby the amount of energy generated is relatively high: one glucose molecule stands for 36 ATP molecules. The body can easily eliminate the by-products produced: water is excreted via the kidneys or evaporated through sweat and carbon dioxide is breathed out through the lungs. This allows muscles to work for long periods without getting tired. However, there are also disadvantages: aerobic metabolism takes a while to get going. The aerobic system is too sluggish for rapid, explosive movements.

Table 12.3 Advantages and disadvantages of aerobic muscle work

Advantages	Disadvantages
Metabolism of carbohydrates and fats (the higher the intensity of activity, the more carbohydrates metabolized; the lower the intensity, the more fats metabolized)	
High energy yield (36 ATP)	Light to medium intensity
Long duration	Delayed effect
"Waste products" water and carbon dioxide can be easily eliminated and do not place a burden on the body.	

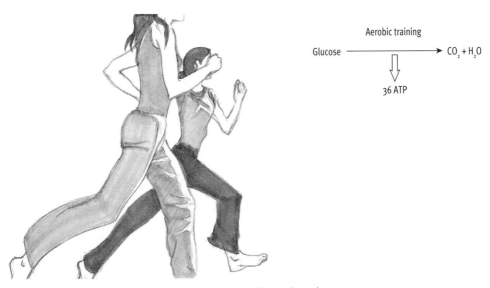

Aerobic training

Glucose ⟶ $CO_2 + H_2O$

36 ATP

Figure 12.5 Aerobic muscle work.

Anaerobic muscle work

Carbohydrates are the source of energy used in anaerobic muscle work. Without the use of oxygen energy can be rapidly generated. However, the efficiency is low: no more than two ATP molecules are produced from one glucose molecule. The produced lactic acid makes muscle work difficult. After just a few minutes the efficiency of the muscle is hampered as it becomes tired and sluggish; coordination is reduced and the risk of injury increases. Lactic acid impedes further anaerobic metabolism. This is known from dance training: the muscles get tired and do not want to work any more. You feel that you have hit a wall. Avoiding high concentrations of lactic acid is important as they also reduce the muscle's ability to recover.

Anaerobic metabolism allows quick and intensive muscle work, but only for a short period. Jump variations that require a lot of power are a typical example of anaerobic work: they involve high intensity over a relatively short period of time.

Aerobic and anaerobic metabolism mechanisms do not work entirely separately from one another. Depending on the intensity and duration of the physical activity, one mechanism or the other will predominate. Usually, at the beginning of an intensive activity, oxygen supply is not sufficient for a primary use of aerobic metabolism, as the body is still in its "rest modus". Therefore anaerobic energy production is the first one to start. The onset of aerobic metabolism comes with delay. Depending on training intensity, it will cover a smaller or larger amount of the total energy production.

Table 12.4 Advantages and disadvantages of anaerobic muscle work

Advantages	Disadvantages
	Only metabolism of carbohydrates
Maximum intensity	Low energy yield (2 ATP)
Rapid effect	Short duration
	Concentration of the "waste product" lactic acid in the muscle increases, limiting its working ability and increasing the required recovery time.

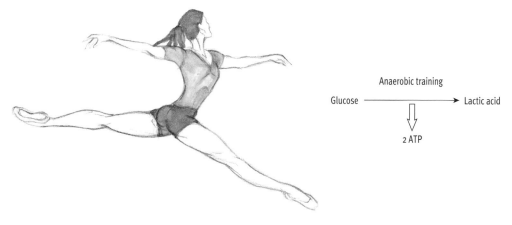

Figure 12.6 Anaerobic muscle work.

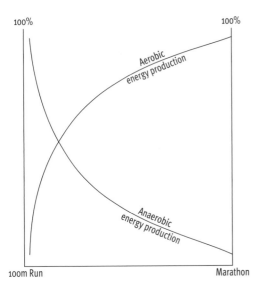

100%   100%

Figure 12.7 The distribution of aerobic and anaerobic
energy production.

Stamina – the Basis for Healthy Dancing

Big jumps, partner work, speedy combinations: many dance steps ask for both speed and strength. To match these demands dancers need a quick supply of energy, and this is what they get from anaerobic energy production. In other words, anaerobic work is important in dance. However, it should be supplemented by a good basic level of fitness, as this improves the overall ability to withstand physical strain. For a dancer with good stamina, the demands on the muscles that would lead to acidosis in a less fit person can be met using aerobic energy production. Supplying sufficient oxygen to the working muscles is the key to aerobic fitness. For this, the cardiovascular system and the breathing play an important role. That is why aerobic fitness is also referred to as *cardiovascular endurance*.

The lungs

The lungs are where gas exchange takes place. In the tiny alveoli, oxygen is uptaken by the blood, while carbon dioxide is simultaneously released

into the air. This happens very quickly: in a quarter of a second, the red blood cells take up oxygen in order to transport it to the periphery of the body, where it is used for aerobic muscle work. While resting, about ten litres of air are inhaled and exhaled each minute. During intense physical activity, this can rise to up to 120 litres. Only approximately 50 litres can be breathed in through the nose. The rest flows through the mouth, which makes the inhaled air drier and cooler. This irritates the lungs and can lead to exercise-induced asthma, a disease that is becoming increasingly common among athletes, including dancers.

In training science, maximum oxygen absorption is used as an important parameter for determining basic endurance. The more oxygen can be absorbed, the higher the basic endurance level and the greater the supply of oxygen to the muscles. But dancers often harm themselves in precisely this respect: as little as two cigarettes a day reduce the blood's ability to transport oxygen by about eight per cent. This is because of the carbon monoxide that attaches itself to the red blood cells, thus blocking the transportation of oxygen. One more good reason not to smoke!

The heart

While resting, the heart pumps about five litres of blood per minute through the body. During intense physical activity, depending on age and gender, blood circulation can rise to 20 litres per minute. This is hard work for the heart, and the pulse rises. A reaction that is not very economic in the long term. An increase in the stroke volume – the blood volume that is pumped into the circulatory system by a single contraction of the heart – is a more efficient adaptation. The heart muscle, like every other muscle, reacts to an increase in stress by increasing its volume: the heart becomes bigger, the heart muscle gets stronger. Fewer beats are now needed to pump the same amount of blood. This can also be seen at rest: the resting heart rate lowers; a typical sign for a dancer with a high level of overall fitness.

The blood vessels

The human body's network of blood vessels is more than 100,000km long. The diameter of the finest blood vessels is barely wider than that of a single blood cell. It is in the capillaries, the smallest of the blood vessels, where exchange takes place: oxygen, building materials and energy supplies are delivered, while waste products are removed. The higher the number of capillaries within the muscle, the quicker the supply and removal of substances, and the better for the metabolism and recovery. Endurance training helps in this respect; the number of capillaries in the muscle can be more than doubled by aerobic training. This also supports anaerobic work as increased capillarization speeds up the removal of lactic acid, and a reduced level of lactic acid in turn increases the muscle's ability to perform.

Good stamina:
- keeps the muscles fit for longer when dancing;
- allows longer periods of concentrated work;
- speeds up regeneration and helps recovery even during short breaks;
- primarily trains Type-I-muscle fibres and thus supports the formation of long, slender muscles;
- reduces the overall risk of injury;
- stimulates the immune system and improves health.

Endurance through (Dance) Training

Levels of activity increase steadily during dance training: relatively static and long exercises with short breaks give way to increasingly dynamic movements with shorter sequences and longer and longer breaks. Overall, the dancer is only active for about 50 per cent of the class. This discrepancy becomes even more pronounced during rehearsals and performances. Here, short combinations of steps and choreographies predominate putting maximum strain on the cardiovascular system, but are often followed by long breaks. Thereby, the dancer's activity usually lasts only a fraction of the total length of rehearsal or performance. This shows clearly that in general, traditional dance training, everyday rehearsals and performances cannot improve dancers' stamina, as the intensity is too high and the duration too short.

But dancers should take advantage of the benefits of good stamina. This can either be achieved through additional endurance training, or by changes to the dance training itself.

Regular endurance training, twice or three times a week for 30 to 40 minutes, will provide a good level of fitness. Depending on each dancer's individual preferences, typical endurance sports such as jogging, cycling, aqua fitness and swimming are all suitable. If endurance training is to be incorporated into dance training, as is sometimes the only option due to time constraints, it is the first part of the training (barre, or warm-up training) that should be adapted. The principle is simply to reduce the breaks. If the entire first part of the training is choreographed, the breaks between exercises used for explanations will be skipped and the duration of activity automatically increases. This allows for training the dancers' stamina. No matter which method of endurance

Suggestions for dance-specific endurance training:
- Two to three blocks of endurance training per season, four weeks each.
- Replacement of regular training with specific endurance training two to three times a week.
- 40-minute-long 'choreographed' session, with all barre and warm-up exercises combined into a single sequence, without breaks. Can be prolonged to include the smaller jumps.
- Medium-intensity exercises.
- Simple movement sequences.

training is used, endurance can only be trained if the muscles are optimally supplied with oxygen. Training intensity should be kept just below the threshold at which energy production changes from aerobic to anaerobic, the so-called *aerobic threshold*. A variety of tests can help to determine one's individual aerobic threshold. Under laboratory conditions maximum oxygen absorption can be tested, while blood tests can measure the lactic acid concentration. All these methods are too laborious and too expensive to be used in general in the dance studio. But a simple and reliable measure can be used instead: one's own heartbeat.

The rule of thumb, "220 minus age in years" can be used to estimate one's maximum heart rate. This indicates one's individual training pulse, depending on the training goal. By training at 70 to 80 per cent of the maximum heart rate, the dancer will remain below the aerobic threshold. For a 25-year-old dancer, that works out as a training pulse somewhere between 136 and 156 beats per minute. One more useful tip is that if you can still have a conversation while doing your endurance training without becoming completely out of breath, you can rest assured that you are well within the aerobic training spectrum.

Resting heart rate and recovery heart rate give an indication of one's basic stamina:

Resting heart rate: The pulse, measured immediately after waking up in the morning, before speaking a single word or getting out of bed.
Resting heart rate 45–60/min = well trained.
Resting heart rate 70–80/min = untrained.

Recovery heart rate: Measure the initial heart rate, then raise the heart rate significantly by 30 seconds of running or jumping on the spot. Measure the time needed for the heart rate to drop down to the initial heart rate.
Initial heart rate reached after two to three minutes = trained.
Initial heart rate reached after more than four minutes = untrained.

Warming Up and Cooling Down

Appropriate warm-up protects against injuries, and regular cool-down speeds up regeneration. This is reason enough to integrate warming up and cooling down into one's daily training programme. However, dancers do not always use the entire spectrum of possibilities. Moreover, although regular stretching is part of every dancer's routine, it is seldom complemented with further useful methods.

Warming Up

For improving performance and avoiding injury, the key phrase is "warming up". Warming up prepares body and mind for the activity that follows. It falls into two categories: general and specific warm-up. **General warm-up** gets the circulation going. It warms up the entire body and prepares the metabolism for the upcoming demands. **Specific warm-up**, on the other hand, specifically prepares the muscle groups that are particularly utilized when dancing.

Different methods for warming-up:
active * passive * mental

A purely "mental" warm-up is appropriate mainly for low-intensity activity. Passive warm-up (such as a hot shower, massage or rub) is only of limited use. Although the body's surface is being warmed, the heat cannot penetrate deeper into the body. This superficial warmth can even be counter-productive: the blood vessels in the skin dilate, leading to increased circulation at the surface. The blood volume flowing through the skin is not available to the muscles. Following passive warming-up the muscles are neither sufficiently warm nor supplied with the amount of blood needed.

The ideal warm-up combines active and mental preparation: this gets body and mind ready to perform at its highest potential.

The effects of warming up

It is remarkable that dancers continue to pay so little attention to efficient warming-up, given the wealth of positive changes brought about by *general warm-up* exercises. As little as five to ten minutes of gentle running are sufficient to raise the body's temperature to the ideal level, and to prepare the body systems for the activity to come. This is clearly a worthwhile investment of time.

Increased metabolic rate: Warming up increases the temperature and speeds up metabolism. This is of great relevance as intense physical training can raise the metabolic rate to almost 200 times its resting rate. The body can hardly cope with this without specific preparation.

Higher oxygen supply: The increased circulation resulting from a higher blood volume being pumped and from the dilatation of the capillaries, leads to the muscles being supplied more quickly with oxygen and nutrients. This improves the muscles' performance.

Better preparation for muscles and joints: Warming up makes muscles, tendons and ligaments more elastic, which in turn reduces the risk of tears. Gently moving the joints stimulates the production of synovial fluid. Like a sponge, the hyaline cartilage soaks up the joint fluid, which thickens the cartilage and makes it more resistant to pressure or shear forces.

Improved coordination: The rise in temperature increases the nerves' excitability. The reaction and contraction time decreases, and the sensitivity of the sensory receptors raise. The skin's sense of touch and the proprioceptive systems of the body are sensitized. This, as well, improves co-ordination.

Higher concentration: The increased circulation within the brain improves concentration.

Activation of central brain structures can have a positive effect on vision. The increasing circulation of the retina improves spatial vision and sense of contrast. Even visual acuity can be improved by up to 0.75 dioptres by actively warming up.

Once the body is sufficiently warmed up by general warm-up exercises, *specific warm-up* will distribute the bloodstream throughout the working muscles. This is most easily achieved by the dance training itself. Depending on the activity to come, 20 to 45 minutes of preparatory training are ideal, either as a warm-up training in the centre or in the form of the classic barre.

If warm-up is not undertaken, the dancer will become tired more quickly. This is hardly surprising: if one does not warm up, the metabolism is still at rest. Not until after one is well into a high level activity does metabolism reach its peak. "Waste products" are not sufficiently eliminated, lactic acid accumulates and the muscle gets tired right from the beginning (see p. 221). This carries a great risk of injury.

Tips for warming up

Although warming-up always follows the same basic principles (general warm-up followed by specific warm-up), length and intensity depend on various factors. The following points should be considered when planning one's individual warm-up:

- The time required to warm up increases with age. Warming-up should become longer and more gentle over time. Children generally need less in the way of warming-up than adults. However, young dancers should be trained to warm up. Firstly, warming-up will improve their performance and lower their risk of injury. And secondly, making warm-up an integral part of training provides the best possible chance that the dancers will continue to pay sufficient attention to warming-up in their future dance careers.
- Duration and intensity of the warm-up depend on the dancer's physical condition. The higher the dancer's level of fitness, the more intensive the warm-up training should be. This is because warming-up should prepare the dancer for the activity that will follow, and this will be more strenuous in the case of a well-trained dancer than for a beginner.
- Body temperature increases over the course of the day, generally reaching its peak at about 3 p.m. This explains why warming-up should be longer in the early morning than in the late afternoon or evening.
- The weather, too, has an impact: the colder and wetter, the longer the body needs to achieve its ideal working temperature. The duration of warming-up has to change accordingly.

Warming up for dancers

1. General warming-up

- Stimulating the cardiovascular circulation (five to ten minutes): On the way to the studio: by cycling, walking quickly, running up stairs. In the dance studio: by running gently, jogging on the spot or doing aerobic exercises.

2. Specific warming-up

- Warm-up for the joints (five minutes): Passive joint mobilization, not weight bearing.
- Activating the skeletal muscles (five minutes): short stretching of the muscles.
- Warm-up training or classical barre (20–45 minutes).

Cooling Down

Dancers who cool down after training reduce their risk of injury. Although this has been clearly shown by studies, almost 60 per cent of dancers go home after training without having done any cool-down at all, a percentage which rises to over 80 per cent after performances. Still, cooling down is essential to a rapid regeneration of body and mind; specific cool-down exercises speed up the onset of regeneration and repair mechanisms. Active cooling down exercises like gentle running, swinging or stretching, speed up the elimination of metabolic waste products by six times compared to passive cooling down such as massages, sauna or a hot shower. This can make all the difference when it comes to feeling ready to get back to dance the following day.

The effects of cooling down

Recuperation is the main point of cooling down; cooling down exercises should not put additional stress on the body. An appropriate cool-down lasts between five and 15 minutes. Gentle running is a common active cool-down, which is important for both the cardiovascular system *and* the muscles. If movement ends abruptly – like when you have danced the last combination with great enthusiasm, and get changed quickly before rushing to the next appointment – the blood "gets stuck" in the muscles. This has two negative consequences: suddenly the cardiovascular system "runs out of blood". The blood supply to the brain is decreased, which can lead to dizziness and nausea. The muscles, too, suffer from abruptly ended movement. Waste products remain in the muscle delaying its recovery.

Gentle muscle work in the form of slow running, swinging or contract-relax stretching keeps the muscle pump going. By the alternation of muscle contraction and relaxation the venous blood is transported towards the heart. This speeds up the elimination of the metabolic waste products from the muscle. The higher heart rate following activity increases the blood circulation: the blood is pumped through the body at up to three times its usual speed. Cooling down uses this rapid "turnover" for eliminating waste products and replenishing building material.

Tips for cooling down

The optimal length of the cooling down depends on various factors:

- The dancer's physical condition determines the length of the cool-down. The fitter the dancer, the longer the cool-down, as winding the body down from a high level of activity takes time.
- The length of the cool-down varies, depending on the time of day. A shorter cool-down is necessary in the morning than in the evening as the body has not yet moved into top gear at this time.
- Warmer temperatures make a longer, but less intensive cool-down advisable.

Cooling down for dancers:

1. Keeping the increased circulation rate (five minutes): gentle running, swinging, mobilizing the joints.
2. Relaxation of the muscles: stretching, e.g. short static or contract-relax stretching of the most important muscles, three to five repetitions each.
3. Mental relaxation supports recovery. Also, passive relaxation methods are supportive, e.g. warm showers, baths, massages, sauna or steam room.

Training – Timing Matters

Good dance training disturbs homeostasis, the body's restful state of balance, and this is as it should be. Activity stimulates adjustment reactions, adaptations of body and mind that gradually prepare the body for the increasing strain. Both the quantity and the quality of the training determine the effect. Monotonous dance training with no variety or progression cannot possibly challenge the body. The training stimulus is lost.

Training Boosts the Body

Training influences the entire body, has an effect on body cells, and alters metabolism, hormone status and the brain. A glance at the adjustment mechanisms of the nervous system provides an indication of the many advantages to be gained from regular training. The experience of generations of dance teachers can also be explained in scientific terms: dance training boosts brain function.

Training-induced adjustments in the nervous system:
- increased blood supply to the brain;
- building up of new nerve cells;
- formation of new synaptic connections;
- enhanced mood as a result of the release of endorphins;
- increase in neurotransmitters;
- increase of growth stimuli for the nerves.

The body's response to training stimuli depends on their intensity. If a stimulus is *below threshold*, it has no effect; if it is *just above*, it will maintain the current physical condition. Stimuli *far above threshold* trigger optimal adjustment responses, both functional and structural. They are ideal for performance enhancement. If stimuli are *too intense*, they damage the function.

Unfortunately there is no universal level that allows us to determine the ideal stimulation intensity, as this depends on age, gender and physical condition, and therefore changes individually from one dancer to the other. Finding the optimal training intensity requires great experience on the part of the dance teacher, mindful self-assessment by the dancer and, most importantly, good communication between the dancer and the teacher.

Figure 12.8 shows how the body reacts to training stimuli well above threshold. The dancer starts at his individual performance level (1). From the moment activity begins (2), fatigue sets in (3). The recovery period (4) starts once the period of activity is over. The effect of training shows at the end of the recovery period when the performance level rises above the pre-training base level. This state of increased performance capacity is known as supercompensation (5), and is the basis for performance enhancement.

In healthy dancers, recovery processes generally outweigh degenerative processes. This explains the body's adaptation to the increasing training intensity. This model can be applied to all substances "used" in training, from muscles to bones and the brain, as well as enzymes and hormones. To enhance performance in the long term, one has to find the optimal time to implement the next training stimulus.

Training at the Right Time

Ideally, dance training increases the dancer's performance. But it can also result in excessive stress or show no effect at all, depending on the timing of the training stimulus. A new training stimulus should be timed precisely during the phase of supercompensation, when the body's performance capacity is at its highest. In this way, repeated training stimuli will lead to a slow, continuous increase in performance (Figure 12.9). If the time between the individual training units is

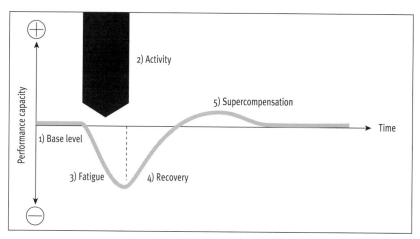

Figure 12.8
The principle of
biological adaptation
to a stimulus above
threshold.

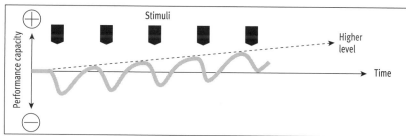

Figure 12.9
Performance
enhancement as
result of optimal
timing of training.

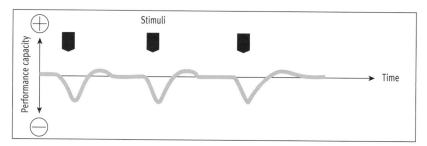

Figure 12.10.
Performance
stagnation as result
of infrequent
training.

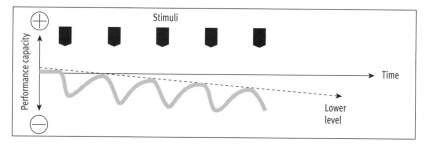

Figure 12.11
Performance
deterioration as
result of excessively
frequent training.

too long, there will be no improvement and performance stagnates (Figure 12.10). On the other hand, if the intervals are too short, the recovery processes are hindered. If the body is strained too early, it has not yet fully recovered, resulting in a decrease in physical performance (Figure 12.11). The models show clearly that optimal timing of activity and recovery will determine the dancer's performance.

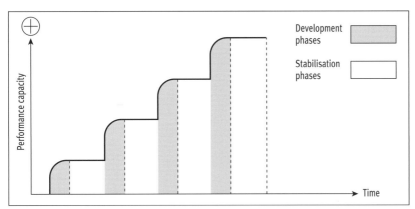

Figure 12.12
Necessary stabilization phases during the course of training.

In establishing a training plan, timing training around muscular recovery time has proven to be the most effective approach. In a well-trained dancer, muscular recovery time is about 24 hours, while in the untrained dancer it can differ from between 48 to 72 hours. Recovery time is much longer in tissue that only has poor blood supply and therefore has to be nourished by diffusion. Thus, while training stimuli may be well timed for muscle tissue, they may overtax the connective and supportive tissue. In order to prevent this, stabilization phases, which keep the training intensity on a constant level, should be part of each training plan. This allows the tissue and systems that regenerate more slowly to catch up.

Overtraining is not Uncommon

High levels of motivation, relatively low basic endurance levels and practising individual sports: these three factors together can easily lead to overtraining; and all three of them often apply to dancers. The situation is aggravated by commonly-held attitudes such as "do more to achieve more" or, even worse, "no pain, no gain". These beliefs have a high impact on the balance between activity and recovery.

This is dangerous as overtraining usually develops from excessive training with insufficient breaks for recovery. The image of the "personal stress pot" of each individual dancer can provide insight into the complex causes of overtraining. Put everything into this pot: training, performance and working conditions, financial situation, private and professional stress, infections, chronic inflammation such as badly-maintained teeth or allergies, nutrition and unfavourable lifestyle factors such as smoking, alcohol and too little sleep. If the sum of all these factors is too great, it only takes one more drop to make the pot overflow. The dancer starts to get overtrained and his performance decreases continuously although the level of activity stays the same.

There are two forms of overtraining: sympathetic and parasympathetic. In *sympathetic* overtraining, symptoms of agitation such as sleeplessness, irritability and loss of appetite predominate. The *parasympathetic* form is more common but also more difficult to recognize as its development is more subtle. Here, depressive symptoms such as great fatigue, weakness and lack of drive are primary, making it difficult for the dancer to get going. Unfortunately, there is no easy indicator for the reliable diagnosis of overtraining. Overtraining should only be diagnosed after making sure that no organic problems (such as iron deficiency, inflammations and myocarditis for example) are causing the symptoms.

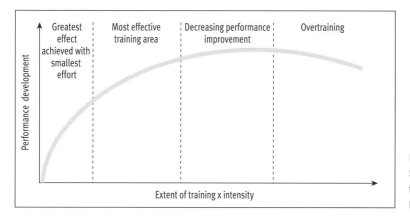

Figure 12.13
Sometimes less is more: too much training can be harmful.

The following symptoms can point to overtraining:

- The body feels heavy and tired during training, often accompanied by excessive sweating.
- Performance during training deteriorates, both subjectively and objectively.
- Training is perceived to be stressful.
- Extreme fatigue, shortness of breath and slow recovery following training.
- A feeling of constant fatigue over a prolonged period of time; tiredness is not relieved by sleep.
- Trouble going to sleep or sleeping without interruption.
- Decreased appetite.
- Small scratches on the skin do not heal easily.
- Increase of infections, headache or allergies.

- Lack of drive, irritation, decrease in ability to concentrate and lethargy that carry over into everyday life.

Important: Overtraining is never diagnosed on the basis of just one symptom. On the other hand, if a number of the listed indicators are present, medical advice should be sought.

The precise dividing line between training and overtraining is difficult to define. The optimal quantity of high-quality dance training, a healthy diet, a healthy balance of fluids, active relaxation and sufficient sleep offer the best protection against overtraining.

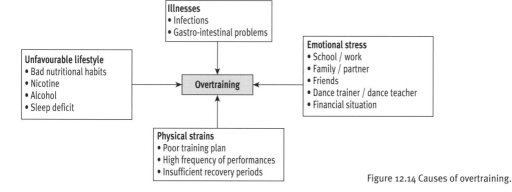

Figure 12.14 Causes of overtraining.

Training and Rehearsal Planning – Tuning in Professional Dance Schools and Companies

Of course every dance teacher considers the subject they teach and the training they provide to be the most important. It goes without saying that each choreographer's rehearsals and performances are of the greatest significance to him. And yet, despite all external pressures, it must be the dancer's health that takes centre stage when it comes to planning and designing the year of training or the performance season. It is not necessary to delve into the theory of training to realize that it cannot be healthy for any dancer to perform at the highest level all year round and without a break. All professional athletes divide their seasons into periods of preparation, competition and transition. Different focuses govern the different phases, alternating between performance enhancement and recovery. This is difficult when it comes to the theatre. The dance company that draws up its schedule to suit its dancers' physical conditions is still a rare thing. In general, entirely different factors determine the timing and number of performances: from the casting to availability of the stage and technical equipment and even the choreographer's schedule. The situation is no better in the freelance dance world. Dancers have to be extremely stress resistant, as their workload ranges from occasional performances with frequently long breaks in between to long-running productions with eight or more performances a week. Planning the training year or season according to the principles of training science remains a rarity in the world of dance to this day.

Planning for professional dance schools

In professional dance education school holidays and term breaks automatically supply a framework for the training year. Even if they cannot be kept entirely free of training, duration and intensity should be reduced during the holidays, as regeneration and recovery periods are essential for the child's or adolescent's growing body. It makes sense to implement different training emphases for certain periods, depending on age and training level. Thematic blocks can help to focus on the same aspect in all dance classes. Body-centred themes (e.g. feet, hips, back) focus on dance technique (e.g. turnout or relevé) or sensitive-artistic elements (e.g. balance, space, expression) can serve as points of interest. Thus all dance classes give insight into different aspects of the same subject and provide the student with a multifaceted understanding of different approaches. Ideally, at the same time, these themes should be echoed in complementary theory lessons.

> **Some helpful guidelines for planning training and training-free days:**
> - At least 1.5 to two training-free days a week.
> - Four training-free weeks in a row, once a year.
> - After 6 weeks (at most), implementation of a recovery period with training reduced in length and intensity.

Tips on planning training in professional dance schools:
- Almost 80 per cent of all accidents happen during rehearsals when repeating well-known choreographies. Two-thirds of these occur at the end of a long day of training. Therefore, remember, less can be more.
- Keeping warm is essential during breaks in between training sessions! Long waits and idle breaks cool the body down. Efficient training and rehearsal planning is therefore indispensable.
- Sufficient leisure time is important for recovery.

Planning for companies

Planning training, rehearsals and performances properly is essential to the prevention of injuries. Two aspects have to be taken into account: firstly, the performance capacity of a dancer varies depending on the time of day, and, secondly, dancers need time for relaxation and regeneration during the dance season.

Daily schedule: One of two forms of daily scheduling is in use at most theatres and dance companies. Both have advantages as well as disadvantages, which must be weighed up against each another.

Continuous rehearsal days: Start at 10 am and end at 6 pm, with a lunch break of between 45 to 60 minutes.

Advantages:
- A lunch break lasting up to one hour allows the body to "stay warm" for the continuing rehearsals after the break.
- The recovery period, including night-time rest, is longer than 12 hours.
- High-level evening performances are required only when actually performing.
- If there is no performance, the evening is kept free. This allows dancers to socialize with people outside the theatre/dance world.

Disadvantages:
- Missing opportunity to get used to the strain of evening performances.
- Short recovery period at lunchtime.

Split rehearsal days: two blocks of four hours, one in the morning and the other in the evening, with a break of four to five hours between blocks.

Advantages:
- Long recovery period in the afternoon.
- Dancers get used to the strain of evening performances by regular evening rehearsals.

Disadvantages:
- The body cools down during the long lunch break and insufficient warm-up before the evening rehearsal increases the risk of injury.
- Short night-time rest period and recovery time between rehearsal days.

- Two commutes per day.
- The evening rehearsals do not take into account the circadian curve in performance capacity.
- Socializing outside the theatre world is more difficult.

Continuity is important in planning the daily schedule, regardless of whether this takes the form of continuous or split rehearsal days. Where a continuous rehearsal-day schedule is adopted, the run-throughs at the end of the rehearsal process should be scheduled at the time of the planned evening performance. This allows the dancers to adapt their bodies to the activity late at night.

Tips on season planning:
- Increasing levels of fitness and training technical skills are the priorities at the beginning of the season. Early premieres/performances at the very beginning of the season should be avoided.
- After about six months, a two-week recovery period is beneficial: one week without any training at all and one week of reduced daily workload with low-intensity training and less intense rehearsals.
- It is no coincidence that premieres are often less successful from a technical point of view than the performances that follow. Studies have shown that dancers are often in a state of overtraining when it comes to the premiere. This results in a noticeable drop in performance capacity. Training science shows, that tuning is essential in dance. It is best to increase activity level up until 14 days before the premiere; to maintain this level from 14 days before until eight days before the premiere; and to reduce the intensity from seven days before the premiere until the day of the premiere itself. The dress rehearsal should be scheduled two days before the premiere. This allows dancers to regenerate and to perform to their highest potential on the day of the premiere.

- Breaks during rehearsals should be kept as short as possible. Waiting for long periods cools the body down and therefore increases the risk of injury.
- Towards the end of the day, demanding movement sequences should be avoided, as approximately two-thirds of all acute injuries happen at the end of the rehearsal day.
- Even if time is running out, there is no point in more than one full run-through a day.

- After long evening performances the beginning of the following day's training should be rescheduled to a later start.
- For adequate regeneration 1.5 training-free days a week are essential! If the performance or rehearsal plan does not allow this, it is important to catch up on these regeneration days as soon as possible.
- There should be a minimum of three training-free weeks in a row at least once a year.

Recovery – After Dancing is Before Dancing

Every physical training is tiring – to varying degrees depending on the individual. Fatigue limits the duration and intensity of the training and is thus an important protective mechanism for the body as it prevents us from entirely exhausting our physical reserves. Regular training pushes our resilience further and further. No matter when fatigue sets in, the subsequent regeneration is decisive when it comes to how and when activity can start anew.

After training, the body needs time to relax, regenerate and to gather power again. Only then can it reach the stage of supercompensation (see p. 228), and only then can performance capacity increase. It is important to note that most adaptations within the body that will increase performance do not happen during the training, but during the regeneration period that follows! Scheduled recovery periods are therefore an important part of every training plan.

Twenty-four hours are usually sufficient for recovery. If dancers train two to three times a day for several days in a row – as is required of any professional dancer – 1.5 to two days of rest per week are needed. In this respect, the findings of a large survey among dancers in the UK is alarming: 11 per cent of dancers stated that they did not have a single training-free day a week, while 44 per cent recorded 0.5 to one training-free day a week. Whether driven by personal ambition or set

training and rehearsal schedules, less than half of all dancers grant their bodies sufficient rest.

The more focused on achievement the dancer is, the more likely he is to ignore the body's signs of fatigue. This can lead to a vicious circle: if performance deteriorates, dancers tend to increase their training intensity hoping that this will prevent a further slump. This strategy backfires as an increase in training reduces the recovery period, the level of fatigue rises and dance performance capacity suffers even further.

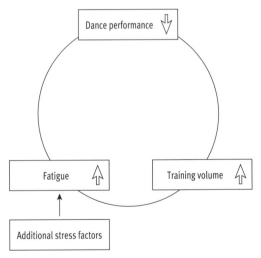

Figure 12.15 Vicious circle resulting from a decrease in dance performance.

One Thing at a Time – Regeneration Takes Place in Stages

All muscle work and every form of dance training is a strain on the body, causing micro-injuries and wearing out of body material: myofibrils are damaged, enzyme particles are destroyed, cell particles perish. Waste products accumulate, a build up of lactic acid leads to acidosis in the muscles and energy reserves are emptied. In order to start all of the necessary repair mechanisms, and to replenish its stores, the body needs time. This regeneration period can last anywhere between a few minutes and several days, depending on the system.

It is clear that there is no such thing as *the* ideal duration when it comes to a recovery time for all structures in need of regeneration. While the cardiovascular system can be put to work again after just a few minutes, the repair of cell particles can take up to ten days. This means that the next training stimulus always takes place during the regeneration of one body system or the other, no matter how well planned the training schedule is. And yet another factor makes it difficult to determine the ideal duration for regeneration: the body's regeneration time varies according to age, gender and physical condition, as well as being dependent on the duration and intensity of the preceding activity.

> In general, the time required for muscular regeneration is used to determine the optimal regeneration period in dance.

Sensible Regeneration Improves Fitness

Depending on the type and duration of activity, regeneration can actually start during training. Dynamic muscle work, the constant alternation between engaging and relaxing, between load and unload, allows the muscle to start regeneration processes while still working. Slow movements

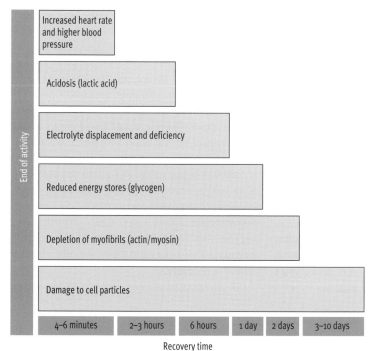

Figure 12.16 The different recovery times required by various systems.

recruit only part of the muscle's motor units (see Chapter 1, p. 14). The idle muscle fibres can recuperate, and are fresh and rested when they take over during the next movement. This increases the possible duration of activity for the particular muscle. In order to allow regenerative processes to take place during activity, work intensity should be well below its maximum in both, dynamic muscle work and during slow movement.

An effective cool-down, both active and passive, supports regeneration (see p. 227). Other factors can also speed up the recovery process: a balanced way of life is considered the most important key to rapid and efficient recovery.

Measures for efficient recovery:
- Cool-down (active and passive)
- Fast replenishment of lost fluids
- Rapid refilling of emptied carbohydrate stores
- Relaxation techniques (e.g. autogenic training, mental training, self-hypnosis)
- Good basic endurance
- Plenty of fresh air
- Adequate sleep

Recuperation does not have to mean enforced idleness. Movement is also welcome during the recovery period, although other forms of activity from those used in the dance studio should be chosen. Low-intensity swimming, cycling, jogging and walking are linked to a number of advantages. They regenerate the muscles, improve the basic endurance and make the dancer go outside and breathe in fresh air.

When rehearsing a particular choreography, the better your practice, the shorter your reaction time. This is the normal effect of training. Scientists have shown that even sleep may

The following are detrimental to recovery:
- Regeneration processes in the body need oxygen. Smoking, however, reduces oxygen uptake. As popular as the idea of having a cigarette to relax may be, smoking immediately after physical activity can seriously impede regeneration.
- Drinking alcohol four hours or less after training increases the time needed for recovery. By hampering hormone synthesis, alcohol impedes the regeneration of numerous body substances.
- Caffeine ties up the body's protective agents and obstructs important repair mechanisms. Coffee is not suitable as a regeneration drink!

shorten your reaction time as the brain continues to practise at night. Participants who were allowed a sufficient amount of sleep after having learned a sequence of movements showed a considerable increase in the automatization of this sequence the following day. On the other hand, participants who were prevented from sleeping did not benefit at all. Sleep can support the learning process. Also sleeping takes care of another task: it structures the newly learned material. Distant neural networks are co-ordinated, and the brain is "defragmented", like a hard drive. Therefore, sufficient sleep has a great impact on the brain's ability to work well. But sleep plays an important role in physical recovery, too: the growth hormone somatotropin is released while we sleep. In addition to its importance in growth and a child's development, somatotropin stimulates cell growth and regenerative processes in adults. In other words, adequate sleep can have a positive effect on the dancer's recovery.

Building Up and Easing Down

"Building up" means a gradual increase of activity level in preparation for periods of greater training intensity. "Easing down" refers to a step-by-step reduction of intensity allowing the body to slowly unwind.

Building Up – the Art of Gradual Increase

Regular training leads to adaptation mechanisms; the body adjusts to what is demanded. However, if the load is increased too rapidly the body's adaptation lags behind. The risk of chronic overload and acute injuries increases. This can be prevented by means of a good training plan.

> **Training science recommends progressively increasing training as follows:**
> 1. Increase the frequency of training sessions (number of dance-trainings per week).
> 2. Increase the duration of the training sessions (by 15 minutes at a time).
> 3. Reduce the duration of the breaks during training sessions.
> 4. Increase the intensity of the training sessions.

Dancers who are "in good shape" and can match the demands of the dance training cannot rest on their laurels. If the regular training stimulus is missing, the body's adaptations are soon reversed. After just a few days, coordination, muscle strength and speed are reduced. Even dancers in good physical shape must adhere to the following rule: after prolonged breaks from training, after holidays or injuries, the body must carefully be reintroduced to training one step at a time.

Building up after a break from training:
- Preparation should begin in plenty of time before the season starts. In the case of a few weeks' summer break, half of the free time should be used to recuperate and relax, and the remaining time to gradually return to form. Endurance training as well as body techniques such as yoga, Pilates, Gyrotonic, Feldenkrais or Alexander Technique are of great help.
- Training intensity should be increased slowly and continuously during the first two weeks after a training break. Do not perform big jumps until the end of the first week at the earliest.
- Extreme stretches, complicated combinations and demanding partner work are best avoided during the first week. After a break from training, the body's limitations are more pronounced than usual.
- After a prolonged break from training the muscles are weak and relaxed. This increases flexibility but fine coordination is also reduced. At the beginning of the training season, care should be taken in combinations that require a high amount of coordination or place great strain on the body.

Easing Down – Step-By-Step Reduction

Problems can occur when a regular training stimulus is suddenly removed. Cardiac arrhythmia and circulatory problems, as well as depressive moods due to endorphin deficiencies, are common symptoms. Changes in diet can affect the hormone balance and the composition of the blood; the fat level of the blood rises. Degeneration of the joints are often not felt until the intensive dance period is over. Then, muscle strength and coordination are reduced, taking away protection and stabilization from the joints. Discomfort grows although the strain is reduced.

Sensible, gradual detraining at the end of an active dance career can prevent these problems. It is helpful to replace dance training with other forms of training during this process.

Easing down at the end of a dance career:
- Before the end of the active dance career one should look out for alternative forms of movement. A wide range of alternatives can make the final break from dance less painful.
- Unfortunately, the advantages of a previously active life are short lived: any positive effects of dance on the cardiovascular system disappear within months of no longer dancing. A new range of physical activities can prevent this.
- Endurance training such as jogging, walking, cycling and swimming are ideal companions in the gradual process of easing down. These activities allow one to freely choose both intensity and duration. Be aware that it is more efficient to train with low intensity for a longer period than intensively and briefly: 45 to 60 minutes, two to three times a week are recommended. If practised appropriately, endurance training not only keeps the cardiovascular system fit, but also helps to maintain one's usual weight.
- Unfortunately, it is not uncommon for injury to lead to a sudden end of the dance career. But dancers must not allow an injury to rob them of their love of movement. An injury that stops one from being a professional dancer need not hamper the practice of other forms of dance, movements or sports. One should continue to engage in an hour of activity two to three times a week.
- Any decisions about the form of easing down have to be made on an individual level. Consultation with a doctor specializing in dance medicine is advisable. As a general rule, the slower the level of activity is reduced, the better for body and mind.

Easing down over the course of 12 months:
First to sixth months: Dance training two to three days a week with a gradual reduction in intensity first and in duration second.
Seventh to twelfth months: Dance training one to two days a week, complemented by other sports such as endurance training or body techniques one to two days a week.

Further Reading

Books

Barringer, Janice and Schlesinger, Sarah, *The Pointe Book: Shoes, Training and Technique*, Princeton Book Company, Pennington 1991.

Brinson, Peter and Dick, Fiona, *Fit to Dance? The report of the national inquiry into dancers' health and injury*, Calouste Gulbenkian Foundation, London 1996.

Buckroyd, Julia, *The Student Dancer: Emotional Aspects of the Teaching and Learning of Dance*, Dance Books, London 2000.

Calais-Germain, Blandine, *Anatomy of Movement*, Eastland Press, Seattle 2007.

Chmelar, Robin and Fitt, *Sally Severy: Diet for Dancers*, Princeton Book, Pennington 1995.

Clippinger, Karen, *Dance Anatomy and Kinesiology*, Human Kinetics, Champaign, IL 2007.

Feldenkrais, Moshe, *Awareness Through Movement: Easy-to-Do Health Exercises to Improve Your Posture*, Vision, Imagination, and Personal Awareness, HarperOne, New York 1991.

Fitt, Sally Severy, *Dance Kinesiology*, Schirmer Books, New York 1996.

Foley, Mark, *Dance floors. A handbook for the design of floors for dance*, Dance UK, London 1989.

Franklin, Eric, *Conditioning for Dancers*, Human Kinetics, Champaign, IL 2004.

Franklin, Eric, *Dance Imagery for Technique and Performance*, Human Kinetics, Champaign, IL 1996.

Franklin, Eric, *Dynamic Alignment Through Imagery*, Human Kinetics, Champaign, IL 2012.

Grieg, Valerie, *Inside Ballet Technique: Separating Anatomical Facts from Fiction in the Ballet Class*, Dance Horizons, Pennington 1994.

Haas, Jacqui, *Dance Anatomy,* Human Kinetics, Champaign, IL 2010.

Hale, Robert Beverly/Coyle, Terence, *Albinus on Anatomy*, Dover Publications, New York 1989.

Hamilton, Linda, *Advice for Dancers*, Jossey-Bass Publisher, San Francisco 1998.

Hamilton, Linda, *The Dancer's Way*, Griffin, New York 2009.

Howse, Justin and Hancock, Shirley, *Dance Technique and Injury Prevention*, A&C Black, London 2000.

Huwyler, Josef, *The Dancer's Body: A Medical Perspective on Dance and Dance Training*, Dance Books, Alton, 2002

Kimmerle, Marliese and Côté-Laurence, Paulette, *Teaching Dance Skills: A Motor Learning and Development Approach*, J. Michael Ryan, Andover 2003.

Koutedakis, Yiannis/Sharp, Craig, *The Fit and Healthy Dancer*, Wiley Verlag, Chichester 1999.

Laws, Helen, *Fit to Dance 2*, Dance UK, London 2005.

Malina, Robert; Bouchard, Claude and Bar-Or, Oded, *Growth, Maturation, and Physical Activity*, Human Kinetics, Champaign, IL 2004.

Mastin, Zerlina, *Nutrition for the Dancer*, Dance Books, Alton 2009.

Peterson, Judith, *Dance Medicine: Head to Toe*, Princeton Book Company, Hightstown, NJ 2011.

Rolf, Ida, *Rolfing: Integration of Human Structures*, Harper Collins, New York 1987.

Ryan, Allan and Stephens, Robert, *The Dancer's Complete Guide to Healthcare and a Long Career*, Dance Books, Alton 1989.

Ryan, Allan and Stephens, Robert, *The Healthy Dancer: Dance Medicine for Dancers*, Princeton Book Company, Hightstown, NJ 1989.

Simmel, Liane, *Dance Medicine, The Dancer's Workplace: An introduction for performing artists.* Unfallkasse Berlin (ed.), 2005, www.unfallkasse-berlin.de.

Solomon, Ruth; Solomon, John and Minton, Sandra Cerny, *Preventing Dance Injuries: An interdisciplinary perspective*, Human Kinetics, Champaign, IL 2005.

Thomas, Emlyn, *Homeopathy for Sports, Exercise and Dance*, Beaconsfield Publishers Ltd, Bath 2000.

Todd, Mabel, *The Thinking Body*, Gestalt Journal Press, Gouldsboro 2008.

Welsh, Tom, *Conditioning for Dancers*, University Press of Florida, Gainesville, 2009.

Willemsen, Ted, *Anatomy and Injuries*, Obey Willemsen, Amsterdam 2007.

Useful websites

www.admrdanse.com
  Bilingual (English and French) website of the *Association Danse Médecine Recherche* (ADMR) an association based in Monaco dedicating their work to the health of dancers.
www.danceuk.org
  Website of the British organization Dance UK. Under the heading "Healthier Dancer Programme" you will find useful information on medical aspects of dance.

www.fitfordance.de
  Bilingual (English and German) website of the Institute for Dance Medicine. "Fit for Dance". Numerous publications on all aspects of dance medicine.
www.iadms.org
  Website of the International Association for Dance, Medicine and Science with various links to useful resources, publications, and conferences.
www.nureyev-medical.org
  Medical website of the Rudolf Nureyev Foundation. Provides a wide variety of dance medical information.
www.tamed.de
  Website of "tamed", Dance Medicine Germany, the German Organization for Dance Medicine. Provides a great deal of health information for dancers.

Index

References in **bold** indicate tables and in *italics* indicate figures.